FAMILIES
OF
HANDICAPPED PERSONS

FAMILIES
OF
HANDICAPPED
PERSONS

Research, Programs, and
Policy Issues

edited by

James J. Gallagher, Ph.D.
Director
Frank Porter Graham
Child Development Center
University of North Carolina at Chapel Hill

and

Peter M. Vietze, Ph.D.
Head
Mental Retardation Research Centers
National Institute of Child Health
and Human Development

·P A U L·H·
BROOKES
PUBLISHING Cº

Baltimore • London

Paul H. Brookes Publishing Co.
P.O. Box 10624
Baltimore, Maryland 21285-0624

Typeset by The Composing Room, Grand Rapids, Michigan.
Manufactured in The United States of America by
The Maple Press Company, York, Pennsylvania.

Library of Congress Cataloging-in-Publication Data
Main entry under title:

Families of handicapped persons.

   Papers presented at a conference sponsored by the Mental
Retardation/Developmental Disabilities Branch of the National Institute of Child
Health and Human Development.

   Bibliography: p.
   Includes index.
   1. Mentally handicapped children—United States—Family relationships—
Congresses. 2. Stress (Psychology)—Congresses. I.   Gallagher, James John,
1926–   . II. Vietze, Peter, 1944–   . III.   National Institute of
Child Health and Human Development (U.S.). Mental Retardation/Developmental
Disabilities Branch.
HV894.F36   1986   649′.151   85-26971
ISBN 0-933716-58-3 (pbk.)

Contents

Contributors

Donald B. Bailey, Jr., Ph.D.
Director of Early Childhood Research
Frank Porter Graham Child Development Center
The University of North Carolina at Chapel Hill
Chapel Hill, NC 27514

Michael Berger, Ph.D.
The Atlanta Institute for Family Studies
61 Eighth Street, N.E.
Atlanta, GA 30309

Marie M. Bristol, Ph.D.
Carolina Institute for Research on Early
  Education for the Handicapped
Frank Porter Graham Child Development Center
and
Division TEACCH
Department of Psychiatry
School of Medicine
The University of North Carolina at Chapel Hill
300 NCNB Plaza 300Q
Chapel Hill, NC 27514

Gene H. Brody, Ph.D.
Associate Professor
Department of Child and Family Development
and
Institute for Behavioral Research
Dawson Hall
University of Georgia
Athens, GA 30602

Mary Jane Brotherson, Ph.D.
Department of Child & Family Development
University of Minnesota
Duluth, MN 55812

Karen Schlueter Budd, Ph.D.
Associate Professor
University of Nebraska Medical Center
Meyer Children's Rehabilitation Center
Omaha, NE 68105

Deborah L. Coates, Ph.D.
Youth Research Center
Catholic University
Washington, DC 20017

Bernard Farber, Ph.D.
Department of Sociology
Arizona State University
Tempe, AZ 85281

Dale C. Farran, Ph.D.
Department Head
Child Development
Kamehameha Schools/Bishop Estate
Center for Development of Early Education
Honolulu, HI 96817

Martha Foster, Ph.D.
Department of Psychology
Georgia State University
and
Atlanta Area Child Guidance Clinic
2531 Briarcliff Road, N.E.
Suite 215
Atlanta, GA 30329

James J. Fox, Ph.D.
Assistant Professor
Department of Special Education
Peabody College of Vanderbilt University
Nashville, TN 37203

James J. Gallagher, Ph.D.
Director
Frank Porter Graham Child Development Center
Highway 54 Bypass West 071 A
Chapel Hill, NC 27514

Laraine Masters Glidden, Ph.D.
Professor of Human Development
Division of Human Development
St. Mary's College of Maryland
St. Mary's City, MD 20686

Stephen Greenspan, Ph.D.
Associate Director
University Affiliated Program in Developmental
    Disabilities
University of Connecticut
Box U-64
Storrs, CT 06268

Barbara Hawes, M.S.
Associate Commissioner
Operational Design and Program Evaluation
New York State Office of Mental Retardation and
    Developmental Disabilities
44 Holland Avenue
Albany, NY 12229

Ann P. Kaiser, Ph.D.
Associate Professor and Chair
Department of Special Education
Peabody College of Vanderbilt University
Nashville, TN 37203

Marty Wyngaarden Krauss, Ph.D.
Director of Social Science Research Department
Eunice Kennedy Shriver Center
and
Lecturer and Senior Research Associate
Florence Heller Graduate School
Brandeis University
Waltham, MA 02254

Ann E. MacEachron, Ph.D.
Professor
School of Social Work
Arizona State University
Tempe, AZ 85287

Joyce Metzger
Technical/Production Editor
Center for Development of Early Education
Kamehameha Schools/Bishop Estate
Honolulu, HI 96817

Iris Tan Mink, Ph.D.
Mental Retardation Research Center
Center for the Health Sciences
University of California, Los Angeles
760 Westwood Plaza
Los Angeles, CA 90024

Ross D. Parke, Ph.D.
Professor
Department of Psychology and School of
    Medicine
University of Illinois at Urbana-Champaign
603 East Daniel Street
Champaign, IL 61820

Denise Pensky, M.S.
Program Specialist
Operational Design and Program Evaluation
New York State Office of Mental Retardation and
    Developmental Disabilities
44 Holland Avenue
Albany, NY 12229

Rune J. Simeonsson, Ph.D.
Professor of Education
and Investigator
Carolina Institute for Research on Early
    Education for the Handicapped
Frank Porter Graham Child Development Center
The University of North Carolina at Chapel Hill
301-C NCNB Plaza 322A
Chapel Hill, NC 27514

Joyce Sparling, M.S., L.P.T, O.T.R.
Special Education
University of North Carolina at Chapel Hill
Highway 54–Bypass West
Chapel Hill, NC 27514

Zolinda Stoneman, Ph.D.
Associate Professor
Department of Child and Family Development
Dawson Hall
University of Georgia
Athens, GA 30602

Jean Ann Summers, B.G.S.
Kansas University Affiliated Facility at Lawrence
Bureau of Child Research
University of Kansas
Lawrence, KS 66045

Ann P. Turnbull, Ed.D.
Bureau of Child Research
University of Kansas
223 Haworth Hall
Lawrence, KS 66045

Peter M. Vietze, Ph.D.
Head
Mental Retardation Research Centers
National Institute of Child Health and Human
    Development
Bethesda, MD 20205

Valora Washington, Ph.D.
Assistant Dean and Associate Professor
Department of Human Development
School of Human Biology
Howard University
2400 Sixth Street, N.W.
Washington, DC 20059

Lynn McDonald Wikler, ACSW, Ph.D.
Assistant Professor
School of Social Work
and
Waisman Center on Mental Retardation and
    Human Development
425 Henry Mall
University of Wisconsin-Madison
Madison, WI 53706

Preface

THIS BOOK ON THE families of handicapped children emerged from a conference sponsored by the Mental Retardation/Developmental Disabilities Branch of the National Institute of Child Health and Human Development (NICHD) in cooperation with the University of North Carolina at Chapel Hill. Each year NICHD picks a topic that has great research potential and popular interest in the field of mental retardation and developmental disabilities and brings together professionals who have been working on this issue (Brooks, Sperber, & McCauley, 1984; Kernan, Begab, & Edgerton, 1983). These scientists, often from multidisciplinary backgrounds, are asked to review current trends and project future productive directions. This volume compiles the conference papers that addressed a wide range of issues concerning the adaptation problems of families who must cope with many pressures, on a daily basis, with their handicapped children.

There is little doubt that the family has become an increasing focus of attention as professionals try to cope with the problem of how to help children with mental retardation and developmental disabilities. In this latter part of the 20th century, the family remains the core unit within the society within which individual crises are most often coped (Turnbull & Turnbull, 1985). This fact remains true despite the undeniable shifting of traditional roles within the family that has taken place in the past century. Scanzoni and Scanzoni (1976) have pointed out the historical evolution of the relationship between husband and wife over the centuries from *owner-property*, to *head-complement*, to *senior partner-junior partner*, to *equilibrium of rights*. Each of these patterns carries a different set of roles for family members to learn and act on. One element of the family-child adaptation to be researched is the nature and perspective of the family unit itself, as well as that of the child—in this case, the handicapped child (Gallagher, Beckman, & Cross, 1983).

The various attempts that are made to cope with the presence of a young handicapped child or individual in the family unit is the focus of this volume. This topic has become increasingly important in the last two generations with the evolution of social policy in the United States regarding handicapped individuals. It is within the living memory of many of us that the predominant and approved response to having a moderately to severely handicapped child was to place him or her out of the family in a large institutional setting that was often built far away from urban centers. The family crisis in those days was how to adapt to the discarding of one of its members (Farber, 1959).

New information and experience from both education and the social sciences provided the basis for a changed societal attitude. One of the fundamental findings was that most of these handicapped individuals were not doomed to a life of dependency or helplessness, but could under proper education and care develop into at least partially self-sufficient human beings (Martin, 1976).

Great social pressures were brought about to bring these individuals back from their isolated and often unstimulating environments into the family unit (a process referred to as deinstitutionalization) and to become a member in full standing of the community and the school. The current high watermark of societal acceptance was the passage of Public Law 94-142, the Education for All Handicapped Children Act of 1975, which provided for equality of educational treatment for handicapped children so that these youngsters could make the maximum use of their capabilities. It also strongly implied that the family responsibility was to keep children with handicaps within the family unit and that the family was supposed to play a significant role in the development of the program for their child. This legislation introduced an entirely new phase of the family coping with the problem, because now the family had to deal with the daily stresses and pressures such a child may bring.

As we explore the adaptation of families to handicapped children and adults, one of the obvious findings from many of the chapters in this volume is the substantial diversity of response and adaptation, family by family (Bristol & Schopler, 1984). Even when we control for the type of handicap or severity of handicap, this diversity makes it difficult to design a single treatment program or to emerge with confident generalizations about family adaptation. When there are multiple variables involved, which certainly is the case here, then some type of multivariate conceptual model has to be constructed if we are to explain or predict what is happening in a particular family. The ABCX model developed by Hill (1949, 1958) and expanded by McCubbin (1979) represents one attempt to specify factors affecting family stress.

The three dimensions proposed by Hill, and modified by McCubbin, deal with the *stressor event* (A), in this case the presence of the handicapped child; (B) the *resources of the family*, the presence of support systems to meet the crisis; and finally, (C) the *definition of the stressor* on the part of the family itself. It appears that some mix or blend of those three major factors plays a role in determining the final level of stress or effective adaptation that the family can make in such circumstances (X).

The careful study of the family reveals that having a handicapped child is not the only stressful event that a family can face nor even the most serious. Families can have members who are terminally ill, or there may be chronic unemployment for all the breadwinners in the family or serious discord interpersonally within the family. All these factors can add arithmetically or geometrically to the stress. What the chapter authors are attempting to do in this book is to try to sort out those dimensions that are particularly relevant to the handicapped child and then to propose some forms of amelioration to those stresses.

The chapters cover a variety of topics, including the history of families of handicapped children, exploration of family typologies and life cycles, and roles played by fathers and siblings in the family, as well as the usual role played by the mother. The implications for public policy are discussed along with future research directions. The editors hope that the reader will find this smorgasbord of topics to be a tasty intellectual meal that will help them think more deeply about this fascinating social issue.

REFERENCES

Bristol, M., & Schopler, E. (1984). A developmental perspective on stress and coping in families of autistic children. In J. Blacher (Ed.), *Families of severely handicapped children: A re-*

view of research. New York: Academic Press.

Brooks, P., Sperber, R., & McCauley, C. (Eds.). (1984). *Learning and cognition in the mentally retarded*. Hillsdale, NJ: Lawrence Erlbaum Associates, Inc.

Farber, B. (1959). Effects of a severely mentally retarded child on family integration. *Monographs of the Society for Research in Child Development, 24*(2, Serial No. 71).

Gallagher, J. J., Beckman, P., & Cross, A. H. (1983). Families of handicapped children: Sources of stress and its amelioration. *Exceptional Children, 50*(1), 10–19.

Hill, R. (1949). *Families under stress: Adjustment to the crisis of war separation and reunion*. New York: Harper & Row.

Hill, R. (1958). Social stresses on the family. *Social Casework, 39*, 139–150.

Kernan, K. T., Begab, M. J., Edgerton, R. B. (Eds.). (1983). *Environments and behavior: The adaptation of mentally retarded persons*. Baltimore: University Park Press.

Martin, E. W. (1976). A national commitment to the rights of the individual—1776–1976. *Exceptional Children, 43*(3), 132–134.

McCubbin, H. (1979). Integrating coping behavior in family stress theory. *Journal of Marriage and the Family, 41*, 237–244.

Scanzoni, L., & Scanzoni, J. (1976). *Men, women, and change: A sociology of marriage and family*. New York: McGraw-Hill Book Co.

Turnbull, H. R., III, & Turnbull, A. P. (Eds.). (1985). *Parents speak out: Then and now* (2nd ed.). Columbus, OH: Charles E. Merrill Publishing Co.

Section

I

FAMILIES OF
HANDICAPPED CHILDREN

Chapter

1

Historical Contexts of Research on Families with Mentally Retarded Members

Bernard Farber

RESEARCH ON FAMILIES with severely mentally retarded members is not an isolated phenomenon. The changes that have occurred in the character of this research cannot be separated from the historical changes that have taken place in the role of the family as a social institution in the United States. Using the approach applied by Thomas Kuhn (1970) in his analysis of changes in scientific research, this chapter describes different periods in the history of the American family; it then suggests how each period seems to have evoked particular kinds of research on families with retarded members.

In his book on scientific revolutions, Kuhn (1970) presents an institutional analysis of radical shifts in the directions of scientific endeavors. These shifts are brought about as new paradigms emerge, which then generate novel streams of research and theory and, in the process, restructure scientific subcommunities.

Kuhn's application of the concept of paradigms has been extensively criticized (e.g., Lakatos & Musgrave, 1970). Yet, despite certain shortcomings, the paradigm concept seems to be a useful heuristic device to portray the exemplars or models that organize scholarly research activity. However, in this chapter, the characterization of how changes occur in research interests differs considerably from that proposed by Kuhn.

Viewing family history from the perspective of exemplars or paradigms implies that the family is similar to the sciences and to the arts in that it too creates "cultural products." (See Clignet, 1979, on paradigms in the arts and the sciences.) As with the arts and sciences, in each particular time period, families are constrained to conform to the exemplars of that era in creating their own "cultural products," that is, the next generation of families.

The position taken in this chapter is that cul-

I gratefully acknowledge the helpful critical commentary by Fred Lindstrom of Arizona State University, Barbara Laslett of the University of Minnesota, James J. Gallagher of the University of North Carolina, and my wife, Rosanna Farber.

tural exemplars or paradigms of family life serve as a means for accommodating contradictions in values and demands between family life and other social domains (as well as internal contradictions) (cf. Douglas, 1975; Schelsky, 1966). As profound changes occur in economic, political, and religious institutions, new contradictions emerge, and family paradigms are revised (Farber, 1975a, 1981). Each new era seems to be marked by modifications in the distribution of power in the society; characteristically, these modifications have been reflected in the broadening of voting rights and their implementation. The author proposes that shifts in the cultural paradigms that define family norms 1) stimulate the development of new policy issues regarding the family and thereby 2) generate fresh frameworks for research on families with retarded members.

However, in contrast to the physical sciences, the rise of a new research framework in the social sciences does not necessarily imply a complete replacement of the old one. Rather, in sociology, as in the arts, paradigms tend to proliferate (Clignet, 1979). In the study of social phenomena, a new paradigm may introduce a fresh strand of research without necessarily dominating research in the entire field. Social and economic concerns that have sustained the old paradigm may persist alongside the new concerns, thereby prolonging the endurance of the old model.

Yet, in a sense, old paradigms hold the seeds of their own destruction. Even as they dominate research hypotheses in any era, efforts are made to discredit the studies that provide their empirical justification. Ordinarily, investigators using the old paradigm are aware of the shortcomings in their studies, but they consider the criticisms to be peripheral to the validity of the paradigm. The critiques that seek to discredit the old cultural paradigm, however, elevate these shortcomings to signs of crucial defects in the evidence supporting the paradigm (cf. Kuhn, 1970). Implied in these discrediting critiques are perspectives that define new paradigms (e.g., Gouldner, 1973).

The division of American family history into time periods refers to general eras, rather than precisely bounded stages. Complexities of the times and conflicts over paradigms are ignored in this chapter for the sake of clarity of the description of each period (e.g., Andrews, 1853). One age overlaps another: Some families are ahead of their time, and family characteristics of earlier eras fade slowly. Consequently, one should regard the dating of these eras merely as signposts, rather than as boundaries. (See Demos, 1979, 1983.) Each of these eras can probably be subdivided further, but for purposes of this chapter, the broad classifications seem sufficient.

In this chapter, the eras are designated as 1) the colonial/revolutionary era, 2) the century of growth, 3) the era of the welfare state, 4) the age of reaction to bureaucratic authority, and 5) the robotized society to come. The general characteristics of each era are presented in Table 1. The table integrates information about the various institutions in the society during each period, and it tries to indicate the overall coherence of the social structure in meeting the major problems—the social contradictions— of the times. The family paradigms are metaphorical statements that describe the basic forms of social organization intended to resolve these problems: the family as "a little commonwealth," as a business firm, as a unit based on companionship, as a pluralistic collectivity, and as an engineered construction. (See such anthologies as Demos & Boocock, 1978; Gordon, 1983; Laslett, 1973, 1977; Tufte & Myerhoff, 1979.)

The sections that follow briefly describe the central concerns relevant to social policies, the predominant family paradigms, and the issues dealt with in research on families with retarded members in each era.

THE COLONIAL/REVOLUTIONARY ERA

The social issues of the colonial/revolutionary era were primarily political. This era saw the emergence of the national state, and much attention was given to the appropriate role of government. The family was regarded as an entity analogous to the state, and the government metaphor seems to have been used exten-

Table 1.   Family models in historical eras

Generality of social entity	Family governance model	Entrepreneurial family model	Companionship family model	Pluralistic family model
Historical era	Colonial / revolutionary (ca. 1620–1820)	Jacksonian / Victorian Era (ca. 1820–1915)	Development of welfare state (ca. 1915–1965)	Reaction to bureaucracy (ca. 1965–now)
Social problem seen as basic	High risks of survival (U.S. Census, 1949)	Constraints on capitalism and national growth (Ryan, 1981)	Inequities and social crises of capitalism (Lasch, 1983)	Inequities in public and private sectors (Schelsky, 1966)
Societal or community domain	Strong sanctions against deviance; firm boundaries between factions (Demos, 1970; Farber, 1972)	Emphasis on competition as prevailing social process (Hofstadter, 1955)	Emphasis on collective security as strategy of organization (Burgess, 1974)	Redress of violations of personal and civil rights (Skolnick & Skolnick, 1971)
Political domain	Control by elite, rooted in Puritan doctrine of elect (Morgan, 1966)	Democratizing process in voting, urban control, and so forth (Degler, 1959)	Extending franchise to women; consensus politics (Lipset, 1960)	Ensuring franchise to minorities; politics of confrontation (U.S. Civil Rights Act)
Economic domain	Organization of both production and consumption problematic; Artisan-apprentice relations model of labor; conflict between artisan and merchant factions (Farber, 1972; Kett, 1971)	Dialectic of production and consumption: paternalism as strategy of control; isolation of production and consumption in home and factory (Hareven, 1982)	Balance of production and consumption; public sector as balancing private sector (Keynesian model)	Confrontations to rectify inequities in productive and consumption systems (as seen by each social class: minority, women, etc.) (Literature of blacks', women's, etc. movements)
Kinship	Centripetal organization, including first cousin marriage (Farber, 1972, 1975a)	Bridge for gap between consumption and production by nepotism and family capitalism (Hall, 1974; Hareven, 1982)	Kin ties as augmenting public sector as support system (Farber, 1971)	Confrontation as focusing on affinal ties as representing opposing interests
Family	Domestic unit used to integrate production and consumption (Greven, 1970; Hall, 1974)	Family economy: pooling members' resources (Hareven, 1982; Scott & Tilly, 1975)	Companionate ties— "togetherness"— as bond (Burgess & Wallin, 1953)	Family as an instrument for achieving personal rights (Orr, 1979)
Marriage	Means for maintaining factions by controlling members (Farber, 1972; Smith, 1973)	Economic security as a basis for marital choice, timing, and stability (Degler, 1983; May, 1978)	Homogamy as a basis for marital consensus (Burgess, 1974)	Fit between couple's demands regarding personal rights, wants, and ambitions (Becker, 1981)
Justification	Family as	Family firm as	Unity of the	Personal

(continued)

Table 1. (continued)

Generality of social entity	Family governance model	Entrepreneurial family model	Companionship family model	Pluralistic family model
	microcosm of the state: the mercantilist model (Demos, 1970; Morgan, 1966)	effective unit in competition: cults of self-made man and of true womanhood as basis for joining loyalty and achievement (Demos, 1979; Welter, 1983)	family through consensus on overall group priorities for welfare of members (Burgess 1974)	relationships as a means for facilitating mutual achievement of self-realization (Orr, 1979; Shorter, 1975)
Discrediting evidence	Demographic growth and economic complexity as obstacles to rigorous controls (Farber, 1972)	Neurotic and obsessive personality disorders; excessive restraints in family life; exposure to poverty and to crisis (Lasch, 1977)	Prevalence of domestic violence and divorce; persistence of power differentials and class deprivations (Gelles, 1972; Laing, 1971; Skolnick, 1979)	Prevalence of loneliness and other indices of unhappiness; uneven self-realization of family members interpreted as exploitation (Otto, 1970)
Sources for characteriz-ing paradigm	Demos, 1979; Farber, 1972; Hall, 1974; Morgan, 1966; Smith, 1978	Demos, 1979; Degler, 1983; Greeley, 1853; Hareven, 1982; Kett, 1971; Miller & Swanson, 1958; St. John, 1848	Burgess & Locke, 1945; Burgess & Wallin, 1953; Folsom, 1943; Lasch, 1977	Orr, 1979; Skolnick & Skolnick, 1971

sively by contemporary writers. One of these writers, Davenport, suggested the importance of men's "Family-Government over their Wives, Children, and Servants" (cited in Morgan, 1966, pp. 142–3), and another author, Gouge, wrote in 1622 that "the family is . . . a little commonwealth" (cited in Demos, 1979, p. 46). The very writings that underlay the American constitution expressed this view of the family. For example, John Locke (1949) had noted in his *Second Treatise of Civil Government* that "A child is born a subject of no country or government. He is under his father's tuition and authority" (p. 17). Moreover, a basic tenet in 18th-century New England was that effective "family-government" was the foundation of social order. Indeed, according to Cotton Mather, "Well-ordered Families naturally produce a Good Order in other So-

cieties" (cited in Morgan, 1966, pp. 143–144). In the earlier Colonial period, "single individuals of whatever age were required by law to place themselves under good family government, and even a few married persons—those whose family government failed—were placed under the jurisdiction of other families" (Towner, 1966, p. 420). However, as the population grew, this practice was abandoned.

With family concerns framed in terms of governance, the chief issues regarding mentally retarded individuals centered around the extent to which families could control their deviant members. In death records, individuals were sometimes described as "non compos mentis," but they did not seem to present any special issues in everyday family life (see Farber, 1972). Because the prevalent political paradigm of the family permitted retarded persons to be viewed in the same framework as other family members, one would expect little research to be undertaken on families into which they were born. (The colonial/revolutionary era is discussed here mainly to provide a contrast to later historical periods.)

THE CENTURY OF GROWTH

A major change in American family ideology was ushered in during the Jacksonian era. As capitalism began to spread, the older hierarchical, Puritan-based order disintegrated. Indeed, Katz and Davey (1978) suggest that "it was not industrialization that had undermined [the institution of apprenticeship and family transmission of crafts], but capitalism. Apprenticeship was incompatible with a system of wage labor which stressed the manipulation of mobile resources in order to maximize profit" (p. 96). During the Jacksonian period, there was a basic shift in the social structure from a political model based on government by elites to one of reliance on economic market mechanisms to maintain social order (Degler, 1983). From the beginning of the Jacksonian era onward, there was a strong movement to expand suffrage by eliminating the holding of property as a qualification for voting (Degler, 1959).

Along with this structural change, the rise of entrepreneurship also instigated revisions in the ideological basis of social order. The reform movements and "religious revivals of the 1830s were part of the struggles of the middle class to fashion new moral codes for a new way of life, to foster self-discipline for their own class, and to inculcate a new work discipline in the workingclass" (Tilly & Cohen, 1982, p. 155; see also Smith-Rosenberg, 1978). Horace Greeley (1853) wrote extensively as editor of the *New York Tribune* about "true" marriage and the "purity" of family life, where abjuring responsibilities serves to "increase the sum of human degradation and wretchedness" (p. 72). At least one commentator in the mid-19th century characterized the middle-class family as "a partnership in business, of which the husband and wife constitute

the firm, the former attending to the external relations of the home, the latter to the internal" (St. John, 1848, pp. 169–170). All of this concern seems to have reflected an increasing emphasis on economic rationality in family life (see May, 1978).

As a result, there was a movement away from the Puritan-derived stress on social control and moral conformity imposed by a benevolent patriarch. Instead, family life was reorganized according to what might be called the entrepreneurial family model (Miller & Swanson, 1958) that called for self-discipline and firm, internalized moral codes. For men, there was the Cult of the Self-Made Man (Demos, 1979), whereas for women, these codes were expressed in the Cult of True Womanhood, an ideology resting on "four cardinal virtues—piety, purity, submissiveness, and domesticity" (Welter, 1983, p. 372). The Cult of True Womanhood

> helped to curtail the employment of native-born women in factories, and as the [19th] century progressed it was immigrant women who constituted an increasingly large percentage of the female work force. . . . The family ideology of the early Victorian era granted the woman authority and responsibility in that arena of social life to which she was in fact being structurally consigned. (Smelser & Halpern, 1978, p. S307)

Beginning with the Jacksonian era, which corresponded roughly to the beginning of the Victorian era, institutions affecting the young

> were more carefully and precisely age-graded . . . than before. . . . Age grading may have been part of an effort to lock-step the child into rigid and predetermined modes of behavior. The change looked not to his benefit, but to the rationalization of childhood so that behavior would become more predictable and manageable. (Rothman, 1971, p. 189)

As the public school system was established in the latter half of the 19th century, there "came the introduction of more specific norms about the behavior expected of children of different ages," and with the consolidation of more uniform expectations, the problems to parents and teachers of children who were off-schedule were noted (Smelser & Halpern, 1978, pp. S304–S305).

8 FARBER

Simultaneously, a change was taking place in the residential patterns of young persons. Whereas in the early 19th century most youths lived in nonparental households, "in the latter part of the century, this pattern changed so that children in their late teens and beyond were remaining in the homes of their parents until marriage and sometimes after their marriages" (Foner, 1978, p. S345; see also Chudacoff & Hareven, 1979, p. 76). This shift meant that children were expected to contribute greatly to the collective family economy that had emerged in the context of the entrepreneurial family model. In fact, Demos (1979) suggests that

> the entire system was infused with a strain of dire urgency. If the family did not function in the expected ways, there were no other institutions to back it up. If one family member fell short of the prescribed ways and standards, all the others were placed in jeopardy. (pp. 54–55)

The rationalization of family norms in the entrepreneurial family paradigm, along with the drive for religious revival and reform, created new issues in dealing with mental retardation. In the Jacksonian era, previous concerns about control of retarded persons were transformed into demands to make them useful. One social reformer interested in retardation was Edouard Seguin, a follower of Saint-Simon, who advocated the application of positive philosophy to guide the evolution of industrializing society on the basis of scientific principles. Seguin's work focused on training children in institutions to return to their families and "yonder world" as useful citizens (Seguin, 1866, p. 243; see also Scheerenberger, 1983). Similarly, Samuel Howe, whose life was devoted to the needy (e.g., the blind, the deaf, the retarded, the imprisoned, and later, the blacks after freedom), legitimated his institutional programs on the basis of economic and social usefulness. In support of his position, he cited a Dr. Woodward,

> the eminent physician of the State Lunatic Hospital, who said: "My opinion is that nearly all idiots can be made better: the physical condition and personal habits of the lowest order can be improved, and those possessing more mind can be trained to usefulness, and some can be taught to

read, write, and labor advantageously, and be useful and happy. (Howe, 1857, cited in Farber, 1968, p. 181)

The optimism of early Jacksonian reformers was shaded by the general conception that biological and social characteristics were intertwined. On the one hand, the concept of racial and national differences guided the work of many of the reformers. For example, Howe distinguished between the creative and imitative races and regarded retarded individuals as analogous to the imitative races. On the other hand, as time went on, explanations of deviance from the entrepreneurial family model were couched in terms of "moral degeneracy." The theory of degeneracy was described by Benedict Morel in 1857, just 2 years before Darwin's *Origin of the Species* (Ackerknecht, 1959, pp. 47–51). Morel had reached the conclusion that all varieties of mental disease, such as insanity and mental deficiency, were related. Regarding these disorders as hereditary, Morel hypothesized that they became more profound with each succeeding generation. This progression was seen as a continual loss of "vital energy" from one generation to the next, until a state of idiocy was reached. Tredgold (1903) noted that

> it is indeed more than likely that many of the conditions of life at the present day, the struggle for place or for mere existence, with its accompanying wear and tear and nervous strain, and often insufficiency of food and fresh air, contribute largely not only to the deterioration of our manners but also of our nervous system. (p. 366)

He further suggested that

> the most reasonable view would seem to be that the germinal plasm shares in the general bodily deterioration which results from the harmful conditions [including "consumption, syphilis, and alcoholism"], and that, therefore, the offspring to which it gives rise is rendered unstable and of diminished vital energy . . .—in other words, a neuropath has been created; should such a person marry another of similar neuropathic tendencies an aggravation of the condition will be the result in the next generation. (cf. Wohl, 1978, p. 366)

The theory of degeneracy stimulated a variety of studies that provided empirical support for the policies of placement in residential institutions and of the sterilization of retarded adults (cf. Wolfensberger, 1975). The earliest of these studies was Richard L. Dugdale's (1877) genealogical analysis of the Jukes family. In his analysis of six generations of blood relatives, Dugdale found "a preponderance of pauperism, harlotry, illegitimate children, syphilis, deformed youngsters, and a higher crime rate among the offspring of those with Jukes blood" in comparison with persons related only by marriage or cohabitation with the Jukes family (Scheerenberger, 1983, p. 115). By implication, based on the theory of degeneracy, it was presumed that many of the Jukes were mentally retarded.

In 1915, Estabrook (1916) did a more extensive analysis of the Jukes genealogy and found that, for the 984 persons for whom data were available, about 30% were educationally retarded 2 or more years, and almost 20% had never attended school. Consistent with the degeneracy theory, Estabrook concluded that licentiousness, pauperism, and criminality were all products of the degeneracy that leads to mental deficiency. (See Scheerenberger, 1983, pp. 151–152.)

Other genealogical analyses provided additional support for the family degeneracy theory. These included reports on the Nams by Davenport (1912), the Hill Folk by Danielson and Davenport (1912), the Dack family by Finlayson (1916), and the "Mongrel Virginians, the Win Tribe" by Estabrook and McDougle (1926). The most influential study was conducted by Goddard (1912) on the Kallikaks, in which the idea of a comparison group was involved. There were two lines of descent from Martin Kallikak—"one characterized by thoroughly good, respectable, normal citizenship, with almost no exception; the other being equally characterized by mental defect in every generation" (Goddard, 1912, p. 116). The signs of familial degeneracy were clear: illegitimacy, sexual immorality, alcoholism, prostitution, criminality, high infant mortality, and "conclusive proof" of feeble-mindedness.

As the rate of urbanization reached its peak at the beginning of the 20th century, threads of functionalism began to weave their way into the fabric of thought about the family (e.g., Lichtenberger, 1909). Increasingly, social Darwinism gave way to an emphasis on the functions that the family performs in contributing to the maintenance of the social order. Hankins (1925) noted in the mid-1920s that in sociology, generally, "there has been a drift away from the early physical and biological terminology [and that] . . . there have appeared hopeful efforts to find some principles of collective life itself" (p. 310).

With these developments in social thought, the theory of familial degeneracy and its supporting evidence was increasingly being questioned, particularly in view of modern genetics and the developments in special education (e.g., Doll, 1924; Wallin, 1914). The 1920s seem to have marked a transition from studies of progressive familial hereditary degeneration to research on familial social degeneration, and from the entrepreneurial family model to the companionship family. This transition to a new paradigm is discussed in the next section.

THE ERA OF THE WELFARE STATE

The next significant paradigm shift in family life occurred in the decades after World War I, as the United States achieved the status of an urbanized, industrialized world power. The pre-World War I era had been dominated by the slogan of survival of the fittest in a competitive struggle for existence. The theories of Herbert Spencer and William Graham Sumner dominated popular social thought. But after World War I, there was a growing emphasis on the slogan that in union there is strength and fulfillment. In family life, this shift was marked by a decline in the entrepreneurial family model, with its emphasis on competitiveness as the basic social process; concomitantly, there emerged the companionship family model that stressed the primacy of mutuality and reciprocity. (From the perspective of social theory, the Comtean view of organic unity had triumphed over Spencerian individualism [cf. Gouldner, 1970].)

A growing suspicion that competitiveness had failed as a basic principle for structuring social institutions brought about this paradigm shift. Although this view had achieved some popularity in the Progressive Era at the beginning of the century, its significance became increasingly apparent after World War I. Many important events suggesting a redistribution of power took place in the postwar era. Immediately after the war, the franchise was extended to women. On the international scene, there was an increasing acceptance of the position that unrestrained competition between countries was a major factor in war and that war was becoming too threatening to mankind; to achieve collective security, the League of Nations was organized. In the economic domain, the fear that only the most ruthless would survive revived the public concern over the evils of monopoly that had emerged in the Progressive Era. In labor relations, whereas paternalistic exploitation had characterized 19th-century family capitalism, the movement toward corporate capitalism brought industry-wide unionism (Hareven, 1982).

In general, the notion gained ascendancy that unbridled competitive struggle for the survival of the fittest posed grave dangers to American society. This notion was given further impetus by the Depression in the 1930s; deficiencies of the traditional, competition-based social order became apparent (Elder, 1974). The government was transformed into a welfare state, seeking a national consensus, as it established new programs pertaining to social security and social welfare.

The decline in the use of competition as a basic organizing principle in social arrangements was reflected in ideas about family relations. Family sociologists tried to capture the major elements of these changes in their conceptualizations. Ernest W. Burgess depicted a shift from external community controls of the "institutional" family to internal interpersonal consensus of the "companionship" family (Burgess, 1926; Burgess & Locke, 1945). Similarly, in an analysis of major social trends, Ogburn (1929) portrayed a decline of family functions until only affection remained as the family's legitimate reason for continued existence. Other social scientists devised similar descriptions based on alternative conceptual schemes (e.g., Parsons & Bales, 1955). Regardless of the particular conceptualization, however, there was agreement among family sociologists that there had been a paradigmatic transformation from the entrepreneurial family model, with its moralistic emphasis on tactics for survival or advancement in a socioeconomic sense, to the companionship family model, with its humanistic emphasis on the dependence of personal welfare of individual members on the unity of the family group (e.g., Folsom, 1943).

Just as the paradigm shift in the Jacksonian era brought into question the traditional ways of handling mentally retarded persons, so apparently did the transformation from the entrepreneurial family model to the companionship family. During the 1930s and 1940s, research was undertaken on the efficacy of public residential institutions (e.g., Skeels, 1942; Skeels & Dye, 1939), and leading proponents of the policy of residential institutionalization changed their positions (Fernald, 1924; Goddard, 1928). There was a pause in research during World War II, but in the postwar years, the questioning of the welfare benefits of institutionalization resumed.

In line with changing policy interests, postwar research centered on two related questions: 1) How does the presence of a mentally retarded child affect family relationships and the lives of parents and siblings—the collective welfare of the family? and 2) How does the family's welfare change (e.g., degree of improvement) if the child is institutionalized? (See Farber, 1959; Fotheringham, Skelton, & Hoddinott, 1971; Mercer, 1965; Saenger, 1960).

The shift in research questions seems to have been related to a corresponding shift in theories of deviancy associated with the cultural paradigms. The 19th-century studies regarded departures from the entrepreneurial family model as reflecting a cumulative hereditary degeneracy fed by environmental insufficiencies; the remedial policy was to isolate and sterilize the degenerate families (or among reformers, to regenerate them as much as possible). However, the mid-20th-century studies saw departures from the companionship family model as social degeneracy (i.e.,poor social and mental health); the remedial policy was then to devise support services to alleviate hardships of family members in their domestic and community relationships.

The research programs undertaken shortly after World War II were, for the most part, stimulated by the increased demand for services for mentally retarded individuals, as well as for other needy groups. This increase in demand required the development of research programs to define and to justify areas of need and to provide new techniques of remediation. Investigations dealt with areas of special concern to policy-makers and to parents: institutional placement versus family residence, the efficacy of special classes for children classified as "trainable," the extent of stress in family life, mental health and economic difficulties, and so on (e.g., Caldwell & Guze, 1960; Farber, 1959; Farber, Jenne, & Toigo, 1960; Kramm, 1963; Saenger, 1960; Schonell, Middleton, Watts, & Rorke, 1959; Tizard & Grad, 1961). Studies of specific family hardships have been summarized by Moroney (1983): financial burdens (Aldrich et al., 1971; Dunlap, 1976; Holt, 1958; Sultz, 1972), stigma (Barsch, 1968; Birenbaum, 1970; Gottlieb, 1975; Kershaw, 1965; Schonell & Watts, 1956), personal care and behavioral problems (Aldrich et al., 1971;Bayley, 1973; Farber, 1960b), interruptions of family routines (Bayley, 1973; Hewett, 1972; Younghusband, 1971), and social isolation and limitations on recreation (Aldrich et al., 1971; Farber, 1959; Holt, 1958; Tizard & Grad, 1961).

Research focusing on the need of families for remedial services presupposed the existence of a norm of a "healthy" family life toward which people strive—the companionship family model. Consequently, the research programs tended to focus on variables that pertained to the departure of family life from this norm: degree of family disintegration, role tension and conflict, personality disorders, psychosomatic illness, inhibition of school and occupational success of parents and siblings, and so forth. A common finding was

that, although parental suspicion of developmental problems evoked some anxiety, the critical point in parental turmoil occurred when the child was actually labeled as retarded (Farber, 1959, 1960b; Hall, 1961; MacKeith, 1973; Meyerowitz & Kaplan, 1967; Rowitz, 1981; Waisbren, 1980).

The concept of family crisis provided a basis for designing much of the research that was undertaken. As formulated by Reuben Hill (1949), the character of the stressor event, in combination with the way in which the family defines that event and the family's resources, determined the extent of family crisis (cf. Horejsi, 1983). In an early study, Farber (1959) defined the character of the crisis faced by families with mentally retarded children as an arrest in the family life cycle, whereby 1) family development is slowed and 2) family roles are thrown out of synchronization with the cohort of families who would ordinarily define the character of family development. Presumably, the greater the asynchronism, the greater the degree of family crisis. Indeed, the weight of evidence suggested that situations in families with severely mentally retarded members become more stressful as the family life cycle proceeds toward its later stages (Birenbaum, 1971; Farber, 1960b; Miller, 1969; Suelzle & Keenan, 1981).

The hypothesis of family cycle arrest also proposed that, regardless of birth order, the social role of the retarded child eventually shifts to that of the youngest child (Farber, 1959). Here too, the findings tended to support this conceptualization (Miller, 1974; Shere, 1955), with the amount of sibling interaction found to have an impact on the adjustment of normal brothers and sisters (except when age differences were large) (Cleveland & Miller, 1977; Farber & Jenne, 1963b; Gath, 1972; Graliker, Fishler, & Koch, 1962; Grossman, 1972). In fact, only a minority of parents of developmentally disabled persons believed that such individuals should be awarded full legal rights as adults (Suelzle & Keenan, 1981).

In brief, studies utilizing the family crisis approach—although particular conceptualizations might vary—discovered that several factors were especially important in evoking stress among family members. These factors included nature of the disability (Cummings, Bayley, & Rie, 1966; Klebanoff, 1959), age and sex composition of the family (Cain & Levine, 1963; Cleveland & Miller, 1977; Farber & Jenne, 1963a; Farber et al., 1960; Fowle, 1968), socioeconomic status of the family (Farber, 1959, 1960a, 1960b; Grossman, 1972), and religion (Bernard, 1974; Farber, 1959; Jordan, 1961; Saenger, 1960; Waterman, 1948; Zuk, 1959; Zuk, Miller, Bertram, & Kling, 1961; Zwerling, 1954).

Within the context of the welfare state, families unable to endure crises provoked by the presence of a retarded child required remedial action, particularly under governmental auspices. The research on the issue of institutional versus familial residence indicated that institutionalization per se does not solve family problems (Farber, 1960a; Fotheringham et al., 1971; Fowle, 1968). It may instead produce other problems (Farber, 1959; Farber & Jenne, 1963a). Consequently, a wide variety of services are necessary. Zimmerman (1979) proposed that

> threats to family equilibrium and adaptation from both internal and external sources . . . suggest the need for the planning and provision of services in all areas—health, education, income maintenance, employment and manpower, housing, and personal social services—adapted to the particular needs of the developmentally disabled and their families. (p. 93)

Hence, the family crisis approach led ultimately to a consideration of issues regarding the development of specialized supportive services to permit home care of retarded individuals (Bruininks & Krantz, 1979; Mercer, 1966).

THE AGE OF REACTION TO BUREAUCRACY AND AUTHORITY

The most recent paradigmatic change has been from the companionship family model, which emphasizes the importance of consensus among family members, to the pluralistic family model, which emphasizes the achievement of members' individual rights.

The decade of the 1960s seems to have marked a turning point in the faith of the American people in the efficacy of the welfare state. The supposedly beneficent welfare state had manipulated the nation into (what was for many citizens) an unpopular war, and the ensuing disillusionment carried with it a replacement of consensual politics with confrontational politics. In addition, the massive government programs established to dispel the ills of society were seen as failing in their mission. These signs of failure included the persistence of poverty, massive cultural "deprivation," delinquency, cumulative educational deficit, and so forth.

In this historical setting, the state was perceived as impeding social justice, rather than promoting it. The attainment of full civil and constitutional rights for all citizens became a central social concern. Early in this era, there was a major movement to reduce constraints on voting among minorities, particularly blacks, through such mechanisms as broadened voting registration drives, elimination of poll taxes, and so forth. Politically, this movement culminated in the passage of the Civil Rights Act. Particular attention was focused on situations in which there had been a history of unequal treatment under the law. Earlier, the issue of equal treatment had been interpreted as referring only to individuals. In the 1960s, however, inequality was reinterpreted as pertaining to social classes (e.g., blacks, Hispanics, women), with the implication that unequal treatment of these classes had cumulative and far-reaching debilitating effects on their members. Because membership in these classes is ascribed by group labels assigned at birth, the interpretation was that the injustices wrought by unequal treatment demanded not individual remedies, but instead broad changes in social institutions. In the vocabulary of the 1960s, the power structure was keeping minorities out of the mainstream, and reforms were needed to end institutional discrimination.

In this context, the companionship family model seemed inappropriate. To operate effectively, the companionship family required an undergirding of support programs. With the decline of the idea that the welfare state was an effective means for dealing with social problems in America, the coordinate companionship family ideology began to be sharply criticized. It became commonplace for social critics to assert that the companionship family had failed. They claimed that its very emphasis on unity often impeded personal development and self-realization, and occasionally its emphasis on expressiveness had even fostered family violence (Straus, Gelles, & Steinmetz, 1980). The gender power differentials and personal alienation in the outside world were seen as having been transported into family relationships. As a result, the very privacy of the household extolled in the companionship family model was devalued.

The remedy proposed was to reconstruct the family along lines that would respect the rights of all family members to reach their full potential, regardless of the specific forms that it may take. The paradigmatic shift subtly replaced an emphasis on personal satisfactions in stable family ties with one on personal rights, regardless of stability of family ties (see Kobrin, 1978). The shift implied a change from a concern with the common interests of the members to a concern about the special interests, the personal rights, of each family member. Just as the societal model moved toward pluralism in its stress on group civil and constitutional rights, so too did the family model become pluralistic.

Since the 1960s, images of the family have changed markedly in the social sciences, as well as in the popular media. In sociological analyses, the hegemony of functionalism has been challenged. Less emphasis is given to the ways that the family as a social institution contributes to maintaining the social order. With that challenge, there has been serious questioning of the universality of the nuclear family as a social form (Adams, 1960; Edwards & Kluck, 1980). In law, "the liberty and autonomy interests of women and children have been recognized and furthered and the costs of family life have been exposed" (Morse, 1979, p. 321). There has been a "dominant shift in family law—increasing autonomy for family members in relation to one another" (Morse, 1979, p. 321). The description of the pluralistic family by John B. Orr (1979), a social ethicist, is typical:

> I believe it is important ... to affirm the integrity of a pluralism of family life styles within the American environment. . . . My bias is toward policies and procedures that insure the civil rights of conventional and deviant families, and that insure as broad a choice of life styles as can be included within the bounds of democratic society. We need, for example, to liberalize laws that relate to nonconventional households and to define more carefully the legal rights and responsibilities of persons who enter into nonconventional family experiments or simple "living-together" arrangements. Choices that should be open to traditionally conceived families need to be extended and protected as well. (p. 386)

When providing support services to retarded individuals is no longer a growing industry, research on families with retarded children tends to be redirected. The pluralistic family paradigm replaced the vocabulary of crisis and maladjustment with one of modes of confrontation. Whereas the previous paradigm evoked research on ways in which the presence of a retarded child produced family deviance, the pluralistic family paradigm focuses on how the family acts to retain the rights of its members— its battle to retain a semblance of normality. This focus is perhaps an outgrowth of social movements—advocacy, normalization, and deinstitutionalization—related to the attainment of civil and personal rights for retarded individuals (Willer, Intagliata, & Atkinson, 1981).

The emergence of the pluralistic family paradigm has been expressed in research on families with mentally retarded children in two ways: in the conceptualization of 1) overall strategies in family organization and 2) the ways that family members cope with outsiders.

Family Organization Strategies

The family crisis perspective led researchers to treat the family as if the presence of the retarded child were the only problematic element in its existence. The pluralistic family model, however, regards the intrusion of the retarded child on family processes as only one more element to be dealt with in organizing domestic life; the parents must still make a living, maintain a domicile, and show a sensitivity to the needs of all family members (Farber, 1979). This model focuses on the fact that, in most ways, the family seeks to provide a normal existence for all its members.

A central element of family organization strategies is the identification of a set of priorities for determining the extent to which family life revolves around the retarded child as compared with other foci. Parents are generally faced with the dilemma of whether to overplay or underplay their child's handicap (Hewett, 1972). Some families turn in on themselves in order to cope with the child, whereas others are able to accommodate a variety of kinship and community activities of interest to individual family members. Family organizational strategies have been conceptualized in different ways, but each approach rests on an assumption that, at least for theoretical purposes, people act rationally.

For example, Farber (1960a) used a model based on the theory of games as described in economic literature. In his investigation, he regarded the parents of the retarded children as antagonists against "Nature." This anthropomorphic fiction of "Nature" as a player provided a framework for evaluating how unfavorable the "moves" of nature—conditions over which families have no control—are for the outcome of the family. For the parents as players, making choices that minimize social costs would be more urgent under a severe challenge by nature than under a moderate challenge. Farber regarded some kinds of strategies as general (i.e., as capable of overcoming a wide range of oppositions by "Nature") and others as specific (i.e., restricted in their usefulness to particular kinds of situations).

In applying the theory-of-games model in his research, Farber found three modes of balancing the contradictory pulls and pressures of caregiving and interests outside the family. He described these as general strategies of family organization: parent oriented, child oriented, and home oriented. In addition, Farber reported a fourth kind of "play" in the game against "Nature"—families who do not develop a consistent strategy of organization, a residual category. Families in the residual category seem to focus their activities on the retarded child and seem most affected in their cohesiveness and in their life chances in the socioeconomic structure (cf. Mink, Nihira, & Meyers, 1983).

Drawing on the theory-of-games conceptualization, Farber (1975b) then developed a processual model to make sense of the range of "moves" by the family with a retarded child in its game against nature. The processual model itself is based on a principle of successive minimal adaptations. This principle implies that, other things being equal, families will make as minimal an adaptation as possible in order to solve their problems (or at least to endure living with them). The model proposes a temporal progression of adaptations from the least disruptive to the potentially fully disruptive modifications in family organization. At any stage, if the family believes that the kind of adaptation it has made has been effective in handling its predicament, it presumably would cease seeking further solutions to its problem and would stabilize its organization (or, in Bayley's [1973] terms, its structures of coping and of living). On the basis of this set of assumptions, Farber's (1975b) processual model describes the various phases in this progression of adaptations.

In contrast to Farber's emphasis on process, the approach by Michael Bayley (1973) stresses structural arrangements in living with a retarded family member. Bayley makes a distinction between "structure of coping" and "structure of living." The structure of coping pertains to the techniques that families develop to handle the often-inordinate needs and demands of the retarded child. Even routines that are typically simple may become gargantuan challenges to families with a severely retarded member, and the parents may require help from kith and kin in order to survive physically and mentally. Bayley notes that it is primarily the reliable, frequent, and regular help and respite provided in informal networks that are effective in alleviating pressure on the family.

Whereas Bayley defines the structure of coping as dealing primarily with the demands of caregiving, the structure of living pertains to the needs of the parents and siblings. The quality of their lives, according to Bayley, depends in part on their freedom from such caregiving. It was important to the parents to belong to organizations, societies, and churches. "The important thing about these contacts was their normality and the friendships to which they gave rise" (Bayley, 1973, p. 287). In assessing the structure of living, he places much emphasis on "the support and acceptance of the neighborhood" (Bayley, 1973, p. 263). Bayley (1973) suggests that "the parents' interpretation of society's attitude to them and to their subnormal child was related to their attitude to social activities in general" (p. 262).

The policy issues with which the family strategy models deal are broader than those dealt with by the family crisis approach. The family crisis perspective focused on the disintegration of family relationships and its consequences for the family members; it was thus the family that required remediation. The family strategy approach, however, in its emphasis on attempts to retain a semblance of normality, involves the interaction between family and community. As a result, this approach suggests that remedial programs should be aimed at the nonretarded community in order to change the social context in which the families with retarded members must survive.

Coping with Outsiders

Investigators who apply a dramaturgic model in their studies emphasize the importance of outsiders to the way of life of families with retarded members. Social scientists using this approach envision efforts by parents to present an appearance that all is "really" normal as a central theme in their adaptation. The viewpoint is based in large measure on the work of Erving Goffman (1959, 1968, 1974). Taking literally the metaphor that "all the world's a stage," Goffman sees a strong motivation for people to sway those with whom they interact to accept their point of view with regard to whatever matters are at hand. This aim is accomplished by giving a believable performance, by acting as political entrepreneurs

(Darling, 1979), and by enlisting enlightened, powerful people to act as their advocates (Hewett, 1972).

In most social relationships, people act in ways that validate (or conform to) the roles in which others cast them (see Goffman, 1974). However, for the person who bears a stigma as a deviant (e.g., a disabled person [Davis, 1961]), or a "courtesy stigma" as a retarded child's parent (Birenbaum, 1970), it is usually against the individual's interests to validate that persona. Rather, the individual is motivated to hide or to disavow the stigma, to transform the stigmatized status into an elevated one, to account for the stigma in a rational way, or otherwise to dissociate it from him- or herself. Hence, in deviance, the task of impression management is that of convincing an "audience" that what it observes at first sight is not the true situation. How this is done constitutes the core of interest in studies using the dramaturgic model (e.g., Birenbaum, 1970, 1971; Booth, 1978; Voysey, 1972, 1975).

Booth (1978) has found that, in the diagnosis of mental retardation, parents are given "little insight into how [they or the child] will fare in the routine world of daily life" (p. 217). In this respect, they differ from parents with normal children. With a child who is labelled as normal, parents can anticipate a set of developmental rules and expectations. However, the social meaning of retardation entails an uncertainty in trends of family interaction. The parents are faced with the task of transforming this anomalous situation into a set of meanings that can be understood by everyone as falling within the realm of "normal" social relations.

The appearance of normality in family relationships depends in part on the age of the retarded child. Birenbaum (1970) reports that, when children are young, mothers can readily simulate a normal-appearing round of activities; at that time, there is only a small discrepancy between the retarded child and the other children with whom the family interacts. As the children grow older, the discrepancy becomes more pronounced, and it is increasingly difficult to maintain the appearance of a normal family life.

The management of interaction is also accomplished by parents' accounting for those differences in family life that do occur as reasonable, " 'what any parent would do' in the circumstances in question" (Voysey, 1975, p. 156). The parents try to "be seen as reconstituting an appearance which is congruent with normal parenthood and family life" (Voysey, 1975, p. 156). (It is, of course, likely that when institutionalization is a socially acceptable solution, parents will try to present their family situation to officials as being abnormal.) An underlying assumption in these studies is that the parents of retarded individuals apply the same appeals to convince themselves and their families of their own normality. The community relationships are thereby regarded as being of crucial significance in enduring the hardships and disappointments of raising a retarded child.

THE AGE OF ROBOTICS

New technological developments can be expected to produce profound structural changes in society, and with these changes, one can expect further transformations in cultural paradigms. In a few generations, it is likely that another shift in family models will take place, and the technological advances themselves may provide the analogue for the emergence of a new family model. For reasons suggested below, the author thinks it reasonable to anticipate that the next major paradigm will be the constructed family model, a conception that families will be able to devise artfully their domestic relationships in ways that meet the particular hardships that they face.

Discussions of postindustrial society see a trend of continual increase in the automation of production. Much of that discussion emphasizes the control over information processing and transmission. There has been less attention to the robotization of the production of goods and services, perhaps because robots are seen merely as more elaborate traditional machines. However, as computers that "think" are developed, so will more robots "think." Eventually, robots will be able to move out of their sheltered, highly restricted workplaces and to perform many kinds of skills now in the hands of "professionals." Thus, in a few generations, one can expect the displacement of human workers by robots to grow at an increasing rate across a wide socioeconomic range.

The anticipated surge in robotics may have significant implications for the general welfare of the society. It is true that "men of no use to production have almost always existed" (Aron, 1966, p. 236); they form a surplus population in the society. "The organizational view of a surplus population implies that there is an optimal size and composition of people to utilize a given machinery of social organization" (Farber, 1968, p. 10). Indeed, according to Farber (1968),

> In one sense, organizationally surplus populations are necessary in modern society as it is now constituted. The efficient use of human beings in the economic, political, family, and educational institutions depends on a good fit between the abilities of persons and the slots they fill in organizations. In order to achieve this fit, there must be a surplus in the population so that the appropriate persons will be selected for any given slot, since a surplus permits a constant rearranging of persons to maximize efficiency. (pp. 13–14)

In all probability, the size and diversity of surplus populations will expand enormously with the robotization of society. Many people will fall into these surplus groups for traditional reasons: old age, poverty, lack of education, developmental disability, severe physical disability, technological unemployment, and so forth. In the future, however, the boundaries of these groups may be expanded to include more unemployables. In addition, new categories of unemployability (or marginal employability) may be invented. Eventually, the number of families with members in a surplus population may greatly exceed the total number of families in the mainstream population.

This expansion in the population surplus may change the character of social structure, politics, and family life in important ways. The expansion will undoubtedly evoke a reaction by government to minimize any potential threat to its stability. As part of this reaction, mass media and service agencies may increase their efforts at constraining deviant actions in these surplus populations, at least partly by emphasizing conformity to a legal family model (cf. Farber, 1973). In the process, one might expect a reversal in voting rights, with a contraction in the franchise—with the justification that voting creates a conflict of interest for surplus populations; that is, because they depend on government for their very subsistence, they are particularly vulnerable to demogogues who cater to their dependency, and as a result, they cannot honestly vote for candidates who would best serve the general welfare of the society.

As now, the diverse segments of surplus population would tend to gather in "colonies" of various sorts: slums of cities, retirement communities, service centers (e.g., senior citizen centers), educational institutions, and so forth. In order to protect their interests, these surplus populations would generally form into subcommunities, just as they do now. And out of this ongoing community activity would emerge numerous subcultures, each one directed against mainstream values and norms. A state of tension would then exist between the surplus-population subcultures and the culture imposed by agencies and the mass media.

Perhaps the major difference between today and the future can be attributed to the anticipated growth of the surplus populations. Surely, if a majority of families were to become surplus, collectively they would represent a major potential for violence. This threat would provide an impetus for establishing policies intended to avoid major disruptions in the social order. These policies would have to accommodate the contradictions between the official, legal culture and the diverse subcultural reactions. As a consequence of this need to reduce (or eliminate) contradictions, the predominant family paradigm in the society would change.

What would the cultural family paradigm be like? The great diversity among surplus-population segments would dictate a wide range of different models that are qualitatively different from the previous cultural paradigms. Whereas family paradigms in previous eras described a focal point in family goals derived from the general culture—governance, entrepreneurship, companionship, or pluralism in personal rights—the new family model would instead depict a range of subcultural focal points. In previous eras, people took the focal point in family models for granted; these focal points crystallized, as changing functions of the family wrought new concerns in creating the next generation of families. Yet, if the family loses its economic and political basis for maintaining an autonomous existence, then it is led to create new functions to sustain its viability. It is the creation of these new functions that will lead to the task of engineering new forms of domestic existence: How does one convert so-called functionless, surplus social relationships into viable systems that will in turn produce a new generation of families? Because of this concern with social methodology in organizing family relationships, rather than social content, the author proposes the term "constructed family model" to describe this paradigm.

The author is not sure exactly which directions that research on families with retarded children will take. In a robotized age, structural changes in society will likely force large segments of surplus populations and their families into alternative living arrangements. If they are to avoid the denigrating life-styles described by Bercovici (1983) in her study of deinstitutionalized retarded persons, they will require a methodology for designing a family life suited to their special circumstances (see Biklen, 1977; Scull, 1977). Today, the emphasis is on normalization of family life, with attention to creating a new generation of families in the present-day economic and political context. But without this context, what is normality? The author suggests that the present-day economic and political context confounds the perplexities in families with severely retarded members. In the robotic age, when superfluousness is normal, the *problems* would provide the focal point for organization; families could then construct their existence precisely to deal with the problems at hand. One would have to assume that the robot would become the key metaphor for organizing social relationships in society. Research would then focus on how to engineer a domestic group appropriate to its task (Farber & Royce, 1977):

1. Alternatives in rearranging personnel: divorce and remarriage, fostering retarded and/or normal children, introducing supplementary support systems, and/or use of multiple domiciles
2. Alternatives in rearranging roles: rearrangement of generational and gender roles, adding or subtracting generations, revising structure of authority, creating therapeutic roles, and/or developing recreational roles
3. Alternatives in establishing external support systems (or avoiding external destructive systems): emergency support, routine formal and informal resources, move domicile, break up family (a new start), and/or establish communities of families with similar problems

Research would then have as its aim the development of a body of findings that would permit the construction of theoretical models of family organization. The effectiveness of these models could be subjected to experimentation in ways not now acceptable according to present-day norms. The application of these models by families in surplus populations would lead to further research on the evaluation and revision of these models. Moreover, because members of the same family could be members of different surplus populations, studies of their interaction would yield further understanding of how a multitude of family organization models works.

CONCLUSION

This chapter has reviewed the history of research in the United States on families with profoundly retarded children. It has examined the proposition that shifts in cultural paradigms that define family norms 1) stimulate new policy issues regarding the handling of retarded children and their families and 2) generate fresh frameworks for research relevant to these policies. It has identified several family para-

digms and the historical eras associated with them: the family government model, the entrepreneurial family model, the companionship family model, the pluralistic family model, and a projected constructed family model. Table 2 summarizes their historical contexts, the policy issues associated with them, and the foci of research they generate.

The depictions of family paradigms in this chapter imply that, in each historical era, contemporary writers described these family models in much the same way as they are presented here. Otherwise, these depictions would be merely analytical reifications, rather than cultural models. Evidence of such writings has been presented in the text.

The analysis of family paradigms in historical contexts raises a question about the effectiveness of policies pertaining to the treatment of retarded persons and their families. For example, presumably policies dealing with deinstitutionalization are predicated on the existence of the companionship family model. If that model is assumed, then one can readily justify bringing retarded individuals (as well as mentally ill persons) home to a haven of nurturance. Yet, if in contemporary society the pluralistic model predominates over the companionship family, then introducing a multitude of additional burdens may be counterproductive for achieving a desirable level of nurturance. The family paradigms of the policy-makers thus may not correspond with those models that guide the family life of the people to whom they are supposed to apply.

The historical paradigmatic shifts discussed above can be regarded as producing a series of transformations in the definition of central social concerns with family deviance: The concern with family governance in preindustrial America was transformed into a concern with cumulative hereditary degeneration under the entrepreneurial family model, which was then transformed into a concern with family crisis as social degeneration under the companionship family model; later the concern with deviance was transformed into modes of overcoming interference with personal rights under the pluralistic family model. The author speculates

Table 2.   Historical contexts and research on families with retarded children

Cultural family paradigms	Historical contexts	Policy concerns	Family research strands generated
Family governance model	Colonial/revolutionary era; pre-industrial period; concern with stability of traditional social order	Maintenance of family control over deviant and dependent members	(No research strands)
Entrepreneurial family model	Jacksonian/Victorian era; concern with the growth of capitalism and urbanization	Handling interference by retarded persons with collective family economy and with conformity to capitalistic moral order: 1) train for usefulness, or 2) isolate in residential institutions	Genealogical studies based on concepts of neuropathy and family degeneration fed by environmental insufficiencies
Companionship family model	Era of the welfare state; concern with collective welfare and security	Handling interference by retarded children with social/emotional family functioning; focus on need for effective governmental support services	Research on family crisis, family disfunctioning, and personal problems induced by the presence of a retarded family member
Pluralistic family model	Era of reaction to bureaucracy and authority; concern with personal rights and rights of traditionally powerless groups	Remedial actions with regard to rights of retarded persons and their families; issues of: advocacy, normalization, and deinstitutionalization	Research on family members' pursuit of their personal rights; studies of: 1) strategies in family organization and 2) maintaining an appearance of normal family life in the face of deviance
Constructed family	A projected age of robotics; concern with constructing a stable social order despite wide range of surplus populations	Construction of subcultural communities, each with its own definition of normality and personal rights in order to dispel "colonization" of the powerless	Studies for designing models of family organization in different subcultures; research on interaction among family members in different surplus populations

that the next major transformation will involve a concern with designs of social reconstruction under the constructed family model. Beyond that point, further predictions cannot be made.

REFERENCES

Ackerknecht, E. H. (1959). *A short history of psychiatry*. New York: Hafner Publishing Co.

Adams, R. N. (1960). An inquiry into the nature of the family. In G. E. Dole & R. L. Carniero (Eds.), *Essays in the science of culture in honor of Leslie A. White* (pp. 35–49). New York: Crowell.

Aldrich, F., et al. (1971). *The mental retardation service delivery system: A survey of mental retardation service usage and needs among families with retarded children in selected areas of Washington State*. (Research Report, Vol. 3). Olympia, WA: Office of Research.

Andrews, S. P. (1853). (Ed.). *Love, marriage and divorce and the sovereignty of the individual*. New York: Stringer & Townsend.

Aron, R. (1966). *Peace and war*. New York: Doubleday.

Barsch, R. H. (1968). *The parent of the handicapped child*. Springfield, IL: Charles C Thomas.

Bayley, M. (1973). *Mental handicap and community care*. Boston: Routledge & Kegan Paul of America Ltd.

Becker, G. (1981). *A treatise on marriage*. Chicago: University of Chicago Press.

Bercovici, S. M. (1983). *Barriers to normalization*. Baltimore: University Park Press.

Bernard, A. W. (1974). A comparative study of marital

integration and sibling role tension differences between families who have a severely retarded child and families of non-handicapped children. *Dissertation Abstracts International, 35*A(5), 2800–2801.

Biklen, D. (1977). The politics of institutions. In B. Blatt, D. Biklen, & R. Bogden (Eds.), *An alternative textbook in special education*. Denver: Love Publishing Co.

Birenbaum, A. (1970). On managing courtesy stigma. *Journal of Health and Social Behavior, 11*, 196–206.

Birenbaum, A. (1971). The mentally retarded in the home and the family cycle. *Journal of Health and Social Behavior, 12*, 55–56.

Booth, T. A. (1978). From normal baby to handicapped child: Unravelling the idea of subnormality in families of mentally handicapped children. *Sociology, 12*, 203–221.

Bruininks, R. H., & Krantz, G. C. (Eds.). (1979). *Family care of developmentally disabled members*. Minneapolis: University of Minnesota.

Burgess, E. W. (1926). The family as a unity of interacting personalities. *The Family, 7*, 3–9.

Burgess, E. W. (1974). *The basic writings of Ernest W. Burgess*. Chicago: Community and Family Study Center, University of Chicago.

Burgess, E. W., & Locke, H. J. (1945). *The family: From institution to companionship*. Cincinnati: American Book Company.

Burgess, E. W., & Wallin, P. (1953). *Engagement and marriage*. Philadelphia: J. B. Lippincott Co.

Cain, L. F., & Levine, S. (1963). Effects of community and institutional school programs on trainable mentally retarded children. *Council of Exceptional Children, NEA, Research Monograph Series* (No. B-1).

Caldwell, B. M., & Guze, S. B. (1960). A study of the adjustment of parents and siblings of institutionalized and non-institutionalized retarded children. *American Journal of Mental Deficiency, 64*, 845–861.

Chudacoff, H. P., & Hareven, T. K. (1979). From the empty nest to family dissolution: Life course transitions into old age. *Journal of Family History, 4*, 69–83.

Cleveland, B. M., & Miller, N. (1977). Attitudes and life commitments of older siblings of mentally retarded adults: An exploratory study. *Mental Retardation, 15*, 38–41.

Clignet, R. (1979). The variability of paradigms in the construction of culture. *American Sociological Review, 44*, 392–409.

Cummings, T., Bayley, H. C., & Rie, H. E. (1966). Effects of the child's deficiency on the mother: A study of mothers of mentally retarded, chronically ill, and neurotic children. *American Journal of Orthopsychiatry, 36*, 595–605.

Danielson, F., & Davenport, C. (1912). *The hill folk*. Cold Harbor, NY: Eugenics Record Office.

Darling, R. (1979). *Families against society*. Beverly Hills: Sage Publications.

Davenport, C. (1912). *The Nams*. Cold Harbor, NY: Eugenics Record Office.

Davis, F. (1961). Deviance disavowal: The management of strained interaction by the visibly handicapped. *Social Problems, 9*, 120–132.

Degler, C. N. (1959). *Out of our past*. New York: Harper & Row.

Degler, C. N. (1983). The emergence of the modern American family. In M. Gordon (Ed.), *The American family in social-historical perspective* (pp. 61–79). New York: St. Martin's Press.

Demos, J. (1970). *A little commonwealth: Family life in Plymouth Colony*. New York: Oxford University Press.

Demos, J. (1979). Images of the American family, then and now. In V. Tufte & B. Myerhoff (Eds.), *Changing images of the family* (pp. 43–60). New Haven: Yale University Press.

Demos, J. (1983). Family home care: Historical notes and reflections. In R. Perlman (Ed.), *Family home care: Critical issues for services and policies* (pp. 161–175). New York: The Haworth Press.

Demos, J., & Boocock, S. (Eds.). (1978). *Turning points: Historical and sociological essays on the family*. Chicago: University of Chicago Press.

Doll, E. (1924). Capabilities of low-grade feeble-minded. *Training School Bulletin, 21*, 65–77.

Douglas, M. (1975). *Implicit meanings: Essays in anthropology*. Boston: Routledge & Kegan Paul of America Ltd.

Dugdale, R. (1877). *The Jukes: A study of crime, pauperism, disease, and heredity*. New York: The Putnam Publishing Group.

Dunlap, W. (1976). Services for families of the developmentally disabled. *Social Work, 21*, 220–223.

Edwards, J. N., & Kluck, P. (1980). Patriarchy. *Journal of Family Issues, 1*, 317–337.

Elder, G. H., Jr. (1974). *Children of the great depression*. Chicago: University of Chicago Press.

Estabrook, A. (1916). *The Jukes in 1915*. Washington, D C : Carnegie Institute.

Estabrook, A., & McDougle, I. (1926). *Mongrel Virginians: The Win tribe*. Washington, D C : Carnegie Institute.

Farber, B. (1959). Effects of a severely mentally retarded child on family integration. *Monographs of the Society for Research in Child Development* (Serial No. 71).

Farber, B. (1960a). Family organization and crisis: Maintenance of integration in families with a severely mentally retarded child. *Monographs of the Society for Research in Child Development* (Serial No. 75).

Farber, B. (1960b). Perceptions of crisis and related variables in the impact of a retarded child on the mother. *Journal of Health and Human Behavior, 1*, 108–118.

Farber, B. (1968). *Mental retardation: Its social context and social consequences*. Boston: Houghton Mifflin Co.

Farber, B. (1971). *Kinship and class: A midwestern study*. New York: Basic Books.

Farber, B. (1972). *Guardians of virtue; Salem families in 1800*. New York: Basic Books.

Farber, B. (1973). *Family and kinship in modern society*. Glenview, IL: Scott, Foresman & Co.

Farber, B. (1975a). Bilateral kinship: Centripetal and centrifugal types of organization. *Journal of Marriage and the Family, 37*, 871–888.

Farber, B. (1975b). Family adaptations to severely mentally retarded children. In M. J. Begab & S. A. Richardson (Eds.), *The mentally retarded and society* (pp. 247–266). Baltimore: University Park Press.

Farber, B. (1979). Developmental disability and sociological ambivalence. In R. H. Bruininks & G. C. Krantz (Eds.), *Family care of developmentally disabled members* (pp. 27–36). Minneapolis: University of Minnesota.

Farber, B. (1981). *Conceptions of kinship.* New York: Elsevier-North Holland.

Farber, B., & Jenne, W. C. (1963a). Family organization and parent-child communication: Parents and siblings of a retarded child. *Monographs of the Society for Research in Child Development* (Serial No. 91).

Farber, B., & Jenne, W. C. (1963b). Interaction with retarded siblings and life goals of children. *Marriage and Family Living, 25,* 96–98.

Farber, B., Jenne, W. C., & Toigo, R. (1960). Family crisis and the decision to institutionalize the retarded child. *Council of Exceptional Children, NEA, Research Monograph Series* (No. A-1).

Farber, B., & Royce, E. (1977). The mentally retarded: Valuable individuals or superfluous population, a futuristic analysis. In P. Mittler (Ed.), *Research to practice in mental retardation* (Vol. 1, pp. 45–51). Baltimore: University Park Press.

Fernald, W. (1924). Thirty years' progress in the care of the feeble-minded. *Journal of Psycho-Asthenics, 29,* 206–219.

Finlayson, A. (1916). *The Dack family: A study in the lack of emotional control.* Cold Harbor, NY: Eugenics Record Office.

Folsom, J. K. (1943). *The family in a democratic society.* New York: John Wiley & Sons.

Foner, A. (1978). Age stratification and the changing family. *American Journal of Sociology, 84,* S340–S365.

Fotheringham, J. B., Skelton, M., & Hoddinott, B. A. (1971). *The retarded child and his family.* Toronto: Ontario Institute for Studies in Education.

Fowle, C. M. (1968). The effects of the severely mentally retarded child on his family. *American Journal of Mental Deficiency, 73,* 468–473.

Gath, A. (1972). The mental health of siblings of a congenitally abnormal child. *Journal of Child Psychology and Psychiatry, 13,* 211–218.

Gelles, R. J. (1972). The violent home: A study of physical aggression between husbands and wives. Beverly Hills: Sage Publications.

Goddard, H. (1912). *The Kallikak family: A study in the heredity of feeblemindedness.* New York: Macmillan Publishing Co.

Goddard, H. (1928). Feeblemindedness: A question of definition. *Journal of Psycho-Asthenics, 33,* 219–227.

Goffman, E. (1959). *Presentation of self in everyday life.* New York: Doubleday & Co.

Goffman, E. (1968). Stigma: Notes on the management of spoiled identity. New York: Penguin Books.

Goffman, E. (1974). *Frame analysis.* New York: Harper & Row.

Gordon, M. (Ed.). (1983). *The American family in social-historical perspective.* New York: St. Martin's Press.

Gouldner, A. W. (1970). *The coming crisis in Western sociology.* New York: Basic Books.

Gouldner, A. W. (1973). Sociologist as partisan. In A. W. Gouldner, (Ed.), *For sociology, renewal and critique of sociology today.* New York: Basic Books.

Gottlieb, J. (1975). Public, peer, and professional attitudes toward mentally retarded persons. In M. Begab & S. A. Richardson (Eds.), *The mentally retarded and society: A social science perspective* (pp. 99–125). Baltimore: University Park Press.

Graliker, B. V., Fishler, K., & Koch, R. (1962). Teenage reaction to a mentally retarded sibling. *American Journal of Mental Deficiency, 66,* 838–843.

Greeley, H. (1853). Mr. Greeley's reply to the foregoing. In S. P. Andrews (Ed.), *Love, marriage and divorce and the sovereignty of the individual* (pp. 69–77). New York: Stringer & Townsend.

Greven, P. J., Jr. (1970). *Four generations: Population, land and family in colonial Andover, Massachusetts.* Ithaca, NY: Cornell University Press.

Grossman, F. K. (1972). *Brothers and sisters of retarded children.* Syracuse, NY: Syracuse University Press.

Hall, P. D. (1974). Marital selection and business in Massachusetts merchant families, 1700–1900. In R. L. Coser (Ed.), *The family, its structures and functions* (pp. 226–240). New York: St. Martin's Press.

Hall, W. T. (1961). *Family disorganization as associated with severity of handicap (by cerebral palsy) of a minor child.* Unpublished doctoral dissertation, University of Minnesota, Minneapolis.

Hankins, F. H. (1925). Sociology. In H. E. Barnes (Ed.), *The history and prospects of the social sciences* (pp. 255–332). New York: Alfred A. Knopf.

Hareven, T. K. (1982). *Family time and industrial time.* New York: Cambridge University Press.

Hewett, S. (1972). *The family and the handicapped child.* London: Allen & Unwin.

Hill, R. (1949). *Families under stress.* New York: Harper & Row.

Hofstadter, R. (1955). *Social Darwinism in American thought.* Boston: Beacon Press.

Holt, K. D. (1958). The home care of a severely retarded child. *Pediatrics, 22,* 746–755.

Horejsi, C. R. (1983). Social and psychological factors in family care. In R. Perlman (Ed.), *Family home care.* New York: The Haworth Press.

Howe, S. G. (1857). *A letter to the governor of Massachusetts, upon his veto of a bill, providing for an increase of state beneficiaries at the School for Idiotic Children.* New Haven, CT: Ticknor & Fields.

Jordan, T. E. (1961). *The mentally retarded.* Columbus, OH: Charles E. Merrill Publishing Co.

Katz, M. B., & Davey, I. E. (1978). Youth and early industrialization in a Canadian city. *American Journal of Sociology, 84,* S81–S119.

Kershaw, J. (1965). The handicapped child and his family. *Public Health, 80,* 18–26.

Kett, J. F. (1971). Adolescence and youth in nineteenth century America. In T. K. Rabb & R. I. Rotberg (Eds.), *The family in history* (pp. 95–110). New York: Harper & Row.

Klebanoff, L. (1959). Parental attitudes of mothers of schizophrenic, brain-injured and retarded, and normal children. *American Journal of Orthopsychiatry, 29,* 445–454.

Kobrin, F. E. (1978). The fall in household size and the rise of the primary individual in the United States. In M. Gordon (Ed.), *The American family in social-historical perspective* (2nd ed.) (pp. 100–112). New York: St. Martin's Press.

Kramm, E. (1963). *Families of mongoloid children.* Washington, DC: Government Printing Office, Children's Bureau Publication No. 401.

Kuhn, T. (1970). *The structure of scientific revolution.* Chicago: University of Chicago Press.

Laing, R. D. (1971). *The politics of the family*. New York: Random House.

Lakatos, I., & Musgrave, A. (Eds.). (1970). *Criticism and the growth of knowledge*. New York: Cambridge University Press.

Lasch, C. (1977). *Haven in a heartless world: The family besieged*. New York: Basic Books.

Lasch, C. (1983). Social pathologists and the socialization of reproduction. In M. Gordon (Ed.), *The American family in social-historical perspective* (pp. 80–94). New York: St. Martin's Press.

Laslett, P. (1973). *The world we have lost*. New York: The Scribner Book Companies.

Laslett, P. (1977). *Family life and illicit love in earlier generations*. New York: Cambridge University Press.

Lichtenberger, J. P. (1909). *Divorce: A study of social causation*. Privately published doctoral dissertation, Columbia University, New York.

Lipset, S. M. (1960). *Political man*. New York: Doubleday & Co.

Locke, J. (1949). Second treatise of civil government. In Social Sciences 1 Staff (Eds.), *The people shall judge* (Vol. 1, pp. 68–118). Chicago: University of Chicago Press.

MacKeith, R. (1973). The feelings and behavior of parents and handicapped children. *Developmental Medicine and Child Neurology, 15*, 524–527.

May, E. T. (1978). The pressure to provide: Class, consumerism, and divorce in urban America, 1880–1920. *Journal of Social History, 12*, 180–193.

Mercer, J. R. (1965). Social system perspective and clinical perspective: Frames of reference for understanding career patterns of persons labelled as mentally retarded. *Social Problems, 13*, 18–34.

Mercer, J. R. (1966). Patterns of family crisis related to reacceptance of the retardate. *American Journal of Mental Deficiency, 71*, 19–32.

Meyerowitz, J. H., & Kaplan, H. B. (1967). Family responses to stress: The case of cystic fibrosis. *Social Science and Medicine, 1*, 249–266.

Miller, D. R., & Swanson, G. E. (1958). *The changing American parent*. New York: John Wiley & Sons.

Miller, L. G. (1969). The seven stages in the life cycle of a family with a mentally retarded child. *Proceedings of Ninth Annual Research Meeting*, (Research Report No. 2). Olympia: WA: Washington Institutions Department.

Miller, S. G. (1974). An exploratory study of sibling relationships in families with retarded children. *Dissertation Abstracts International, 35B*(6), 2994–2995.

Mink, I. T., Nihira, K., & Meyers, C. E. (1983). Taxonomy of family life styles: I. Homes with TMR children. *American Journal of Mental Deficiency, 87*, 484–497.

Morgan, E. S. (1966). *The Puritan family*. New York: Harper & Row.

Moroney, R. M. (1983). Families, care of the handicapped, and public policy. In R. Perlman (Ed.), *Family home care: Critical issues for services and policies* (pp. 188–212). New York: The Haworth Press.

Morse, S. J. (1979). Family law in transition from traditional families to individual liberty. In V. Tufte & B. Myerhoff (Eds.), *Changing images of the family* (pp. 319–360). New Haven: Yale University Press.

Ogburn, W. F. (1929). The changing family. *Publications of the American Sociological Society, 23*, 124–133.

Orr, J. B. (1979). The changing family: A social ethical perspective. In V. Tufte & B. Myerhoff (Eds.), *Changing images of the family* (pp. 377–388). New Haven: Yale University Press.

Otto, H. A. (1970). *The family in search of a future*. New York: Appleton-Century-Crofts.

Parsons, T., & Bales, R. F. (1955). *Family, socialization and interaction process*. New York: The Free Press.

Rothman, D. J. (1971). Documents in search of a historian: Toward a history of childhood and youth in America. In T. K. Rabb & R. I. Rotberg (Eds.), *The family in history* (pp. 179–189). New York: Harper & Row.

Rowitz, L. (1981). A sociological perspective on labeling in mental retardation. *Mental Retardation, 19*, 47–51.

Ryan, M. P. (1981). *Cradle of the middle class: The family in Oneida County, New York, 1790–1865*. New York: Cambridge University Press.

Saenger, G. (1960). *Factors influencing the institutionalization of mentally retarded individuals in New York City*. New York: State Interdepartmental Health Resources Board.

St. John, J. A. (1848). Introduction to "Doctrine and Discipline of Divorce." In J. A. St. John (Ed.), *Collected prose works of John Milton* (Vol. 3, pp. 168–171). London: Henry G. Bohn.

Scheerenberger, R. C. (1983). *A history of mental retardation*. Baltimore: Paul H. Brookes Publishing Co.

Schelsky, H. (1966). The German family and opposed developmental tendencies in industrial society. In B. Farber (Ed.), *Kinship and family organization* (pp. 83–87). New York: John Wiley & Sons.

Schonell, F. J., Middleton, I. G., Watts, B. H., & Rorke, M. W. (1959). First and second surveys of the effects of a subnormal child on the family unit. Brisbane, Australia: University of Queensland Papers.

Schonell F. J., & Watts, B. H. (1956). A first study of the effects of a subnormal child on the family unit. *American Journal of Mental Deficiency, 61*, 210–219.

Scott, J. W., & Tilly, L. A. (1975). Women's work and the family in nineteenth century Europe. In C. E. Rosenberg (Ed.), *The family in history* (pp. 145–178). Philadelphia: University of Pennsylvania Press.

Scull, A. T. (1977). *Community treatment and the deviant—a radical view*. Englewood Cliffs, NJ: Prentice-Hall.

Sequin, E. (1866). *Idiocy and its treatment by the physiological method*. New York: William Wood.

Shere, M. O. (1955). Socioemotional factors in families of one twin with cerebral palsy. *Exceptional Children, 22*, 197–199, 206, & 208.

Shorter, E. (1975). *The making of the modern family*. New York: Basic Books.

Skeels, H. (1942). A study of the effects of differential stimulation on mentally retarded children: A follow-up report. *American Journal of Mental Deficiency, 46*, 340–350.

Skeels, H., & Dye, H. (1939). A study of the effects of differential stimulation on mentally retarded children. *Journal of Psycho-Asthenics, 44*, 114–136.

Skolnick, A. (1979). Public images, private realities: The American family in popular culture and social science. In V. Tufte & B. Myerhoff (Eds.), *Changing images of the family* (pp. 297–315). New Haven: Yale University Press.

Skolnick, A. S., & Skolnick, J. H. (1971). *Family in transition.* Boston: Little, Brown & Co.

Smelser, N. J., & Halpern, S. (1978). The historical triangulation of family, economy, and education. *American Journal of Sociology, 84,* S288–S315.

Smith, D. B. (1978). Mortality and family in colonial Chesapeake. *Journal of Interdisciplinary History, 8,* 403–427.

Smith, D. S. (1973). Parental power and marriage patterns: An analysis of historical trends in Hingham, Massachusetts. *Journal of Marriage and the Family, 35,* 419–428.

Smith-Rosenberg, C. (1978). Sex as symbol in Victorian purity: An ethnohistorical analysis of Jacksonian America. *American Journal of Sociology, 84,* S212–S247.

Straus, M. A., Gelles, R. J., & Steinmetz, S. K. (1980). Behind closed doors: Violence in the American family. New York: Doubleday & Co.

Suelzle, M., & Keenan, V. (1981). Changes in family support networks over the life cycle of mentally retarded persons. *American Journal of Mental Deficiency, 86,* 267–274.

Sultz, H. (1972). *Long-term childhood illness.* Pittsburgh: University of Pittsburgh Press.

Tilly, L. A., & Cohen, M. (1982). Does the family have a history? *Social Science History, 6,* 131–179.

Tizard, J., & Grad, J. C. (1961). *The mentally handicapped and their families.* New York: Oxford University Press.

Towner, L. W. (1966). The indentures of Boston's poor apprentices: 1734–1805. *Publications of the Colonial Society of Massachusetts, 43,* 417–468.

Tredgold, A. F. (1903). Amentia (idiocy and imbecility). *Archives of Neurology from the Pathology Laboratory of the London County Asylums, 2,* 363–391.

Tufte, V., & Myerhoff, B. (Eds.). (1979). *Changing images of the family.* New Haven: Yale University Press.

U.S. Census. (1949). *Historical statistics of the United States.* Washington, DC: GPO.

Voysey, M. (1972). Impression management by parents with disabled children. *Journal of Health and Social Behavior, 13,* 80–89.

Voysey, M. (1975). *A constant burden: The reconstitution of family life.* Boston: Routledge & Kegan Paul of America Ltd.

Waisbren, S. E. (1980). Parents' reactions after the birth of a developmentally disabled child. *American Journal of Mental Deficiency, 84,* 345–351.

Waterman, J. H. (1948). Psychogenic factors in parental acceptance of feebleminded children. *Diseases of the Nervous System, 9,* 184–187.

Wallin, J. E. W. (1914). Cited in F. Kuhlmann, "Dr. Wallin's reply to my review of his 'Mental health of the school child.' " *Journal of Psycho-Asthenics, 19,* 154–170.

Welter, B. (1983). The cult of true womanhood. In M. Gordon (Ed.), *The American family in social-historical perspective* (3rd ed.) (pp. 372–392). New York: St. Martin's Press.

Willer, B. S., Intagliata, J. C., & Atkinson, A. C. (1981). Deinstitutionalization as a crisis event for families of mentally retarded children. *Mental Retardation, 19,* 28–29.

Wohl, A. S. (1978). Sex and the single room: Incest among Victorian working classes. In A. S. Wohl (Ed.), *The Victorian family: Structure and stresses* (pp. 197–216). New York: St. Martin's Press.

Wolfensberger, W. (1975). *The origin and nature of our institutional models.* Syracuse: Human Policy Press.

Younghusband, E. (1971). *Living with handicap.* London: National Children's Bureau.

Zimmerman, Z. L. (1979). Families of the mentally disabled. In R. H. Bruininks & G. C. Krantz (Eds.), *Family care of developmentally disabled members* (pp. 87–94). Minneapolis: University of Minnesota.

Zuk, G. H. (1959). The religious factor and role of guilt in parental acceptance of the retarded child. *American Journal of Mental Deficiency, 63,* 139–147.

Zuk, G. H., Miller, R. L., Bertram, J. B., & Kling, F. (1961). Maternal acceptance of retarded children: A questionnaire study of attitudes and religious background. *Child Development, 32,* 525–540.

Zwerling, I. (1954). The initial counseling of parents with mentally retarded children. *Journal of Pediatrics, 44,* 469–479.

Chapter

2

Classification of Families with Mentally Retarded Children

Iris Tan Mink

PRIOR TO FARBER'S series of monographs (Farber, 1959, 1960; Farber, Jenne, & Toigo, 1960), there was little research on families with mentally retarded children. Since that time, there has been a growing body of research dealing with these families; however, much of it is at the descriptive level. Although this research adds to the understanding of the family, if a field is to attain scientific maturity, it must progress from this first stage of development, "adequate description," to the next stage, the establishment of theories (Hempel, 1961).

Classification may be considered an interim step between these two stages—a step away from pure description toward theoretical formulation. Typologies, which are higher-order classificatory procedures, may even be considered a first stage in theory-building. This chapter reviews some of the family typologies found in the general literature; it also reports on two typologies developed by the author's research group, relates these to the literature, and suggests some directions for future work.

WHAT THE LITERATURE TELLS US

There are two types of classifications or typologies: heuristic and empirical (Hempel, 1961; Winch, 1947). Both enable the observer to establish order among the chaotic diversity of experience. The heuristic typology proceeds from a theoretical base; its purpose is to enhance the view of the investigator, not to explain research findings. To the degree that it relates to data, it focuses on the extremes of relevant characteristics. Ideal or extreme types are posited (Hempel, 1969). Heuristic typologies stand logically "between theory and the test of theory" (Winch, 1947, p. 68).

In contrast, the empirical typology emerges from data, rather than from theory. Its purpose is to summarize observations, and the focus is not on extremes but on the average. Natural or classificatory types are posited (Hempel, 1969). Empirical typologies are placed logically "between observation and the reformulation of theory" (Winch, 1947, p. 68).

Research reported here was conducted under a grant from the National Institute of Child Health and Human Development (Grant No. HD-05540). The author wishes to thank Kazuo Nihira, C. E. Meyers, James Gallagher, and J. R. Newbrough for their support and helpful comments.

An early heuristic family typology was that of Burgess (Burgess & Locke, 1945; Burgess, Locke, & Thomes, 1971). From his study of nonproblem families, Burgess proposed two types of family systems: traditional and companionship. In the *traditional family*, which is usually patriarchial, authority is vested in the father, and all other family members are subordinate. This system is buttressed by powerful sanctions from mores, religion, and the law. In contrast, the *companionship family* operates from a democratic base. The family is united by love, congeniality, and common interests. Family members enjoy a high degree of freedom, and decisions are reached by consensus between husband and wife, with children participating according to their degree of maturity.

Another heuristic typology was proposed by Ackerman and Behrens (1956). Working with families attending a development center, they formulated eight different types of families. The "true" family is internally integrated, stable, and cohesive, with compatible family members sharing common realizable goals. There are seven types of deviant families that are characterized by their deviation from the "true" family type; these are the externally isolated, the externally integrated, the internally unintegrated, the unintended, the immature, the deviant, and the disintegrated or regressed.

Farber (1960) classified families with severely mentally retarded children according to the strategies they employed to maintain integration. His heuristic typology specified three types. In the *child-oriented family*, both parents are inclined to high social mobility, traditional rather than companionate values prevail, and children are valued for their potential achievement. In the *home-oriented family*, social mobility is not emphasized, values are companionate, and children are valued intrinsically. *Parent-oriented families* value high social mobility, but have companionate rather than traditional values; children must learn the skills necessary for achievement and advancement.

In a paper on the American lower classes, Miller (1964) devised a heuristic family typology based on two dimensions: economic security and familial stability. The resulting four types were: *the stable poor,* characterized by economic and familial stability; *the strained,* where there is a low but steady income and a great deal of internal strain; *the copers,* where families have economic difficulties but are familially stable; and *the unstable* who have neither economic nor familial stability and often a multiplicity of problems.

A few other widely regarded heuristic family typologies are those of Minuchin, Montalvo, Guerney, Rosman, and Schumer (1967) identifying disengaged, enmeshed, peripheral male, nonevolved parent, and juvenile parent families; Kantor and Lehr (1975) describing closed, open, and random family systems; and Olson and his colleagues (Olson, Russell, & Sprenkle, 1983; Olson, Sprenkle & Russell, 1979) specifying 16 family types that can be reduced to three more global types: balanced, mid-range, and extreme.

Working with multiproblem families, Voilland (1962) and Voilland and Buell (1961) developed an empirical typology based on psychosocial disorder in the family. Four types are identified: In the *perfectionistic family,* expectations for "good" social conduct are too high, success becomes the supreme ideal and failure the greatest sin; in the *inadequate family,* there is immaturity and reliance on others for the solution of problems in everyday living; the *egocentric family* is characterized by selfishness, family members are valued only if they enhance status and prestige, and conflict is the predominant tone; the *unsocial family* is chaotic, there are few rules, and impulses are acted on immediately, often with resulting delinquent behavior.

Riskin and Faunce (1970a, 1970b, 1970c) produced an empirical typology based on their observational study of task solution in problem and nonproblem families. Among their five profiles are three with specified problems: the *multiproblem family* that is unable to communicate clearly, is not supportive of family members, and has a distinct unfriendly atmosphere; the *constricted family* that has an unfriendly, depressive, compulsive atmosphere with the parents supportive of each other but not the children; and the *family with official child-labelled problems* in which members are argumentative, uncooperative, and nonsupportive, and the atmosphere is tense with covert power struggles. In the nonproblem families, there are "questionable" families that show no consistent pattern but that are judged nonoptimal for child rearing, and "normal" families that provide a friendly, supportive atmosphere and allow spontaneity from members.

In their study of community families, Moos and Moos (1976) established an empirical typology employing cluster analysis. They identified six clusters based on the families' orientation toward expression, structure, independence, achievement, moral-religious emphasis, or conflict.

Studying parenting practices occurring during the adolescence of mildly retarded adults, Zetlin, Turner, and Winick (in press) developed an empirical typology. They identified three family types: *supportive,* in which parent-child relations are close and warm, with parents remaining a stable and consistent resource for their grown children; *dependency-producing,* in which parent-child relations are also close and warm, but parental support and regulation of grown children allow for little independence; and *conflict-ridden,* in which parent-child relations are tense and lacking in warmth, with a decrease in parental support but continuation of control as the children advance in age.

Several related typologies focus on subsystems of the family, rather than on the family as a unit. Studying enduring marital relationships, Cuber and Harroff (1965) describe five recurring marital configurations: the conflict-habituated, the devitalized, the passive-congenial, the vital, and the total. In their model of parent-child interaction, Vietze and Anderson (1981) propose eight styles of behavior for each member of the parent-child dyad, resulting in 64 potential styles of interaction. In style 1, which is viewed as an optimal style, parental behavior is maximally flexible, with the parent able to respond to the child in a variety of ways. In contrast, style 8 parental behavior is the least desirable, with the parent generally unable to respond to the child's needs. Between these two extremes are styles in which parental behavior varies in degree of flexibility and responsiveness. Mitchell (1983), studying individual values and life-styles, devised a double hierarchy that includes nine life-styles: survivor, sustainer, belonger, emulator, achiever, I-am-me, experiential, societally conscious, and integrated.

There are both similarities and differences of type across these family typologies. Except for typologies that focus exclusively on deviant families, all posit at least one family type that could be termed growth-promoting. For example, the companionship family (Burgess & Locke, 1945), the "true" family (Ackerman & Behrens, 1956), the home-oriented family (Farber, 1960), the open family (Kantor & Lehr, 1975), the balanced families (Olson, Russell, & Sprenkel, 1983; Olson et al., 1979), the "normal" family (Riskin & Faunce, 1970a), the independence-oriented family (Moos & Moos, 1976), and the supportive family (Zetlin et al., in press) provide family environments that respect and support all members.

Most of the aforementioned typologies have at least one, and often several, types that could be termed growth-defeating for family members. Inflexibility and conflict characterize these types.

It is noteworthy that growth-promoting and growth-defeating types appear in most typologies and have somethat similar definitions. Disparity in types is greatest in the gradations between these extremes. It is here, perhaps, where several factors become important determinants of the resulting types. Most important may be the philosophical or theoretical intent of the investigator. From that prepossession derives the selection of the study variables and the sample. If the investigator neglects to include variables that have "systematic import"—that is, variables that reflect uniformities in the subject matter under study (Hempel, 1961, p. 14)—the resulting typology will have limited explanatory values, and the types may be unique to that study and perhaps trivial. Selection of whom to study also determines types. For example, if the focus is only on disadvantaged, delinquent families (see Minuchin et al., 1967), it is highly unlikely that a growth-promoting type will emerge. It is also important to consider the social conditions prevailing at the time of the study. Mitchell (1983) reports that one of his types, I-am-me, came to prominence only during the decade of the 1960s.

WHAT WAS DISCOVERED AND ITS RELATIONSHIP TO THE LITERATURE

Some of the early studies of the author's research group (Nihira, Meyers, & Mink, 1980; Nihira, Mink, & Meyers, 1981) revealed the importance of family environment in the retarded child's development. Unfortunately, the nature of the analytical procedures employed only allowed specification of trends for the total sample and did not allow for a focus on differential patterns within the samples. Such patterns were indicated by the research group's familiarity with the families from repeated interviews and participant observation.

The research group felt that these patterns or combinations of family environment variables were related to adjustment of the child; however, a quantitative method for discovering potentially meaningful patterns was needed. Cluster analysis was deemed an appropriate method, allowing specification of patterns. With such patterns, it would be possible to relate the nature of the family environment to the child's adjustment and also assess the differential impact that children have on their families. A further benefit would be that the knowledge of family patterns would enable a treatment program to be designed for those families in need that would be consistent with family functioning style and thus be more effective. Finally, a theory of family functioning could begin to be constructed.

Why was a previously specified typology not employed? The answer is two-fold: First, it was felt that families with retarded children differ from multiproblem and unselected families in important ways (Begab, 1966; Fowle,

1968; Grossman, 1972). Second, the existing typologies of families with mentally retarded children focused on specific aspects of family functioning, and it was the research group's belief that, in order to understand the relationship between family environment and child outcome, it was important to develop a typology based on the total psychosocial environment of the family.

As mentioned, the research group's approach to the classification of families with mentally retarded children was empirical and utilized a quantitative cluster analytic procedure. The clustering variables used were measures in three areas: 1) environmental process (Bandura, 1969; Bandura & Walters, 1964; Mischel, 1968), 2) psychosocial climate (Murray, 1938), and 3) child-rearing attitudes and practices (Baldwin, Kalhorn, & Breese, 1949; Baumrind, 1971; Kagan & Moss, 1962; Schaefer, 1959; Schaefer & Bell, 1958; Sears, Maccoby, & Levin, 1957; Yarrow, Campbell, & Burton, 1968). These areas of investigation have been influential in the study of child development and were judged particularly relevant in assessing the home environment of mentally retarded children.

Environmental process refers to the reinforcement aspects of the environment. This approach, from social learning theory (Bandura, 1969; Bandura & Walters, 1964), focuses on the processes whereby social behavior is acquired and modified. Most of the work in this area is experimental, but there are several available assessment instruments. Among the better known is the Home Observation for Measurement of the Environment (HOME-preschool; Bradley & Caldwell, 1979). The preschool version of the HOME, developed for nonhandicapped children age 3–6, provides measures of the quality and quantity of the social, emotional, and cognitive support available within the home. The research group's study included two samples of families, those with children in trainable mentally retarded (TMR) classes and those with slow-learning children in educable mentally retarded or educationally handicapped classes. Through pretesting, HOME was judged to be at the appropriate level for the TMR sample. Its level of assessment was too low for the slow learners; for this sample, the Henderson Environmental Learning Process Scale (HELPS; Henderson, Bergan, & Hurt, 1972) was employed. Developed for nonlabelled elementary school children, HELPS measures aspiration level of the home, parental reinforcement practices, and educational opportunities available to the child.

The study of *psychosocial climate* evolved from Murray's (1938) work on environmental press, in which press was defined as the environmental determinants of behavior. Murray further differentiated press into alpha press, those characteristics of the environment that exist objectively, and beta press, environmental characteristics as perceived by the participants within the environment. The investigation of beta press has been pursued by Moos and his colleagues (Moos, 1973, 1975; Moos, Insel, & Humphrey, 1974; Moos & Moos, 1981). Within this framework, Moos developed scales to measure various environments. Of these, the one appropriate for the research group's study is the Family Environment Scale (FES: Moos et al., 1974) that assesses the social climate of families and focuses on the measurement of interpersonal relationships among family members, the directions of personal growth emphasized by the family, and the organizational structure of the family.

The association between *child-rearing attitudes of parents* and adjustment of children has been explored over an extended period of time. This research may be traced from works by Baldwin et al. (1949) to Schaefer and Bell (1958), down to Baumrind (1971). Although there are several salient dimensions, three seem especially applicable to the study of the retarded child: acceptance versus rejection, restrictiveness versus permissiveness, and concern for development versus detachment. A review of the existing instruments measuring these dimensions revealed that none adequately assessed the sense of love and attachment, the concern for appropriate discipline, and the involvement with ascertaining reason-

able norms for development that were expressed by supportive parents of retarded children. Therefore, the research group developed the Home Quality Rating Scale (HQRS; Meyers, Mink, and Nihira, 1977). Factor analysis of this instrument revealed five factors that differed somewhat from the three basic child-rearing dimensions.

Variables from these three major areas were employed to determine a classification system:

1. **Environmental process of reinforcement aspects of the home**
   Home Observation for Measurement of the Environment
   Stimulation through toys, games, and reading material
   Language stimulation
   Physical environment: safe, clean, and conducive to development
   Pride, affection, and warmth
   Stimulation of academic behavior
   Modelling and encouraging of social maturity
   Variety of stimulation
   Physical punishment
   Henderson Environmental Learning Process Scale
   Extended interests and community involvement
   Provision of a supportive environment for school learning
   Educational expectations and aspirations

2. **Psychosocial climate of the home**
   Family Environment Scale
   Expressiveness
   Achievement orientation
   Moral-religious emphasis
   Control
   Cohesion, independence, and organization versus conflict
   Intellectual-cultural and active-recreational orientation

3. **Child-rearing attitudes and practices**
   Home Quality Rating Scale
   Harmony of the home and quality of parenting

Concordance in parenting and marriage

Openness and awareness of the respondent

Quality of the residential environment

Quality of the residential area

Nineteen variables measure families with TMR children, and 14 variables measure families with slow-learning children. The cluster analytic procedure employed to develop the taxonomies was the *k*-means (Engleman, 1979), which sorts cases into clusters based on the Euclidean distance between cases and the centers of clusters.

Because there is no mathematically unique solution in deriving a classification system with cluster analysis, it is particularly important that the investigator using this statistical tool provide additional evidence that the solution offered is not an artifact of the analysis itself. To that end, the research group determined differences between clusters on some child and family variables *not* employed in the formation of clusters. This process, called external validation or criterion analysis, also helps in understanding the nature of the clusters.

In the criterion analysis, the variables included basic demographics, indices of adjustment for the family and child, a measure of stressful life events (Holmes & Rahe, 1967), and a measure of adaptive behavior (Nihira, Foster, Shellhaas, & Leland, 1974). Also obtained were teacher ratings of classroom behavior, adaptive behavior, self-esteem (Coopersmith, 1975), and self-concept (Agard & Kaufman, 1973; Muller & Leonetti, 1974).

In addition to these analyses, ethnographic material on several families, selected before data analysis, was collected. After analysis, indepth interview data were collected on another subsample of families. Thus, extensive information regarding experiences, frustrations, and family interactions on subsamples of the families was available.

As previously mentioned, the subjects included two sets of families: 115 families with children in trainable mentally retarded classes (TMR), and 218 families with slow-learning children in educable mentally retarded (EMR) and educationally handicapped (EH) classes. An overall description of these families on selected variables can be found in the two "total" rows of Table 1.

In the following description of clusters, clustering and criterion variables are mentioned if they were highest or lowest relative to the other clusters; occasionally, the second highest or lowest variables are mentioned. Findings for each cluster are related to relevant research. Readers are referred to two papers (Mink, Meyers, & Nihira, 1984; Mink, Nihira, & Meyers, 1983) for detailed presentation of profiles and statistics. Note that the terms "child" or "children" refer to the retarded child in the family.

Families with Trainable Mentally Retarded Children

Among families with TMR children, it was found that a five-cluster solution provided the best theoretical and statistical description (Mink, Nihira, & Meyers, 1983). These family clusters were: 1) cohesive, harmonious; 2) control-oriented, somewhat unharmonious; 3) low-disclosure, unharmonious; 4) child-oriented, expressive; and 5) disadvantaged with low morale (see Table 1 for a brief description of these types). In general, names for the family types were taken from the high or low scores for each cluster on the clustering variables. In a few cases, ethnographic material influenced the final name given to the cluster.

Cluster 1: Cohesive, Harmonious (35 families) The families in the first cluster scored high on the clustering variables of cohesion and harmony, somewhat above average on moral-religious emphasis, and quite low on language stimulation. Criterion analysis revealed no children having a negative influence on existing marital relationships, few mothers working, and a significantly low occurrence of stressful life events. At school, these children were highest on all measures of self-concept. Almost two-thirds of the children had Down syndrome.

Table 1. Selected descriptor variables for family types

Family type	Family variables					Child variables			
	Number of families	% With father figure	% Mother employed	Mean SES level[a]	Mean stressful life events	% Down syndrome	% Male	White	Mean IQ
Trainable mentally retarded (N = 115)									
1. Cohesive	35	82.9	31.4	48.5	56.4	65.7	45.7	65.7	40.7
2. Control-oriented	34	91.2	67.7	52.3	62.5	38.2	82.4	88.2	41.9
3. Low-disclosure	7	100.00	57.1	49.4	122.3	42.9	28.6	85.7	47.4
4. Child-oriented	27	66.7	46.2	47.9	84.0	44.4	51.9	96.3	42.3
5. Disadvantaged	12	91.7	33.3	34.8	86.3	33.3	41.7	50.0	36.9
Total	115	83.5	47.4	48.0	71.8	47.8	56.5	79.1	41.5
Slow learners (N = 218)									
A. Child-oriented	23	87.0	47.8	36.3	100.6	—	65.2	73.9	66.3
B. Learning-oriented	58	69.0	41.4	41.2	103.9	—	39.7	77.6	69.6
C. Low-disclosure	19	89.5	36.8	37.0	138.7	—	84.2	57.9	74.6
D. Disadvantaged	18	83.3	50.0	31.4	149.2	—	55.6	61.1	70.6
E. Achievement-oriented	39	76.9	48.7	36.3	103.2	—	61.5	53.8	68.5
F. Expression-oriented	27	70.4	51.9	37.7	93.1	—	66.7	74.1	71.2
G. Outer-directed	34	70.6	38.2	40.6	147.7	—	64.7	58.8	69.5
Total	218	75.7	44.5	38.0	115.7	—	58.7	66.5	69.8

[a]Social class categories utilizing Duncan scale: Lower, 0–29; middle, 30–59; upper, 60–96.

Ethnographic data underscore the growth-promoting atmosphere in these homes.

Sara Isaacs, a Down syndrome child, lived with her parents and older adopted brother in a pleasant, middle-class neighborhood. Mr. Isaacs, a business manager, had rejected a promotion because it involved transferring to a city where he determined that the educational program was inferior to the one that Sara presently enjoyed. Mrs. Isaacs worked at home part-time as a bookkeeper. Sara was 10 and attractive, and she enjoyed considerable freedom in the neighborhood where she walked her dog and played with neighborhood children. The ethnographer noted the considerable amount of time that Sara's parents spent with her and also the parents' patience, warmth, and affection. They were aware of her limitations, knew she would not be independent, and would require a sheltered workshop.

Sara scored 36 on the Stanford-Binet; her major problem was expressive speech. Her speech therapist believed that daily therapy would improve her articulation and that Sara, of all the children in her school, had "one of the better chances for being able to do something with her life." Sara did well at school and was in the highest achievement group for each activity. Her teacher reported that Sara's only problems were incomprehensible speech and occasional stubbornness. She was "the only child on the unit . . . at peace with herself." The teacher attributed her lack of emotional problems to the attention and affection received at home.

In terms of stability and adjustment, the families in this cluster resemble the "true" family of Ackerman and Behrens (1956), the "home-oriented" family of Farber (1960), the "normal" family of Riskin and Faunce (1970a, 1970b, 1970c), and the "supportive" family of Zetlin et al. (in press). Parent-child interaction in these families closely resembles that described as style 1, an optimal style, in the Vietze and Anderson model (1981). Families may be described as warm, caring, and supportive. Parents are realistic about their child's abilities and are flexible in response to child behavior. There is generally a close marital relationship. Children have good adaptive behavior, high self-esteem, and good peer acceptance.

Cluster 2: Control-Oriented, Somewhat Unharmonious (34 families) On the clustering variables, the distinguishing features in cluster 2 families were high scores on physical environment, demand for social maturity, and control, offset by the use of physical punishment, unharmonious relations, and a home environment rated as nonsupportive of child development. In the criterion analysis, all fathers were reported to assist with child care, over two-thirds of the mothers were employed, and family socioeconomic level was significantly high. Children were predominantly male and white. Adaptive behavior scores at home and school were low, and teachers rated these children low on self-esteem measures.

An ethnographic report of the Jones family captures the underlying disharmony in this family type.

Charles Jones was a retarded 10-year-old, good-looking boy with dark brown hair; he was friendly and apparently bright, but had unclear speech, faulty memory, and an IQ of 48. His brother Anthony was 13, not as good-looking, but bright and straightforward in manner, active in sports, and had problems controlling his temper. There was considerable sibling rivalry. Mr. Jones, a deliveryman, appeared to do well financially; the cars, house, and furnishings were of good quality. He was described as being hard on Anthony, expecting the boy to be "the ideal son." Mrs. Jones was reported to be "a pleasant and genuinely kind woman . . . [who] seems hard-working, but is [quite] disorganized."

As an infant, Charles had scarlet fever; Mrs. Jones says "she didn't attend to it quickly despite, or because of, her mother's urgings that this was something more than just a cold." When Charles was finally hospitalized, the doctors said that there might be damage from the high fever. He was diagnosed as retarded at age 3. Mrs. Jones voiced regret that Charles did not look retarded, because people expected him to act normally and became impatient when he did not. Charles's appearance and frequent normal conversations appeared to confuse Mrs. Jones. This, coupled with her apparent guilt over Charles's condition, led her on a constant search for some type of treatment that she felt would allow "Charles a better chance for developing his potential."

Mr. Jones was not sympathetic to his wife's search for treatment; he felt that she developed false hopes and that each search ended in disappointment. Mrs. Jones described her husband as "inflexible and nonempathetic." The father and Anthony had a strained relationship, and Anthony felt that his mother favored Charles over him. The ethnographer concluded that, despite an active social life and family participation in sports, harmony was only on the surface.

This family type resembles Ackerman and Behrens's (1956) internally unintegrated family in which a failure in internal unity and conflict between the parents may be accompanied by the union of a parent and child in opposition to the marital relationship. The type also resembles Farber's (1960) child-oriented family where children are valued for their potential achievement, and there are certain similarities to Voilland's (1962) egocentric family with its lack of intimacy and emphasis on material objects.

Cluster 2 families may be described as unharmonious, inflexible, and unsupportive of child development. The home atmosphere is tense, and conflict may be openly displayed. Fathers are traditional, marital relations are often strained, and there is a tendency for the mother to form a coalition with one child. Parents make high demands on the child for social maturity. The child displays poor adaptive behavior, some maladjustment, and low self-esteem.

Cluster 3: Low-Disclosure, Unharmonious (7 families)   Families in the third cluster had extremely high or low scores on almost all clustering variables. The most distinguishing feature was the exceptionally low score on openness and awareness of the child's disability. Scores were very low on achievement orientation, physical punishment (i.e., they used it), and control. Low scores were also obtained on cohesion versus conflict (i.e., high conflict), harmony, and physical environment. High scores were obtained on all measures of stimulation, moral-religious emphasis, and concordance in parenting. In the criterion analysis, all families had fathers present, and all fathers were reported to assist with child care. Interviewers rated the child to have a negative influence on the marriage. Stressful life event occurrence was the highest of all clusters. Retarded children were predominantly female and had the highest IQ scores; they were also rated as having the highest adaptive behavior and very high self-esteem.

From an interviewer report comes this description of Natalie Bolsky.

Natalie is a nice-looking 12-year-old girl with prominent Down syndrome features and an IQ of 41. The Bolsky family lived in an old, rundown section of a small city. The home, although in need of upkeep, was uncluttered and clean. Mrs. Bolsky was an unattractive woman both in appearance and manner. Although never rude, she was uncooperative during the 4 years of the study. Mr. Bolsky, a construction worker, was never seen and was reported as "always working." Natalie's two older brothers were married and had families of their own.

The interviewer reported Mrs. Bolsky to be the most difficult interviewee she had ever encountered. Whenever there was a question about Natalie's disability, Mrs. Bolsky would leave the room ostensibly to do something. She was described as "uncomfortable with questions and defensive in her answers." During the entire interview, she never mentioned that Natalie had Down syndrome or attended TMR classes. In the annual interviews, Mrs. Bolsky gave the impression that she resented Natalie's disability. The interviewer also felt that Mrs. Bolsky gave socially desirable answers to questions.

No analogue could be found for this type of family. It is the study group's impression that families of this type do not often participate in research studies and that, when they do, because their number is so small, they are often lost in a general analysis. Because many parental responses to questions have a high social desirability component, investigators need to exercise caution.

An adequate description of these families cannot be made. It is apparent that the families, although dissembling, felt some need to cooperate on a long-term basis with a study dealing with children in special education classes. Thus, there is a high probability that parental unwillingness to disclose information stems from an inability to confront the child's retardation, rather than a deliberate attempt to mislead the interviewer. Children in this cluster were high functioning both cognitively and adaptively relative to the total group.

Cluster 4: Child-Oriented, Expressive (27 families)   Cluster 4 families scored high on clustering variables concerned with child well-being: pride, affection and warmth, language stimulation, little use of physical punishment, and provision of a supportive environment for child development. Scores were also high on expressiveness, achievement orientation, and intellectual-recreational orientation. Low scores were on concordance (this variable penalizes single-parent families), control, and moral-religious emphasis. In the criterion analysis, this cluster had the lowest percentage of father figures present. Almost all children were white and had the highest home personal self-sufficiency scores and the lowest self-concept scores.

An ethnographic report describes Evan, a 14-year-old retarded boy, and his mother, Mrs. Thomas.

> Evan was tall and thin with a smooth and almost expressionless face. Although he was not physically attractive, he had a pleasant and engaging manner. His IQ was 38. Mrs. Thomas, an attractive, competent woman with many outside interests, was employed as a sales representative of a small company. She was divorced from Evan's father, who never accepted his son's disability. The father visited about twice a month, but was not otherwise concerned with parenting.
>
> Mrs. Thomas is described as "good with Evan and genuinely likes him." She encouraged him to do his best and was not overly protective. Evan was able to ride a two-wheel bicycle and a skateboard. This competency allowed him to participate in games with neighborhood children. The ethnographer noted that Mrs. Thomas would like to remarry but that she was hampered by Evan who takes it on himself to "cross-exam" her dates. She is good-natured about this.

As with Cluster 1, these families bear some resemblance to the "true" family of Ackerman and Behrens (1956), the "normal" family of Riskin and Faunce (1970a, 1970b, 1970c), and the "supportive" family of Zetlin et al. (in press).

The picture of these families is not as clear as that in Cluster 1, perhaps because one-third of the families are single-parent families. This characteristic may also account for Cluster 4 families' emphasis on expressiveness and the use of extrafamilial outlets for recreational and cultural activities. Parents appear caring and supportive of child development. In the mother-only homes, a considerable amount of time

and energy is spent on the retarded child. These children tend to be self-sufficient, but have poor self-concepts.

Cluster 5: Disadvantaged with Low Morale (12 families)   Cluster 5 families had low scores on all clustering variables. Particularly low were residential area; stimulation through toys, games, and reading materials; intellectual-recreational orientation; and expressiveness. The only elevated variable was achievement orientation. Criterion analysis revealed the lowest percentage of father figures assisting with child care, the lowest socioeconomic level, and the poorest attitude to child impact. This cluster had the lowest percentage of white children and children with Down syndrome. Children had the lowest IQ scores and the lowest adaptive behavior and social adjustment at home. They also were rated lowest on self-esteem.

An interviewer report depicts the Larson family.

> Andrew is a thin, unattractive child with Down syndrome, poor coordination, and poor receptive and expressive language. His IQ is 27. The Larson home was rundown and needed both indoor and outdoor repairs. Mr. Larson managed a department in a discount store; his hard-of-hearing wife was a homemaker. Both parents were older; they appeared kind and warm, but were somewhat passive.
>
> Although Andrew was not muscular nor hyperactive, his mother reported that he had been violent and had struck out at others. He had hit children who teased him and sometimes his mother when she tried to punish him. He had no close friends; his only recreation was solitary swinging in the backyard. He was not allowed out into the neighborhood because his parents were afraid he would get lost. The parents rarely took Andrew on outings for fear that he would become uncontrollable. He also was not taken grocery shopping; one parent almost always stayed home with him. The family life-style was severely limited; socializing occurred only occasionally with the three older daughters who lived away from home. Although both parents cherished Andrew, they had few ideas and sought no outside help regarding his care.

In the literature, Ackerman and Behrens's (1956) externally isolated family—characterized by excessive isolation from the community, few or no friends, and little or no contact with the extended family—resembles this cluster. The strained family of Miller (1964) that has reasonable economic stability but poor coping abilities is also similar to this type. With regard to the somewhat elevated score on achievement orientation, Wortis, Bardach, Cutler, Rue, and Freedman (1963), in a study of child-rearing practices in a low socioeconomic group, found that mothers valued achievement, but had little knowledge of what it entailed. They concluded that this value was part of the mothers' desire for a better life situation for their children.

These families may be characterized as both economically and emotionally disadvantaged. Parents are generally unable to cope with the demands of rearing a retarded child. The children are thus unsocialized and often uncontrollable; the parents' response is to restrict the children to the home, thereby exacerbating their isolation. Adding to this isolation is the parents' own social isolation from community and family support networks. These children tend to display low adaptive behavior, high maladaptive behavior, and low self-esteem.

Families with Slow-Learning Children

Children were termed slow learners if they were in school programs for educably mentally retarded or educationally handicapped students. Among families with slow learners, a seven-cluster solution provided the best theoretical and statistical description (Mink et al., 1984). These family types were: A) child-oriented, cohesive; B) learning-oriented, high residential quality; C) low-disclosure, unharmonious; D) disadvantaged, noncohesive; E) achievement-oriented, low-residential quality; F) expression-oriented with few sociocultural interests; and G) outer-directed with little achievement orientation. A brief description of these family types on selected variables can be seen in Table 1.

Cluster A: Child-Oriented, Cohesive (23 families) The outstanding features of Cluster A families were very high scores on concordance, provision of a supportive environment for school learning, harmony, and cohesion.

Low scores were obtained on residential environment, educational expectations, intellectual-recreational orientation, and community involvement. Criterion analysis revealed a positive parental attitude to the child's impact on the family and a relatively low occurrence of stressful life events. Children had the lowest IQ scores of all clusters, but high psychological and social adjustment. At school, these children were rated low on community self-sufficiency and potential to benefit from further education.

An ethnographic report depicts the Harding family whose son Michael is 12 years old, thin, and hyperactive but quite self-sufficient.

> Michael's IQ is 58. Mr. Harding, an aircraft machinist, is "a definite and strong figure who is quite comfortable in his traditional role as father and husband." Mrs. Harding is a "physically and emotionally sturdy person, capable of effecting good growth and harmony." Both parents have a healthy and supportive attitude toward Michael; they do not focus on him, but they also do not ignore his handicap. Their philosophy is "to establish and stick to firm rules which are well-defined, but [also] to let their children have the flexibility to grow to their own limits. . ." Growth demands made on Michael are not apparent, but "his good manners, ability to do multiplication tables, reading skills, physical coordination, and personal neatness are evidence of parental support and realistic 'press' for achievement." The ethnographer concludes ". . . this is a very nice, well-adjusted family of modest means . . . quite satisfied with their life and appreciative of it."

This cluster compares favorably with the "true" family (Ackerman & Behrens, 1956), the "child-oriented" family (Farber, 1960), the "normal" family (Riskin & Faunce, 1970a, 1970b, 1970c), the "supportive" family (Zetlin et al., in press), and the TMR "cohesive harmonious" family. As in the TMR family type, parent-child interaction is similar to that proposed by Vietze and Anderson (1981) as style 1, an optimal style.

Families in this cluster may be described as traditional, but warm, caring, and supportive of family members. Children are provided with support to achieve their potential, and parents are flexible in response to child behavior. The marital relationship is sharing and close. The children, who have the lowest IQ of all slow-learner types, are well adjusted both personally and socially.

Cluster B: Learning-Oriented, High Residential Quality (58 families) Cluster B families scored fairly high on the clustering variables of educational expectations, provision of an environment supportive of school learning, and residential environment. The low score was on concordance (this factor penalizes single-parent families). On criterion variables, these families had the lowest percentage of father figures present, but the highest percentage of families with good parent-child relations. Average family socioeconomic status was the highest of all clusters. Children were predominantly female and white. They demonstrated high adaptive behavior at school.

Information was obtained from an ethnographic report on Andrea Johnson.

> Andrea is 10 years old, black and lives with her parents in an ethnically mixed suburban neighborhood. Andrea, tall, slender, well dressed and groomed, has an IQ of 68. "Quiet and self-contained," she was quick to learn in new situations with the ethnographer. She spontaneously does simple household chores and light cooking; however, she does "know her limits" and does not attempt complex tasks. She likes school, knows numbers and how to read, and checks books out of the library.
>
> Mrs. Johnson, heavy-set, friendly, and casual, treats Andrea with "natural ease." She appears realistic, recognizes Andrea's need for special classes, but does not like any reference to her disability. She expects Andrea to get a job, "maybe in a restaurant," when she finishes school. Mrs. Johnson is a nurse's aide, but has not worked since Andrea started "a small fire" in the house. Mr. Johnson, a machinist, tall and slim, appears much younger than his wife. He "seems the disciplinarian, stern but consistent." The family defers to him.
>
> Mitchell, the younger son, has a close relationship with Andrea, braiding her hair and playing with her. Alex, the older son, is rarely home, although he does take his mother and sister shopping and on excursions. This is the source of contention in the home. The ethnographer reported that, although the family seemed "tranquil enough," she suspected some "underlying ten-

> sions resulting from Mr. Johnson not taking his wife and Andrea anywhere."

This family type is somewhat difficult to characterize. There appears to be a certain flatness to family life, although there are material comforts and resources for child development. Some of the marital relationships could be termed "utilitarian," that is, "the marriage is useful . . . for reasons outside of personal considerations" (Cuber & Harroff, 1965, p. 109). In other marriages, there is closeness between mates, but without the level of intimacy found in Cluster A families. Children demonstrate high adaptive behavior at school.

Cluster C: Low-Disclosure, Unharmonious (19 families) Outstandingly low scores on the clustering variables are found on openness and awareness of the child's disability and on harmony. High scores are evident on residential area and control. In the criterion analysis, father figures were present in almost all families, and few mothers were employed. Parent-child relations were the poorest of all types. Children were mostly male and had the highest IQ. Parents rated children highest on psychological adjustment. At school, children were rated lowest on two indices of adaptive behavior, but highest on potential to benefit from further education.

Interviewer reports illustrate this type of family's lack of openness with the interviewer.

> Each year, when the interviewer contacted Mrs. Smith and made arrangements for the interview concerning her son Robert (age 12 with an IQ of 81), Mr. Smith always insisted on being present. During each interview, he would interject, "Education is not important." He was a draftsman in an architect's office, whereas his own mother was a professional with a doctorate. It appeared to the interviewer that he resented his mother's achievement. Nothing else was noteworthy about the first two interviews.
>
> In the third year, the interviewer, a substitute teacher, mentioned the planned interview to Robert's teacher. The teacher expressed surprise because it was her understanding that the parents were separating. The interviewer kept the interview appointment. Both parents were present, but no mention was made of marital unhappiness or separation, even in response to direct questioning. In the fourth year of the study, only Mr. Smith

was present at the interview. He had custody of the children and said that his former wife had remarried.

On the Home Quality Rating Scale, this cluster had a similar profile pattern and elevation to the TMR low-disclosure, unharmonious type. As with that type, the research group found no family descriptions in the literature that matched this cluster. Given the relatively high IQ of these children, attention should be paid to Willner and Crane's (1979, p. 33) description of a group of parents whose children are minimally handicapped: ". . . parents who deny the most . . . are those whose children have a marginal handicap, since their children are almost, but not quite normal functioning, they are subject to chronic disappointment." As with the TMR family type, the research group believes that these families are distressed and in need of counseling and parent training. Their children with relatively high IQ scores, whose adaptive behavior is rated low by teachers but not by the parents, may also need guidance.

Cluster D: Disadvantaged, Noncohesive (18 families) This family type had exceptionally low scores on almost all clustering variables; particularly low variables were cohesion, moral-religious emphasis, educational expectations, and control. Only intellectual-recreational orientation was high. In the criterion analysis, this type had the lowest scores on percentage of father figures assisting with child care and on socioeconomic level. A high percentage of mothers were employed, and occurrence of stressful life events was the highest of all types. Children were the oldest in the sample and had the lowest psychological and social adjustment. Relations between the retarded child and siblings were poorest. At school, children had the highest social self-concept.

Interviewer reports describe one of these families:

> Gwendolyn Harris, an 11-year-old black girl with an IQ of 63, lives with her mother, Mrs. Baylis, and three younger siblings in a high-crime area. During the 4 years of data collection, they had lived "in one poor place after another," often in incredible squalor. There is also impermanence in father figures. Most of the men stay for a short time and do not work. The few household rules are only erratically enforced. Family interaction is described as "one constant row," with much shouting and fighting. When things get too bad, Mrs. Baylis delegates responsibility for "straightening things out" to one of the children.
>
> Gwendolyn is disruptive at home and school. Her teacher reports lack of motivation. In the third interview year, her disruptive behavior resulted in suspension. In the fourth year, family life improved. A male companion who worked had stayed for almost a year, housekeeping seemed "a bit better," and Gwendolyn performed better at school and was less disruptive.

This cluster resembles the disadvantaged family with low morale in the TMR taxonomy. Except for the clustering variable of intellectual-recreational orientation, where the TMR score is low whereas that for the slow learner is fairly high, the profiles for both clusters are highly similar. The source of the score disparity may be found in the exceptionally low functioning of children in the TMR cluster, which could preclude parents from obtaining child care or taking children to extra familial functions.

In the family literature, this type resembles the "disintegrated family" (Ackerman & Behrens, 1956, p. 76) with its "lack of integration, immaturity, excessive conflict, lack of compatibility, mutual attack, mutual isolation, and inappropriate and unclear goals." There is also some resemblance to the "disengaged family" (Minuchin et al., 1967) in that mothers feel overwhelmed, have poor self-esteem, are depressed, and are often unable to establish control and guidance over the children. Although this family type is not as pathological as the "unsocial family" (Voilland, 1962), similarities do exist, particularly in maternal care that is often haphazard with mixed responses of hostility and overprotectiveness. Another aspect of the unsocial family is the high intensity of sibling rivalries and jealousies. Finally, this family type showed similarities to the "conflict-ridden" family (Zetlin et al., in press) and to style 8, the least desirable, parent-child interaction (Vietze & Anderson, 1981).

This family type may be described as problematic. The mother appears to have minimum concern for the child's developmental needs, and she is often overwhelmed by the demands of motherhood and reduced economic circumstances. Children may display poor psychological and social adjustment, and it is not unusual to discover intense sibling rivalries.

Cluster E: Achievement-Oriented, Low Residential Quality (39 families) On the clustering variables, Cluster E families display elevated scores on achievement orientation and control and low scores on residential environment and residential area. In the criterion analysis, this type had the highest number of children residing at home and the highest percentage of nonwhite families. Children scored near the average in adjustment and adaptive behavior measures.

An ethnographic report depicts the open and casual climate of the Davis family whose 13-year-old son Harold has an IQ of 64.

> The home is in need of external repair, while the household may be described as "carelessly disheveled." During the 4 months of observation, Mrs. Davis usually wore the same long, faded dress and had her hair in rollers. She was casual and accepting of her three children and made no unrealistic demands on Harold, although she felt he had potential and that the school should develop it. Mr. Davis, a mechanic who had been blinded at work and was presently unemployed, was somewhat distant and appeared to favor his two daughters over Harold.
>
> Harold, though, was never at a loss for companionship. He was well coordinated, rode a bicycle, and played with the neighborhood children; he was also seen with his father's buddies who were often at the house drinking beer. On one visit, the ethnographer encountered a friendly, drunken neighbor, a sister who was baking a cake, Mr. Davis and his buddy, the two daughters who watched TV and danced around the house, and Mrs. Davis's brother, in addition to Mrs. Davis and Harold. The atmosphere on that visit was very sociable and casual, with "many people, in and out, talking and joking, eating and drinking. . . ." The ethnographer concluded that this "household seems well integrated with respect to Harold's disability. There is recognition that it exists but nothing is done to cater to it."

This family type shows some resemblance to the "random-type family" (Kantor & Lehr,

1975) and the "achievement via independence" family subcluster (Moos & Moos, 1976). The families in this cluster expressed a desire for achievement, although there was little provision for learning at home. This finding also has been reported by Meyerowitz and Farber (1966) and Wortis et al. (1963) in lower social-class families. Elaborating on these families, Wortis and his colleagues state that the desire for achievement is most likely a generalized desire for a better life situation. They contend that there are some beneficial aspects to this environment; namely, that the child is permitted to grow at his or her own pace and, if unable to perform, is not criticized or pressured to do better.

Although this is not one of the best family environments for the developing retarded child, it may not be overly harmful. Generally, the child is permitted to develop without parental pressure; however, there is also a lack of consistent discipline and an absence of household rules. Parents tend to be nonjudgmental and reasonably caring. Children are more or less untroubled and have average adaptive behavior.

Cluster F: Expression-Oriented with Few Sociocultural Interests (27 families) On the clustering variables, families in Cluster F score high on expressiveness and particularly low on intellectual-recreational orientation and provision of a learning environment at home. They are also fairly low on achievement orientation, moral-religious emphasis, and control. In the criterion analysis, father figures were absent in many families, but if present, all assisted with child care. Occurrence of stressful life events was lowest of all types. Children were at or near the average on measures of adjustment and adaptive behavior. School social self-concept was lowest of all clusters.

An ethnographic report describes Greg Finley.

> Greg is a nice-looking 12-year-old hyperactive boy who lives with his parents, older half-sister, older sister, and 6-year-old brother, Buddy. Greg must take Ritalin on schedule, or he "goes out of control." He has good coordination, indistinct speech, and an IQ of 71. The ethnographer found

him neat and ingratiating. Mr. Finley, a pipe fitter, often works 12-hour shifts; Mrs. Finley works full-time as a salesclerk. Thus the children are often unsupervised, although Mrs. Finley's mother comes over several times a week to assist with child care and housecleaning. When he is not sleeping, Mr. Finley also assists with child care. The Finleys, who often appeared weary, try to go on family outings several Sundays a month. Their daily recreation is watching TV game shows and situation comedies.

Strife between siblings is rampant, particularly between Greg and Buddy. Buddy, who also has a speech problem, is considered bright, but a behavior problem by his first-grade teacher. Buddy's grandmother considers him "ornery" and "bad"; he often teases and pummels Greg who then "snitches" to his mother. The numerous arguments between Buddy and his mother often end in a "strapping." After one of these episodes, Mrs. Finley said she would like to put Buddy on Ritalin also, even though he's not diagnosed as hyperactive, just as "very active."

There were no types analogous to this cluster in the family typology literature. It may be that this family type is related to maternal unavailability, a high percentage of these mothers worked and many families were single-parent families. Likewise, MacKinnon, Brody, and Stoneman (1982) found that the home environments of children whose mothers were divorced and working were less cognitively and socially stimulating than those of intact homes. As in their study, the "minimal parenting" concept (Zussman, 1980) appears appropriate here; that is, the overworked mother who must attend to the competing responsibilities of job, home, and child care has little time and energy left to provide a growth-enhancing environment for her children.

More study of these families is needed to arrive at an adequate description. For the present, it can be said that there appears to be a lack of cognitive and social stimulation in these homes, that discipline of the children is often a problem, and that mothers sometimes appear overwhelmed by their multiple responsibilities. The children do not seem responsible for their parents' problems, and their adjustment and adaptive behavior are average. The one problem area for these children is poor social self-concept.

Cluster G: Outer-Directed with Little Achievement Orientation

(34 families) On the clustering variables, the only elevated score for Cluster G families is community involvement; low scores are found on achievement orientation, expressiveness, and control. The criterion analysis shows a relatively high family socioeconomic level and few mothers employed. Parental attitude to child impact is the most negative of all clusters, and frequency of occurrence of stressful life events is second highest. The children are near the total sample average on measures of adjustment and adaptive behavior.

Data collected from interviewer reports describe Alexis Marcus, an unattractive 12-year-old girl who lives with her parents and an 8-year-old sister.

Mr. Marcus, an aircraft assembler, is sympathetic to Alexis, helps her with her homework, and cares for her in the evenings. Mrs. Marcus, who was pregnant with Alexis before she married, deeply resents her. She is "so out of tune" with her daughter, and her hostility is so great that she told the interviewer, "I dislike her so, I can't even touch her."

Alexis is quite quarrelsome and has continual fights with her younger sister, who refuses to bring her friends home to play. Her mother says that Alexis misbehaves so much that she can't get a sitter. In the EMR classes, Alexis' temper keeps her in constant trouble. There is high conflict in the family over Alexis. Mr. Marcus feels that his wife should change her attitude and behavior toward Alexis. Mrs. Marcus refuses. She feels that "nobody can help me. I've tried."

This is potentially a problematic family type although more study is needed before an adequate comparison can be made to other family typologies. There is some resemblance to the "externally integrated family" (Ackerman & Behrens, 1956) and the "conflict-ridden family" (Zetlin et al., in press).

A tentative characterization of this family type comes from ethnographic and interviewer reports. In many families, there is overt rejection or abuse of the retarded child by one parent. When this occurs, the other parent attempts to compensate and help, but is generally ineffectual. Conflict and tension are high in the home. Marital difficulties often arise from the problems between the rejecting parent and the child. Some children have difficulties at school.

STABILITY OF CLASSIFICATION OVER LIFE-CYCLE STAGES

The above taxonomies were developed from data collected when the children in these families were in late childhood. An important question therefore is whether these taxonomies are specific to this stage in the family life cycle, or are they stable over the total life cycle.

Family life-cycle theory postulates that, as the family unit continues along a time line, it passes through different stages that have different developmental tasks for the family members (Carter & McGoldrick, 1980; Duvall, 1957, 1977; Olson, Russell, & Sprenkle, 1983; Turnbull, Summers, & Brotherson, 1983). From this theoretical position, one should expect change in the structure of the taxonomies; that is, different clusters will arise at different stages in the life cycle. One should also expect some change in family cluster membership, especially if reciprocal effects between the child and the family are considered (Nihira, Meyers, & Mink, 1983; Nihira, Mink, & Meyers, 1985; Sameroff & Chandler, 1975). For example, when a child has a high impact on the family, parenting practices and attitudes may change and affect cluster membership.

Currently, these families have moved from the stage of families with school-age children to that of families with adolescents in the home to that of launching families (Olson, Russell, & Sprenkle, 1983). Follow-up work with these families has begun, and indications are that the frequency of occurrence of stressful life events has increased, harmony in the home has decreased, and parental attitude has darkened. It appears that the chronicity of the child's disability has begun to affect family life. This effect becomes evident when parents are questioned regarding plans for the retarded adolescent's future: work, living situation, and relations with the opposite sex. Many parents appear dispirited and report few future plans (Mink, Nihira, & Gilkey, 1983).

With the current data, the research group cannot say whether the taxonomic structure will shift with different life-cycle stages. When measures of family environment variables were repeated, there appears to be negligible shifting, with the exception of harmony, which moved downward. It may be that the home environment or clustering variables will not shift.

CONCLUSION

These two classification systems should be viewed as tentative. They are developed from data collected on two samples: families with school-age TMR children, and those with slow-learning school-age children. There is still much work to be done. First, in the area of replicability, it must be demonstrated that the reported types, or at least some of them, appear in other populations, notably an unselected population with school-age children. There is also a need to chart changes, if any, in the psychosocial environment of the family over the life cycle; such changes may result in the emergence of different types. In addition, one must entertain the possibility that some families may change whereas others may not.

Second, the types that were discovered need to be validated. It should be demonstrated that the types develop differently and/or that they respond differently to the same treatment. It should also be shown that these types adequately account for individual family differences, so that professionals in the field are confident about the assignment of families to types. Unless this problem is addressed, classification systems, no matter how statistically elegant, will not be utilized and will fail to lead to more effective treatment of family problems.

Finally, consideration needs to be given to the possibility that no single classification system may be adequate for all families; perhaps there should be one primary classification with additional miniclassification systems. This brief review of family typologies and the findings from the group's research indicate that there are certain basic family types that exist, regardless of the child's level of retardation. Thus, there is some evidence that additional research may yield a standard classification system. At this point, miniclassification systems are mostly conjecture. However, research on reciprocal relations within the family unit, with the child shaping the family environment as much as the parent and family environment

shaping the child, presages the emergence of disability-specific types.

A classification system using a multidimensional typological model is subject to criticism; some would prefer a unidimensional model (Strauss, 1973). Given the complexity of dynamics in families with mentally retarded children, however, this model appears a proper way to proceed. The typological model allows investigators to postulate and validate family types while building a coherent theory of family functioning.

REFERENCES

Ackerman, N. W., & Behrens, M. D. (1956). A study of family diagnosis. *American Journal of Orthopsychiatry, 26,* 66–78.

Agard, J. A., & Kaufman, M. J. (1973). *About you and your friends: Project PRIME.* Austin: University of Texas, Data Analysis Unit.

Baldwin, A., Kalhorn, J., & Breese, F. (1949). The appraisal of parent behavior. *Psychological Monographs, 63*(4, Whole No. 299).

Bandura, A. (1969). *Principles of behavior modification.* New York: Holt, Rinehart & Winston.

Bandura, A., & Walters, R. H. (1964). *Social learning and personality development.* New York: Holt, Rinehart & Winston.

Baumrind, D. (1971). Current patterns of parental authority. *Developmental Psychology Monograph, 4,* No. 1.

Begab, M. J. (1966). The mentally retarded and the family. In I. Phillips (Ed.), *Prevention and treatment of mental retardation* (pp. 71–84). New York: Basic Books.

Bradley, R. H., & Caldwell, B. M. (1979). Home observation for measurement of the environment: A revision of the preschool scale. *American Journal of Mental Deficiency, 84,* 235–244.

Burgess, E. W., & Locke, H. J. (1945). *The family: From institution to companionship.* New York: American Book Co.

Burgess, E. W., Locke, H. J., & Thomes, M. M. (1971). *The family: From traditional to companionship.* New York: Van Nostrand Reinhold Co.

Carter, E. A., & McGoldrick, M. (1980). The family life cycle and family therapy: An overview. In E. A. Carter & M. McGoldrick (Eds.), *The family life cycle: A framework for family therapy* (pp. 3–20). New York: Gardner Press.

Coopersmith, S. (1975). *Coopersmith self-esteem behaviors.* San Francisco: Self-Esteem Institute.

Cuber, J. F., & Harroff, P. B. (1965). *The significant Americans: A study of sexual behavior among the affluent.* New York: Appleton-Century.

Duvall, E. (1957). *Family development.* Philadelphia: J. B. Lippincott Co.

Duvall, E. M. (1977). *Marriage and family development* (5th ed.). Philadelphia: J. B. Lippincott Co.

Engleman, L. (1979). K-means clustering. In W. J. Dixon & M. B. Brown (Eds.), *BMDP Biomedical Computer Program P-Series* (pp. 648.1–652.1). Berkeley: University of California Press.

Farber, B. (1959). Effects of a severely mentally retarded child on family integration. *Monographs of the Society for Research in Child Development, 34* (No. 2).

Farber, B. (1960). Family organization and crisis: Maintenance of integration in families with a severely mentally retarded child. *Monographs of the Society for Research in Child Development, 25* (No. 1).

Farber, B., Jenne, W. C., & Toigo, R. (1960). Family crisis and the decision to institutionalize the retarded child. *Council for Exceptional Children, NEA, Research Monograph Series,* No. A-1.

Fowle, C. M. (1968). The effect of the severely mentally retarded child on his family. *American Journal of Mental Deficiency, 73,* 468–473.

Grossman, F. K. (1972). *Brothers and sisters of retarded children: An exploratory study.* Syracuse, New York: Syracuse University Press.

Hempel, C. G. (1961). Introduction to problems of taxonomy. In J. Zubin (Ed.), *Field studies in the mental disorders* (pp. 3–22). New York: Grune & Stratton.

Hempel, C. G. (1969). Ideal types in social science comply with covering law requirements: Typological methods in the social sciences. In L. I. Krimerman (Ed.), *The nature and scope of social science: A critical anthology* (pp. 445–456). New York: Appleton-Century-Crofts.

Henderson, R. W., Bergan, J. R., & Hurt, J., Jr. (1972). Development and validation of the Henderson environmental learning process scale. *Journal of Social Psychology, 88,* 185–196.

Holmes, T. H., & Rahe, R. H. (1967). The social readjustment rating scale. *Journal of Psychosomatic Research, 11,* 213–218.

Kagan, J., & Moss, H. A. (1962). *Birth to maturity: A study in psychological development.* New York: John Wiley & Sons.

Kantor, D., & Lehr, M. (1975). *Inside the family.* San Francisco: Jossey-Bass.

MacKinnon, C. E., Brody, G. H., & Stoneman, Z. (1982). The effects of divorce and maternal employment on the home environments of preschool children. *Child Development, 53,* 1392–1399.

Meyerowitz, J. H., & Farber, B. (1966). Family background of educably mentally retarded children. In B. Farber (Ed.), *Kinship and family organization* (pp. 388–398). New York: John Wiley & Sons.

Meyers, C. E., Mink, I. T., & Nihira, K. (1977). *Home quality rating scale.* Pomona, CA: UCLA/Neuropsychiatric Institute-Lanterman State Hospital Research Group.

Miller, S. M. (1964). The American lower classes: A typological approach. In F. Reissman, J. Cohen, & A. Pearl (Eds.), *Mental health of the poor* (pp. 139–154). New York: The Free Press.

Mink, I. T., Meyers, C. E., & Nihira, K. (1984). Taxonomy of life styles: II. Homes with slow-learning children. *American Journal of Mental Deficiency, 89,* 111–123.

Mink, I. T., Nihira, K., & Gilkey, L. (1983, August). *From childhood to adolescence: TMR families confront new problems.* Paper presented at the 91st annual convention of the American Psychological Association, Anaheim, CA.

Mink, I. T., Nihira, K., & Meyers, C. E. (1983). Taxonomy of family life styles: I. Homes with TMR children. *American Journal of Mental Deficiency, 87,* 484–497.

Minuchin, S., Montalvo, B., Guerney, B. G., Rosman, B. L., & Schumer, F. (1967). *Families of the slums: An exploration of their structure and treatment.* New York: Basic Books.

Mischel, W. (1968). *Personality and assessment.* New York: John Wiley & Sons.

Mitchell, A. (1983). *The nine American lifestyles: Who we are and where we are going.* New York: Macmillan Publishing Co.

Moos, R. H. (1973). Conceptualizations of human environments. *American Psychologist, 28,* 652–665.

Moos, R. H. (1975). *Evaluating correctional and community settings.* New York: John Wiley & Sons.

Moos, R. H., Insel, P. M., & Humphrey, B. (1974). *Family, work and group environment scales manual.* Palo Alto, CA: Consulting Psychologists Press.

Moos, R. H., & Moos, B. S. (1976). A typology of family social environments, *Family Process, 15,* 357–371.

Moos, R. H., & Moos, B. S. (1981). *Family environment scale manual.* Palo Alto, CA: Consulting Psychologists Press.

Muller, D. G., & Leonetti, R. (1974). *Primary self-concept inventory.* Austin: Learning Concepts.

Murray, H. A. (1938). *Explorations in personality.* New York: Oxford University Press.

Nihira, K., Foster, R., Shellhaas, M., & Leland, H. (1974). *AAMD Adaptive Behavior Scale.* Washington, DC: American Association on Mental Deficiency.

Nihira, K., Meyers, C. E., & Mink, I. T. (1980). Home environment, family adjustment, and the development of mentally retarded children. *Applied Research in Mental Retardation, 1,* 5–24.

Nihira, K., Meyers, C. E., & Mink, I. T. (1983). Reciprocal relationship between home environment and development of TMR adolescents. *American Journal of Mental Deficiency, 88,* 139–149.

Nihira, K., Mink, I. T., & Meyers, C. E. (1981). Relationship between home environment and school adjustment of TMR children. *American Journal of Mental Deficiency, 86,* 8–15.

Nihira, K., Mink, I. T., & Meyers, C. E. (1985). Home environment and development of slow-learning adolescents: Reciprocal relations. *Developmental Psychology, 21,* 784–794.

Olson, D. H., McCubbin, H. I., Barnes, H., Larsen, A., Muxen, M., & Wilson, M. (1983). *Families: What makes them work.* Beverly Hills: Sage Publications.

Olson, D. H., Russell, C., & Sprenkle, D. (1983). Circumplex model of married and family systems: VI. Theoretical update. *Family Process, 22,* 69–83.

Olson, D. H., Sprenkle, D., & Russell, C. (1979). Circumplex model of marital and family systems: I. Cohesion and adaptability dimensions, family types and clinical applications. *Family Process, 18,* 3–28.

Riskin, J., & Faunce, E. E. (1970a). Family interaction scales: I. Theoretical framework and method. *Archives of General Psychiatry, 22,* 504–512.

Riskin, J., & Faunce, E. E. (1970b). Family interaction scales: II. Data analysis and findings. *Archives of General Psychiatry, 22,* 513–526.

Riskin, J., & Faunce, E. E. (1970c). Family interaction scales: III. Discussion of methodology and substantive findings. *Archives of General Psychiatry, 22,* 527–537.

Sameroff, A. J., & Chandler, M. J. (1975). Reproductive risk and the continuum of caretaking casualty. In F. D. Horowitz (Ed.), *Review of child development research* (Vol. 4, pp. 187–244). Chicago: University of Chicago Press.

Schaefer, E. S. (1959). A circumplex model for maternal behavior. *Journal of Abnormal and Social Psychology, 59,* 226–235.

Schaefer, E. S., & Bell, R. O. (1958). Development of a parental attitude research instrument. *Child Development, 29,* 339–361.

Sears, R., Maccoby, E., & Levin, H. (1957). *Patterns of child-rearing.* Evanston, IL: Row & Peterson.

Strauss, J. S. (1973). Diagnostic models and the nature of psychiatric disorder. *Archives of General Psychiatry, 29,* 445–449.

Turnbull, A. P., Summers, J. A., & Brotherson, J. J. (1983, September). *Family life cycle: Theoretical and empirical implications and future directions for families with mentally retarded members.* Paper presented at the NICHD conference on research on families with retarded children, University of North Carolina, Chapel Hill.

Vietze, P. M., & Anderson, B. J. (1981). Styles of parent-child interaction. In M. J. Begab, H. C. Haywood, & H. L. Garber (Eds.), *Psychosocial influences in retarded performance: Vol. 1. Issues and theories in development* (pp. 255–283). Baltimore: University Park Press.

Voilland, A. L. (1962). *Family casework diagnosis.* New York: Columbia University Press.

Voilland, A. L., & Buell, B. (1961). A classification of disordered family types. *Social Work, 6,* 3–11.

Willner, S. K., & Crane, R. (1979). A parental dilemma: The child with a marginal handicap. *Social Casework: The Journal of Contemporary Social Work, 60,* 30–35.

Winch, R. C. (1947). Heuristic and empirical typologies: A job for factor analysis. *American Sociological Review, 12,* 68–75.

Wortis, H., Bardach, J. L., Cutler, R., Rue, R., & Freedman, A. (1963). Child-rearing practices in a low socioeconomic group. *Pediatrics, 32,* 298–307.

Yarrow, M., Campbell, J., & Burton, R. (1968). *Childrearing.* San Francisco: Jossey-Bass.

Zetlin, A. G., Turner, J. L., & Winick, L. (in press). Socialization effects on the adult adaptation of mildly retarded persons living in the community. In S. Landsman-Dwyer & P. M. Vietze, (Eds.), *Impact of residential settings on behavior.* Baltimore: University Park Press.

Zussman, J. U. (1980). Situational determinants of parental behavior: Effects of competing cognitive activity. *Child Development, 51,* 792–800.

Chapter

3

Family Life Cycle

Theoretical and Empirical Implications and Future Directions for Families with Mentally Retarded Members

Ann P. Turnbull, Jean Ann Summers, and Mary Jane Brotherson

FAMILY LIFE CYCLE THEORY focuses on the growth and transitions of families as they move through time historically, developmentally, emotionally, and socially (Neugarten, 1976). Family life cycle is more comprehensive than the milestones of individual members; rather it represents a synthesis of psychological theory on developmental tasks and needs and sociological theory on family processes, dynamics, and stress (Carter & McGoldrick, 1980; Hill, 1964). Within the field of sociology, life-cycle theory is a rather new theoretical perspective developed over the last 3 decades. An excellent historical review of the conceptual chronology of formulating family life-cycle theory is provided by Hill and Rodgers (1969).

There are three major purposes of this chapter. The first is to present a family systems conceptual framework within which life-cycle concepts are linked to other dimensions of family dynamics. The second purpose is to review theoretical and empirical literature on the life-cycle needs of families with mentally retarded

members. The final purpose is to suggest future research, intervention, and policy directions aimed at strengthening family adaptation over the full life cycle.

FAMILY SYSTEMS CONCEPTUAL FRAMEWORK

Historically, research and interventions related to the adaptation of families with mentally retarded members have largely ignored the theoretical contributions of the family systems literature (Benson & Turnbull, 1986; Berardo, 1980; Broderick, 1971; Holman & Burr, 1980; Olson, Russell & Sprenkle, 1980b). Thus, much research has tended to be of an atheoretical nature and to focus on variables in an isolated fashion without regard for the way that they reverberate intended and unintended influences on other aspects of the family system. To address this theoretical gap, a programmatic research effort is currently underway at the Research and Training Center on Independent Living at the University of Kansas. Two phases of the research program have been completed: 1) a comprehensive review and synthesis of two bodies of literature—family systems theory and family impact of mentally retarded persons and 2) a naturalistic study of 12 families (6 with mentally retarded members and with orthopedically handicapped members) involving in-depth interviews with the mother, father, handicapped person, nonhandicapped sibling, and in some cases members of the extended family to analyze family impact from a systems perspective (Skrtic, Summers, Brotherson, & Turnbull, 1984; Turnbull, Brotherson, Summers, 1985; Turnbull, Summers, & Brotherson, 1984). The third phase, currently in process, is an analysis of coping strategies that are a facet of ideological style characteristics (McCubbin et al., 1980; Olson et al., 1984) of families who have successfully completed the launching stage of the life cycle.

A family systems conceptual framework was the major outcome of the first phase of the research effort. This framework, depicted in Figure 1, represents the four dimensions of structure, interaction, functions, and life cycle. As indicated by the arrows, changes in one dimension create changes in others.

This framework incorporates the biologically derived premise (Von Bertalanffy, 1968) that all living systems are composed of interdependent parts and that the interaction of these parts creates properties not contained in any of the separate entities. As applied to families, behavior and needs of individual family members cannot be accurately and fully understood by focusing on individual members in isolation. Rather, the family is "more than the sum of its parts" (Carter & McGoldrick, 1980, p. 4). There are properties of the family that can be understood only by studying the relationships among members and interactions among its different dimensions.

The empirical or hypothetical relationships of variables can be conceptualized within the family systems framework. This framework conceptualizes structure as the resources or characteristics of the family and its individual members. These resources and characteristics are the *inputs* shaping family interaction, which is the *process* by which families fulfill their functions. Functions are the activities that the families must perform to meet their individual and collective needs. These functions are the *outputs* of the system. Finally, the system as a whole (input, process, and output) is in a continual state of *change* as the family moves through the life cycle. This section presents a concise overview of three dimensions—structure, interaction, and functions—followed by a more indepth analysis of life cycle in the next section.

Family Structure

Family structure emphasizes the uniqueness and diversity of families. The almost infinite variety of membership characteristics, cultural styles, and ideological styles (see Table 1) renders every family unique. These unique structural inputs in turn shape the interactional process. Mental retardation is only one of the numerous inputs into family interaction.

Membership Characteristics The first component, membership characteristics, includes an array of elements related to the quantitative and qualitative constellation of the family. A major gap in the family systems and mental retardation literature is an operational definition of family. Researchers and family members alike have idiosyncratic definitions of what is a family. A finding from the authors' naturalistic study is that different families described their membership in highly alternative ways (e.g., only people living in household at the current point in time, multiple stepparents and stepgrandparents, extensive array of extended family separated by wide geographical distance, inclusion of nuclear family member dead for over 20 years whose influence strongly pervades current family ideology, unrelated persons who are significantly involved in affectional relationships). A substantial portion of the literature on families with retarded members is based on the erroneous assumption of family homogeneity. It is important for researchers, service providers, and policymakers to recognize the heterogeneity of fami-

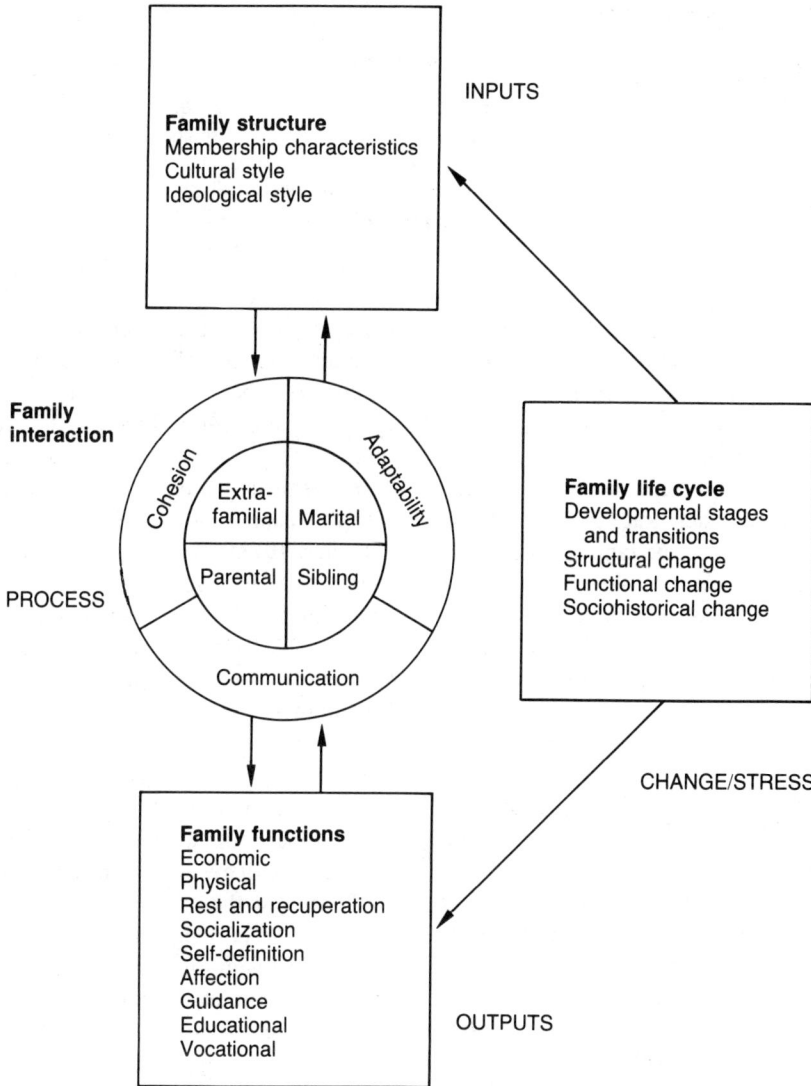

Figure 1. Family systems conceptual framework. (Reprinted with permission from Benson, H., & Turnbull, A. P. [1986]. Approaching families from an individualized perspective. In R. H. Horner, L. H. Meyer, & H. D. Fredericks (Eds.), *Education of learners with severe handicaps: Exemplary service strategies*. Baltimore: Paul H. Brookes Publishing Co.)

lies and respect the unique definition that each family formulates for itself.

Membership characteristics of families with retarded members have been studied in the research literature (e.g., Grossman, 1972; Holroyd & McArthur, 1976; Wadsworth & Wadsworth, 1971). However, little attention has been paid to the relationship of these elements to successful interaction in families. Membership characteristics change across the developmental stages of the family, because developmental transitions involve the entry, increased autonomy, and exit of members. Therefore, research should be conducted within a life-cycle framework, with a focus on the impact of changing membership characteristics on successful family interaction.

Cultural Style Research on family structure has also focused on cultural style, primarily on the elements of race (Dunlap & Hol-

Table 1. Family structure

Membership	Cultural style	Ideological style
Individual characteristics	Ethnic	Beliefs and values
Family size	Racial	Coping styles
Nature of extrafamilial system	Religious	
	Socioeconomic status	
	Geographic location	

lingsworth, 1977), religion (Farber, 1962), and socioeconomic status (Farber, 1962). These elements are possibly the most static component of the family systems framework, yet they can be influential in shaping the family's ideological style, interactional pattern, and functional priorities. Race and social class have been identified in the family systems literature as variables related to the timing of life events (Kerckhoff & Campbell, 1977; Neugarten & Hagestad, 1977). Research should focus on the relationships of different cultural resources in families with mentally retarded members to successful family functioning over the life cycle.

Ideological Style   The ideological style of families is based on their beliefs, values, and coping behaviors. Ideological characteristics are strongly influenced by cultural style. For example, working-class families, due to financial instability and a perceived lack of control over their environment, have a decreased value on future planning (Rubin, 1976). Jewish families tend to place a high value on learning and intellectual achievement, whereas Italian families emphasize family closeness and affection to the point that going away to college is perceived as a threat to family solidarity (McGoldrick, Pearce, & Giordano, 1982). Upper middle-class parents exercise control over their children by developing internal control and initiative, rather than by demanding strict obedience to authority (Lee, 1982). All these characteristics have potential implications for the reciprocal perspectives of the way in which a mentally retarded person affects the family and the way in which the family affects the development of the retarded individual.

Coping is a critical dimension of ideological style that can strongly influence the ability of families to function successfully over the life cycle. Coping is used here to refer to any response designed to reduce stress, either by changing the situation or by changing the perceived meaning of the situation (Pearlin & Schooler, 1978). The coping styles of families can be classified into internal and external strategies based on the work of McCubbin and Patterson (1981). The specific coping patterns associated with each type of strategy include the following:

Internal coping strategies
   Passive appraisal: an avoidance response to problems based on the premise that problems will resolve themselves over time
   Reframing: the ability to identify conditions that can be successfully altered and initiate problem solving; the ability to identify conditions beyond one's control and make attitude adjustments to live with them constructively

External coping strategies
   Social support: ability to acquire and use resources from extended family, friends, and neighbors (extrafamilial subsystem)
   Spiritual support: ability to acquire and use spiritual interpretations, advice from religious leaders, and participation in religious activities
   Formal support: ability to acquire and use community resources and professional assistance

The data from Olson et al. (1984) indicate that, in a sample of 1,000 families, the most important coping strategy was seeking spiritual support (it should be noted, however, that the sample was selected from a religious-related organization). The second most often-reported strategy was reframing, used both to minimize and prevent problems. The least used strategy was passive appraisal. Other pertinent findings of the study include the stage differences in using particular coping strategies across the life cycle (e.g., spiritual support is a more useful strategy for older rather than younger couples; social support is lowest at launching stage) and the disparate perceptions of family coping strategies reported by husbands, wives, and adolescents. There have been no life-cycle studies of coping in families with mentally retarded members. This is a priority area for the future. In particular, the effectiveness of passive appraisal and reframing as coping strategies for dealing with changes throughout the life cycle is a key area for research and intervention.

Family Interaction

Family interaction, conceptualized in the circle of Figure 1, is the core of the systems model. The basic premise is that the behavior among members of the family is interrelated such that changes in an individual or group relationship effect change throughout the total system. In the process of interaction, each member is affected and influenced by every other member and by the system as a whole.

Table 2 outlines the four components of the interactional system: subsystems, cohesion, adaptability, and communication. The family consists of definable subsystems. These subsystems interact according to rules or boundaries governed by the family's level of cohesion, adaptability, and communication style.

Subsystems Each individual family member belongs to two or more subsystems and has a different role in each subsystem. An extension of the work of Minuchin (1974) has led to the four subsystems represented in this framework: 1) marital (husband/wife interactions), 2) sibling (child/child interactions), 3) parental (parent/child interactions), 4) extrafamilial (nuclear family interactions with extended family and networks of social/community/professional support). The constellation of subsystems is greatly influenced by the membership characteristics of families (e.g., single-parent, number of children, size of extrafamilial network) and by the current family life-cycle stage.

Mentally retarded family members affect all four subsystems. Furthermore, an intervention targeted on one subsystem (e.g., parental) will have spillover effects on the other three. Con-

Table 2. Family interactional system

Subsystem	Cohesion	Adaptability	Communication
Marital subsystem	Closeness	Power structure	Closed
Sibling subsystem	Support	Role relationships	Open
Parental subsystem	Decision making	Relationship rules	Random
Extrafamilial subsystem			

Cohesion

low			high
disengaged	separated	connected	enmeshed

Adaptability

low			high
rigid	structured	flexible	chaotic

Communication

closed	open		random

sider the example of a mother who has agreed to work on a home training program in the area of feeding with her severely retarded child. Allowing her child to feed himself triples the time involved in each meal. While the mother is working with the child on feeding, her dinner conversation with her husband and other children is substantially limited. After the other family members finish dinner, the father cleans the kitchen and siblings proceed to their homework, all feeling that some of their needs have been overlooked. Meanwhile, the mother is feeling isolated from the rest of her family and frustrated about all the tasks to which she must attend before midnight. Typically, home intervention has focused only on the developmental gains of the child (e.g., feeding skills). A much broader research, intervention, and policy agenda is needed to examine the systemic impact of intervention on total family interaction. Thus, family outcomes need to be operationalized and analyzed in addition to child outcomes. The needs of all family members should be taken as seriously as the needs of the child (Terkelsen, 1980).

Cohesion, Adaptability, and Communication   Three dynamic elements characterizing the way that the subsystems interact are cohesion, adaptability, and communication (Olson, Russell, & Sprenkle, 1980a). Cohesion is defined as the degree of balance between the emotional bonds among family members and their individual autonomy. Cohesion can be conceptualized on a continuum, with extreme ends representing enmeshment and disengagement (Minuchin, 1974). Enmeshment or disengagement can occur within one subsystem or in a combination of subsystems. An example of enmeshment is the overinvolvement of a mother in an early intervention program for her retarded child so that the mother's self-esteem is defined by the progress of the child and her emotional and physical interactions with other family members are severely curtailed. The unintended consequences of such enmeshment can result in disengagement between the mother and her husband (marital subsystem) and the mother and other children (parental subsystem). Healthy family cohesion is charac-

terized by clear boundaries between subsystems and the balance of unity and individuation in relationships (Minuchin, 1974).

Family adaptability refers to the ability of members to change the familial power structure, role relationships, and relationship rules in response to life-cycle changes resulting from developmental, structural, functional, or sociohistorical catalysts (Olson et al., 1980a). As is discussed in the section on life cycle, the ability of families with retarded members to adapt according to normative and nonnormative changes is a key element influencing the quality of family interaction. As with cohesion, the most viable families are able to maintain a balance between stability and change (Olson, Sprenkle, & Russell, 1979).

The final dynamic element in the family interaction model is communication. The communication element can be described as the process by which information is transmitted in families (Kantor & Lehr, 1975). Important aspects of family communication skills are effective listening, sending clear messages, and providing feedback. Again, communication, as with cohesion and adaptability, falls on a continuum, with the center being most viable for successful family interaction. At one extreme of this continuum, families have closed communication, characterized by little or no discussion, and avoidance of emotion. At the other extreme all topics are discussed and emotionalized (Kantor & Lehr, 1975). One finding of the authors' naturalistic study was that some families avoid communication on issues related to retardation. Quotes from several families illustrate this point (Turnbull et al., 1985):

Father: We didn't talk to our son about the fact that he's retarded. I presume he has figured it out. He never asked questions.

Mother: I have more or less worked out my adjustment on my own. My husband isn't communicative.

Sister: My brother's wife asked me about the genetic implications of Rachel's handicap before they got married. She didn't want to bring it up with my brother. I told her that, as far as we know, it is not genetic. It was probably caused by an outside influence, maybe a flu shot. She was relieved.

Two key concepts related to all three elements—cohesion, adaptability, and communication—are change and balance. Life-cycle changes act as catalysts to modify the nature and quality of family interactions (Carter & McGoldrick, 1980). Families who successfully interact are those who maintain a balance through that change between emotional unity and support of autonomy, between a sense of stability and reaction to change, and between closed and random communication (McCubbin et al., 1980; Olson et al., 1984). Future research is needed to identify the characteristics of families who demonstrate successful interaction at each stage of the family life cycle. These characteristics should then be analyzed to identify intervention strategies for implementation and evaluation.

Family Functions

As indicated in Figure 1, nine functions have been included in the conceptual framework (Caplan, 1976; Leslie, 1976). These are eco- nomic, physical, rest and recuperation, socialization, self-definition, affection, guidance, educational, and vocational. Table 3 outlines specific tasks associated with each function.

Functions are conceptualized as products or *outputs* of family interaction, because they represent the results of interaction in terms of the ability to meet the individual needs of the family's members. The family can be conceptualized as a resource exchange network (McCubbin et al., 1980). Carrying out functions successfully is the essential purpose for the existence of the family and requires interdependence between the family and its extrafamilial network (Terkelsen, 1980).

Families vary in the value and priority that they attach to different functions and to their role allocation in carrying out functions. The interrelationships of the dimensions of structure (e.g., membership, cultural style, and ideological style), interaction (e.g., cohesion, adaptability), and life cycle (e.g., developmental stage) require further investigation to determine how families are influenced to carry out functions in certain ways.

Table 3. Family functions

Economic	Physical	Rest and recuperation
Generating income	Food purchasing and food preparation	Individual and family-oriented recreation
Paying bills and banking	Clothes purchasing and preparation	Setting aside demands
Handling investments	Health care and maintenance	Developing and enjoying hobbies
Overseeing insurance and benefit programs	Safety and protection	
Earning allowance	Transportation	
Dispensing allowance	Home maintenance	

Socialization	Self-Definition	Affection
Interpersonal relationships	Establishing self-identity and self-image	Nurturing and love
Developing social skills	Recognizing strengths and weaknesses	Companionship
	Sense of belonging	Intimacy
		Expressing emotions

Guidance	Educational	Vocational
Problem-solving	Continuing education for parents	Career choice
Advice and feedback	School work	Development of work ethic
Shaping basic beliefs and values	Homework	Support of career interests and problems
Transmitting religious values	Cultural appreciation	

Several themes were apparent from the authors' literature review and naturalistic interview data related to family functions. First, mentally retarded children and youth, particularly those with severe handicaps, increase the consumptive demands on families in functional areas (Birenbaum, 1971; Boggs, 1979; Bristol & Schopler, 1983; Dunlap & Hollingsworth, 1977; Gallagher, Cross, & Scharfman, 1981; McAndrew, 1976; Moroney, 1981) without proportionately increasing its productive capability (e.g., contributing to family income, caring for younger siblings, assisting with household maintenance). Placing many retarded persons in the least restrictive environment of their family has the unintended consequence of creating a highly restrictive environment for family members in carrying out their functions (Turnbull et al., 1985). The implications of these restrictions over the life cycle is a worthy area for future research and policy analysis.

Second, there has been extremely limited recognition in the literature that mentally retarded persons can make positive contributions to fulfilling family functions. Data from the authors' naturalistic study indicated that families perceived the major positive contribution of the retarded member to be related to the more intangible functions of guidance, affection, and self-definition; for example, parents were guided in the development of certain values by the experiences they shared with the retarded member. Parents and siblings describe the values that they had learned as follows (Turnbull et al., 1985):

"Learning to love"

"Looking past a lot to look inside"

"To be more self-confident and to ignore what other people think"

"To value people who are different—whatever their difference is"

"To rely on myself to solve problems"

Although intangible, these contributions had substantial value attached to them. An important area for future research is the analysis of positive contributions by mentally retarded persons to family functions and the impact of positive contributions on the family's ability to cope successfully over the life cycle.

The third functional theme is the overwhelming emphasis placed in the professional literature on the role of parents as teachers of their child (Altman & Mira, 1983; Baker, 1983). Education is only one of nine functions. The following quote from Sondra Diamond (1981), a psychologist and disabled adult, raises a frequently overlooked perspective on an unintended consequence of the parent-as-teacher role:

> Something happens in a parent when relating to his disabled child; he forgets that they're a kid first. I used to think about that a lot when I was a kid. I would be off in a euphoric state, drawing or coloring or cutting out paper dolls and as often as not the activity would be turned into an occupational therapy session. "You're not holding the scissors right," "Sit up straight so your curvature doesn't get worse." That era was ended when I finally let loose a long and exhaustive tirade. "I'm just a kid! You can't therapize me all the time! I get enough therapy in school every day! I don't think about my handicap all the time like you do!" (p. 30)

Important issues warranting empirical documentation include: 1) the impact of the parent-as-teacher role on the degree of cohesion within and across subsystems, 2) the opportunity costs for other functions when parents increase the amount of time that they devote to the educational function and 3) the influence of the heavy emphasis on the parent-as-teacher role at earlier life-cycle stages on the priority given to this role over the full life cycle.

FAMILY LIFE CYCLE

The fourth dimension of the family systems framework and the primary focus of this chapter is family life cycle. Life cycle is the dynamic element of the family system. As a family moves through time, normative and nonnormative *change* alters its structure and/or its functional priorities; these in turn produce change in the way the family interacts. As indicated in Figure 1, life cycle incorporates four components: developmental stages and transitions, structural changes, functional changes, and sociohistorical changes. The elements of each of these components are outlined in Table 4.

Change is the unifying theme of family life-cycle literature. Life events are considered to be "stressors" when they require a change in the stabilized life pattern or routine of the family system (Hill, 1949; McCubbin, 1979; McCubbin et al., 1980). Stress is the psychological and physiological response to stressors resulting from the dissonance between life changes and the capability to respond (Olson et al., 1984). Thus, a major outcome of life-cycle changes is the production of stress. Another key source of stress often overlooked in the family systems and mental retardation literature is conditions that do not change but rather make a chronic demand on the family. Thus, families with mentally retarded members are placed in the paradoxical position of dealing with both change and chronicity. This section examines both of these sources of stress according to the four components of family life cycle.

Theoretical Perspectives of Developmental Stages and Transitions

Developmental Stages Eight stages of the family life cycle were originally proposed by Duvall (1957). These stages have been modified by sociologists and extended to as many as 24 (Rodgers, 1960). Seven stages have been incorporated into the family systems framework patterned after the work of Olson

et al. (1984). These stages include: couple, childbearing, school age, adolescence, launching, postparental, and aging. Variations in family structure (e.g., membership characteristics, cultural style, ideological style) may produce modifications in developmental stages or different stage-appropriate expectations (Colon, 1980; Falicov & Karrer, 1980). Families may also dissolve or become reconstituted before some stages occur (Hubbell, 1981a, 1981b; Sager et al., 1983). These seven stages do generalize, however, to the majority of families in society.

Developmental stages can be visualized as a series of relatively level plateaus. In each stage, different functions have particular priority, and specific developmental tasks and responsibility assumed by different individuals or subsystems of the family change. Some functions are highly age related. Young children as compared to teenagers require more emphasis on physical care, whereas teenagers require more emphasis on vocational preparation.

Specific tasks associated with functions change throughout stages. Parental affection, for example, is typically expressed to infants through intimate physical contact and bonding characterized by high levels of cohesion. As infants grow and eventually become adolescents and young adults, parental affection is expressed to the same individual at different points in time through communication, respect for individuality, and "letting go."

Table 4. Family life cycle

Developmental stages and transitions	Structural change	Functional change	Sociohistorical change
Couple	Membership	Economic	Cultural trends
Childbearing	Cultural style	Physical	Economy
School age	Ideological style	Rest and recuperation	Political trends
Adolescence		Socialization	Formative events
Launching		Self-definition	
Postparental		Affection	
Aging		Guidance	
		Educational	
		Vocational	

Shifts also occur in the responsibility for functions. In the developmental stage of child-bearing, parents or other care providers usually assume primary responsibility for carrying out functions. Life-cycle progression represents the increasing shifting of responsibility from parents to their offspring and their offspring's extrafamilial system. Thus, a key aspect of developmental stages is the change required within families in the way they carry out functions.

Developmental stages are grounded in age-role expectations and are defined in terms of the oldest child (Hill & Rodgers, 1969), based on the assumption that it is this child's advancing developmental needs that require a major reallocation of priority, tasks, and responsibility for carrying out functions. Routines are established during developmental stages that contribute to stability and lower levels of stress. The relevance of a developmental stage perspective in working with families was stated by Hill (1970):

> [A]ny researcher or clinician who seeks to generalize about families without taking into account variations resulting from the stage of development will encounter tremendous variance for which they will not be able to account. (p. 190)

Developmental Transitions Developmental transitions are the periods characterized by change and discontinuity that occur when families are in the process of shifting from one stage to another. In contrast to developmental tasks, which are learning requirements within the established roles of a developmental stage, developmental transitions involve a major shift in family interaction marking movement to a new stage. Transitions are classified as normative changes because transitional events and changes are "*ubiquitous* (they occur to most families), *expectable* (families can anticipate their occurrence at certain scheduled points in the family life cycle), and *short-term* (not chronic)" (McCubbin et al., 1980, pp. 860, 858).

Transitions have frequently been identified as a major point of family stress and dysfunction (Carter & McGoldrick, 1980; Haley,

1973; Minuchin, 1974; Terkelsen, 1980). They primarily involve changes in family interaction based on two factors (Carter & McGoldrick, 1980): 1) entry, increased autonomy, and exit of members (structural change: a new baby is born, young adult leaves home), leading to 2) expansion, contraction, and realignment of subsystems (impact of structural change on family interaction). Examples of subsystem expansion and contraction required by transitions into new developmental stages are outlined below:

Transition to New Stage
   Childbearing
   School age
   Launching

Subsystem Expansion
   Parental
   Extrafamilial
   Marital

Subsystem Contraction
   Marital
   Parental
   Parental

The results of Olson et al.'s (1984) national study of families of nonhandicapped children indicated that, as compared to all other stages, transitions required for launching created the greatest amount of family stress. Family satisfaction, marital satisfaction, and quality of life were rated lowest at this time.

Transitions require systemic changes in social and emotional roles (Neugarten, 1976; Weeks & Wright, 1979), and changes are stressful for most people. Failure to adapt to transitions results in the family moving ahead chronologically but not interpersonally (Hughes, Berger, & Wright, 1978). However, family theorists suggest that even greater stress is created when transitions occur off-time (Haley, 1973; Neugarten, 1976), resulting in a disruption of the expected life rhythms. Variations in structural composition (Carter & McGoldrick, 1980; McGoldrick & Carter, 1982), interactional system (Minuchin, 1974), and functions (Turnbull, Brotherson, Summers, 1985) influence the types and levels of stress at transition points.

Applications of Theoretical Perspectives to Families with Mentally Retarded Members

Developmental Stages In applying developmental stage theory to families with a mentally retarded member, several sources of stress for families are apparent.

The presence of a mentally retarded member creates additional responsibilities for families at every developmental stage beginning with childbearing. Table 5 outlines examples of stressors for families. These are synthesized from the literature and the authors' naturalistic research with families and are organized according to developmental stages. Although developmental stage theory suggests a gradual shift of responsibility from parents to their offspring for carrying out functions, parents with retarded members must continue to assume a substantial degree of responsibility for functions. From a life-cycle perspective, an important research issue is the impact of the chronicity of the retarded member's dependence on

Table 5. Stressors arising from developmental stages and transitions

Childbearing	School age
Dealing with fears and worries of an abnormal birth	Adjusting emotionally to educational implications of handicap
Obtaining an accurate diagnosis	Clarifying personal ideology on mainstreamed vs. specialized placements
Making initial emotional adjustments	
Informing siblings and the extrafamilial subsystem	Participating in IEP conferences
Locating services	Dealing with the reactions of the peer group
Asking "ultimate" questions	
Clarifying a personal ideology to guide decision making	Locating community resources
Seeking to find meaning in the handicap	Arranging for extracurricular activities
Establishing new interaction patterns within the family	
Identifying priority family functions	
Establishing routines to carry out family functions	

Adolescence	Launching
Adjusting emotionally to chronicity of handicapping condition	Adjusting emotionally to the adult implications of the handicap
Identifying issues surrounding emerging sexuality	Deciding on an appropriate residence
Dealing with peer isolation and rejection	Initiating vocational involvement
Making role readjust-	Dealing with issues of sexuality

(continued)

Table 5. *(continued)*

Adolescence	Launching
ments based on skill development	Recognizing needs for continuing family responsibility
Future planning for vocational development	Dealing with continued financial implications of dependency
Arranging for leisure-time activities	Lack of socialization opportunities outside the family for handicapped member
Participating in IEP conferences	
Dealing with physical and emotional changes of puberty	Planning for guardianship

Postparental	Aging
Reestablishing one-to-one relationship with spouse	Planning for care or supervision of handicapped member after death
Interacting with handicapped family member's vocational service provider or employer	Clarifying personal ideology on the need for "permanent" (e.g., institution) vs. "quasi-permanent" (e.g., group home) residences
Interacting with handicapped member's residential service provider	
Adjusting to handicapped family member's interest in dating, marriage, and childbearing	Transferring parental responsibilties to other family subsystems and/or service providers
Establishing new interests and self-identity for parents	
Planning for long-term financial security of handicapped member	

the family's successful functioning across developmental stages.

Families with a severely retarded child are faced with the challenge of readjusting their expectations and assumptions. They must adapt to the increasing independence of their nonhandicapped children as they pass through their developmental stages and at the same time cope with the continued dependence of the severely retarded member (Fotheringham & Creal, 1974). Thus, they have two family life cycles to negotiate. Another theoretical contrast is the specification of family life-cycle stage according to the age-role expectations of the oldest child (Hill & Rodgers, 1969). Particularly if the retarded child is the oldest child in the family, increased adaptability is required for all family members when siblings younger in chronological age become more developmentally advanced than the retarded member (Farber & Ryckman, 1965; Wikler, 1981). The retarded sibling fails to maintain his or her hierarchical position in the family, and this revision of age roles causes stress for younger siblings, especially for males who are less than 2 years younger than the retarded child (Breslau, 1982).

As compared to the recent emphasis in the sociological literature on later years of the family life cycle (McCubbin et al., 1980), research on the impact of mentally retarded members on families has mostly focused on the childbearing stage. Most of the adjustment literature has been time-bound within this early stage (Wolfensberger, 1970), ignoring the adjustments that parents must make at each developmental stage. Wikler, Wasow, and Hatfield (1981) reported that approximately two-thirds of the parent and social worker respondents in their study believed that parents experience chronic sorrow across developmental stages. An interesting finding was that social workers tended to overestimate how upsetting the parents' early experiences were (e.g., time when child would have normally learned to walk, entry into special rather than regular class) and to underestimate the upsetting impact of later experiences (e.g., the child's 21st birthday,

which was symbolic of attaining independence from the family) (Wikler, 1981).

Bristol and Schopler (1983) report the following findings that justify directing more attention to the needs of families at later developmental stages: 1) Older autistic children cause more stress than younger ones, 2) both community acceptance and services are lessened as children grow older, and 3) the potential exists for parental burnout. These findings were corroborated by a life-cycle study of families with mentally retarded children in which it was found that parents of older children, as compared to younger ones, were less supported, more isolated, and more in need of expanded services (Suelzle & Keenan, 1981). An important future direction is greater emphasis on research and intervention at older life-cycle stages. A major need exists for documenting high-stress periods for the subsystems of the family within and between developmental stages.

Developmental Transitions As previously reported, transitions are viewed as normative events and have been described by McCubbin et al. (1980) as ubiquitous, expectable, and short term. What is the impact of nonnormative development, in both intellectual functioning and adaptive behavior of the retarded member, on the normative transitional events of families?

This question cannot yet be answered; a void exists in the mental retardation literature on the impact of stage transitions on successful family functioning. There are no data on the quantitative or qualitative aspects of transitional periods for families with retarded members. For example, what are the marker variables for families of severely retarded youth related to his or her entrance into adolescence? This issue is complicated by dissonance of low developmental skills and emerging physical maturity. At what time should a retarded member be launched from the family? Families lack the normative rituals of high school/college graduation, self-sufficiency in a job, or marriage (Friedman, 1980) to demarcate the transitional period for launching. Families with retarded children do not have access to the same "punctuation marks along the life cycle'' (Neugarten, 1976, p. 18) available to families with nonhandicapped children. Although systematic inquiry into transitional periods becomes more complex for families with a retarded member, it is a priority area for future research.

Off-time transitions frequently occur in families with mentally retarded members, particularly at the launching stage (Turnbull et al., 1985). In some cases, parents or siblings may be eager for the retarded member to be launched from the family, but the individual may not have the prerequisite skills for independent living, or supervised community residential alternatives may be unavailable. In other cases, the retarded member may be eager to leave the family, but enmeshment may prevent the parents from letting go. Several families in the authors' naturalistic study were faced with this transitional resistance. It is interesting to note that all these families had been urged at the time of initial diagnosis to institutionalize their child. They resisted institutionalization vehemently and reared their child with only minimal professional support and community services. In a sense, keeping their child at home substantially shaped their ideological style, family interaction, routines for carrying out functions, and self-definition. Whether enmeshment was the outcome of this parental devotion or whether it was a motivating factor in keeping the child at home in the first place is irrelevant. Enmeshment either resulted from the decision to keep the child at home or prevented institutionalization of the young retarded child, but paradoxically, it also prevents community living outside the home for the retarded adult.

An increasing concern among policymakers and service providers is the dilemma that sometimes occurs when retarded adults live with their elderly parents. On the one hand, there is a major problem when the parents die before any transitional preparation for relocating the retarded adult is completed. On the other hand, several families in the authors' naturalistic study reported that maintaining the retarded member in the home over the life cycle contributed to the functions of socializa-

tion (e.g., companionship) and self-definition (e.g., purpose in life) for the elderly parents. Research and intervention should be directed toward the analysis of factors and development of services related to the off-time transition of launching. Specifically, research efforts need to identify the contributions that retarded adults make to their elderly parents. Competing equities are involved when a retarded adult is prevented from living and working with peers in the community in order to assist elderly parents in carrying out functions in the home environment, thus enabling the parents to avoid placement in a nursing home. The outcome is the placement of middle-age retarded adults in a more restrictive environment in order to maintain their elderly parents in a less restrictive one. An interest analysis from a policy perspective is needed to explicate the potential or actual conflicts of interest (Turnbull, 1981).

A highly consistent finding in the literature is a pervasive worry about the future (Birenbaum, 1971; Bristol & Schopler, 1983; McAndrew, 1976; Minde, Hackett, Killou, & Silver, 1972; Turnbull et al., 1985). A major coping strategy for many families of retarded children is passive appraisal, which involves maintaining a strong present rather than future orientation and taking one day at a time. Although systematic future planning may appear to be a strategy for alleviating concern, it may actually create stress for some families. The effects of passive appraisal and reframing on the ability of families to make successful transitions need to be illuminated through research.

To ameliorate the stress of developmental transitions, more research is needed on the types of interventions that are most supportive of families. A potentially fruitful type of intervention warranting investigation is future forecasting and planning to prepare family members for transitional change. In one intervention model currently being implemented at the University of Kansas, parents and siblings of severely mentally retarded youth complete ecological inventories (Sailor & Guess, 1983; Wilcox & Bellamy, 1982) of adult environments—residential, vocational, recreational. An analysis of the ecological inventories will yield to the specification of critical skills needed to function successfully in the future adult settings. Skills will then be assigned a priority rating by the family and incorporated into the individualized education program (IEP) for the retarded adolescent. A concomitant training model will provide group sessions and written materials for parents, siblings, other significant family members, and community resource persons (e.g., lawyers, trust officers, physicians, insurance counselors, rehabilitation specialists, special education teachers) on future planning from a programmatic, ethical, and legal perspective. Specific topics to be covered include federal and state financial benefits, estate planning, guardianship, consent to service, family law (marriage, contraception, sterilization), and juvenile/adult offenders.

Structural Changes

The remaining three components of family life cycle—structural, functional, and sociohistorical changes—are classified as nonnormative. As distinguished from the normative classification of developmental transitions, nonnormative changes are precipitated by life events or hardships unrelated to passage through developmental stages (McCubbin et al., 1980). Nonnormative changes are stressful when they are of sufficient magnitude to require a shift in family interaction.

Structural changes requiring a shift in family interaction may involve one or more changes in the elements of membership characteristics,

cultural style, and ideological style. Early sociological research of family stress largely focused on structural changes created by war separation (Hill, 1949).

Table 6 is a synthesis of structural stressors identified in the authors' naturalistic study. A major source of structural stress for families identified in this research and supported in the literature surrounds the points of initial institutionalization and deinstitutionalization. An assumption is sometimes made that institutionalizing a mentally retarded family member is an extreme form of disengagement and emotional detachment. On the contrary, the authors' qualitative data indicated intense stress in cohesive families at the time of institutionalization. One mother described this stress as follows:

> There were no programs for children under five [at that time], and those years are so important, we felt we owed her an education—the same philosophy as with the other children. Giving her up at three years of age was the hardest thing I've ever done, other than my husband's death. They were both like deaths.

The Pennhurst longitudinal study of deinstitutionalizational impact of families (Keating, Conroy, & Walker, 1980) reported Likert scale ratings from families on the degrees of stress created by 14 normative changes (e.g., age at which talking and walking were expected, placement in school, adolescence, 21st birthday) and nonnormative changes (e.g., diagnosis, medical or behavioral crisis, institutionalization, initial discussion of deinstitutionalization). As compared to all other stressors, institutionalization was rated as

Table 6. Stressors arising from structural change

Membership	Cultural style	Ideological style
Isolation	Racial/ethnic discrimination	Questioning beliefs
Unemployment	Poverty	Frustrated expectations
Occupational demands	Moving	Value conflicts among members
Negative community reactions	Rural isolation	Ambiguous values
Alcohol or drug dependency	Child or spouse abuse	Value rigidity
Lack of extended family support	Dual careers	Insufficient coping strategies
Too many or too few children		Conflict of coping strategies
Reconstituted family relationships		among family members
Institutionalization/deinstitutionalization		

"very stressful" by the highest percentage of parents. The second and third items, respectively, were diagnosis and initial discussion of deinstitutionalization. The potency of structural stressors, as compared to normative ones, is noteworthy.

A major conflict currently exists between policy preferences in favor of deinstitutionalization and parental resistance to it (Keating et al., 1980; Klaber, 1969; Meyer, 1980; Payne, 1976). The Pennhurst study indicated that 75% of the respondents reported that their retarded family member had reached his or her highest potential; thus, they anticipated the chronicity of dependence and the lack of change. They perceived Pennhurst to be a haven of permanence and security, with over 80% of the families indicating satisfaction with the services. Some families preferred the known problems of Pennhurst to the uncertainty of deinstitutionalization, as illustrated by this parental comment:

> My child had a broken arm and a tooth knocked out. I wonder what will happen next. But at least I know what it's like here. At least there's some control. What would it be like on the outside? He could wander off and get hit by a car. Who would know; Who would care? (Keating et al., 1980, p. 43)

A portion of families in the original Pennhurst study were reassessed after their retarded family member had been deinstitutionalized for 6 months. The findings indicated a significant positive increase in attitudes toward community placement; however, the pervading concern was still lack of future security. One parent described this concern as follows:

> This community living is great. But what happens when this nice young family wants their own family? There might be a psychological let-down if they let them (retarded residents) go. At least Pennhurst was there. It will not crumble. (Conroy & Latib, 1982, p. 8)

Research guided by life-cycle theory should identify factors contributing to structural stress associated with institutionalization and deinstitutionalization. The issues of change and chronicity and their relationship to future security are key areas for intervention. Research at the intervention level should be directed to assist families in lifelong planning and adaptation. At the policy level, research should determine the need for incorporating the valuative criteria of security and permanence into the formulation of family policy.

Functional Changes

Functional changes requiring shifts in family interaction are a result of sudden, sometimes temporary, changes in family members' needs or a gradual realization that someone's needs are not being met. An example of sudden functional change is a mother's hospitalization for surgery; during that period, other family members must assume her usual tasks, as well as additional tasks, such as visits to the hospital, informing relatives, and coping with their own fears and worry about the illness. An example of gradual change is the cumulative neglect of the needs of a nonhandicapped family member over time as parents attend to the demands of care for a retarded child. Table 7 presents a synthesis of stressors arising from functional change identified from the authors' naturalistic study.

Functional stressors often involve practical issues of financial, time, and physical demands on the family, which are the stressors most often reported by families (Dunlap & Hollingsworth, 1977). This finding has positive implications for research and intervention because family functions are often more directly observable and interventions may be less threatening to basic family ideologies.

One potentially fruitful intervention is the use of time management to alleviate functional stressors in families with retarded members. The efficacy of this intervention has not been objectively analyzed. Time management strategies should include assisting families in setting priorities for functions based on their own family situation, the type and degree of the retardation, the family's ideology, and the family's current life-cycle stage. The time management plan produced should help families recognize the need to balance interests of individual family members and family subsystems according to functions and to recog-

Table 7. Stressors arising from functional change

Economic	Physical	Rest and recuperation
Poor budgeting skills Lack of financial planning skills Conflict over allocation of resources among family members Problems dealing with public or private insurance programs	Chronic health problems Extreme time demands for care Lack of medical and allied health services Buying or remodeling home Poor time management Poor nutrition	Lack of respite care or use of respite care Inaccessible recreational facilities Lack of leisure-time activities (boredom) Poor relaxation skills

Socialization	Self-Definition	Affection
Poor social skills Lack of opportunity for social interaction Lack of close friendship Conflict over level of socialization needs Stares and inappropriate public reactions Sibling embarrassment	Comparing handicapped member to nonhandicapped Guilt and shame Loss of sense of control over life Low self-esteem	Sibling jealousy and resentment Inability to express emotions Lack of sibling companionship Failure to establish parent-child bond Lack of privacy

Guidance	Educational	Vocational
Behavior problems of children Engaging in problem-solving Inappropriate feedback Inability to transmit basic values and beliefs	Lack of information about handicapping condition Expectations for home intervention programs Lack of educational services Sacrificing of educational opportunities	Dissatisfaction with career choice Lack of vocational services Lack of support for career interests and problems Sacrificing career opportunities for handicapped family member Job promotion

nize that everyone's needs are legitimate. Emphasis should be placed on considering short-range versus long-range benefits in terms of time investment. For example, the effort to teach a retarded child to dress himself or herself in the morning may require a greater time investment and consequently greater stress in the short-run, but in years to come should involve greater payoff in time saved and independent living skills gained.

Another avenue for research and intervention in the alleviation of functional stressors is the effective use of support systems to increase resources available to fulfill family functions and to reduce functional stressors. Research has indicated in general that support serves as a moderator of life stress (Dean & Lin, 1977) and that parents who feel supported are more involved with their children (Barnard & Kelly, 1980). Families with higher levels of positive

support are reported to experience less stress in raising handicapped children (Nevin & Mc-Cubbin, 1979). Paradoxically, families with handicapped children are at risk for isolation (Korn, Chess, & Fernandez, 1978). Given these findings, the next step in research and intervention is to assist families in using support systems to alleviate functional stressors. More specifically, families should be assisted in matching formal and informal supports to the unique needs of their child and the family as a whole. For example, parent training programs are a valuable resource to eliminate maladaptive behaviors that have been shown to be a significant source of stress (Holroyd & McArthur, 1976). Another important area for research is the identification of barriers to the utilization of support systems. For example, a family may not take advantage of respite care services because the stresses associated with gaining access to the service (e.g., time to locate and arrange it, invasion of privacy, fear of social rejection, violating ideological values surrounding "taking care of our own") are greater than the stresses associated with not using the service.

Sociohistorical Changes

Sociohistorical change represents the societal influences on the family system that shape role expectations (Hill & Rodgers, 1969), the structural composition of families (Hareven, 1982), length of time in developmental stages (Hareven, 1982; McGoldrick & Carter, 1982), and the availability of resources for coping. These changes can exert stress on families as they move through the life cycle. Table 8 includes examples of stressors arising from sociohistorical changes identified in the authors' naturalistic study. Four areas of sociohistorical change have been identified: cultural trends, the economy, political trends, and formative events. The first three of these sociohistorical components are self-explanatory. Formative events are more idiosyncratic events related to an individual's personal involvement with social movements (e.g., participation in civil rights or war protests, being a prisoner of war, growing up in the Depression). Formative events often have a profound impact on shaping the individual's perspective of the world.

A significant cultural trend for families with older mentally retarded family members is the rapid growth of the normalization principle as a service delivery philosophy. Parental stress associated with deinstitutionalization can be interpreted within this sociohistorical perspective (Avis, 1985):

A bit of deinstitutionalization jet lag came with letters parents received several years ago when old forms of admission were changed to reflect new types of admission status. A most carefully worded letter explaining the patient's status, voluntary or otherwise, and his accompanying rights to ask to leave an institution couldn't cover the gap, of course. Many parents expressed wonderment and confusion that their now-adult child, duly labelled as in need of life-time protection and lacking in judgement, was now granted the status to make such important decisions. The person who was now an adult was viewed as capable of making choices when the family had been assured that theirs was an eternal child. (p. 174)

The current political climate resulting in the denial or reduction of services to handicapped persons creates stress for families and likely exacerbates their fear of the future. Interventions aimed at assisting families in using internal and external coping strategies to enhance their ability to live constructively with uncertainty is a worthy area of pursuit. Because family members cannot control the uncertainty emanating from many sociohistorical changes, they can learn to use reframing coping strategies to control their response to uncertainty (Pearlin & Schooler, 1978).

SUMMARY AND RECOMMENDATIONS

A family systems theoretical perspective generates a wealth of important research, intervention, and policy directions. The framework discussed in this chapter includes four dimen-

Table 8. Stressors arising from sociohistorical change

Cultural trends	Economy	Political trends	Formative events
Women's movement	Unemployment	War	Natural catastrophes
Independence movement	Inflation	Political climate denying or reducing services to handicapped populations	Guidance from mentor
Emphasis on self-fulfillment during postparental and retirement years			
Normalization			

sions of family dynamics: structure, interaction, functions, and life cycle. Family structure consists of the descriptive characteristics of the family in the areas of membership, cultural style, and ideological style. These characteristics are the *input* to the interactional system and can be viewed as the resources shaping the way that the family interacts and the manner in which they carry out their functions. Important areas for future research related to structural variations include investigating the impact of membership characteristics and cultural resources and the effectiveness of alternative coping strategies on life-cycle adaptation.

Family interaction, the hub of the family system, is the *process* of individual and group relationships within the family. It includes the different subsystems (i.e., marital, parental, sibling, extrafamilial) within the family and the rules (i.e., cohesion, adaptability, communication) by which the subsystems interact. Recognizing *all* subsystems within the family suggests that research, intervention, and policy agenda should operationalize family or subsystem outcomes in addition to child outcomes. The elements of cohesion, adaptability, and communication are key determinants of successful family interaction. The characteristics of families demonstrating strength in these areas should be identified through systematic investigation and used as the basis for planning functional and relevant interventions.

Family functions are the *output* of the interactional system and represent the essential purpose for the existence of families. Research is needed on the positive and negative impact of persons with mental retardation on the family's ability to carry out functions. The positive contributions that mentally retarded persons make to their family is a particularly important area for future research because it has to date been virtually ignored. Another important direction is investigating the intended and unintended consequences of the parent-as-teacher role.

From a developmental perspective, life cycle interjects *change* into the family system.

The fundamental life-cycle issue for families with mentally retarded members, however, is learning to adjust constructively to *change,* of both a normative and nonnormative nature, as well as to the *chronicity* of retardation or to the conditions beyond their ability to change. Research and intervention efforts focused on this complex issue and conducted within a family system conceptual framework have potential for substantially enhancing the quality of life for mentally retarded persons and their families. Particular interventions that are important to pursue include effective use of alternative coping strategies (e.g., passive appraisal, reframing, spiritual support, social support, formal support) for maintaining balance in family interaction future forecasting and planning, time management, stress management, and the use of reframing as a coping strategy to solve problems that can be remedied and to learn to live with problems that cannot be eliminated.

In addition to the specific future directions discussed throughout this chapter, other recommendations of a more general nature include the following:

1. Increased collaboration among researchers, practitioners, and consumers in the specification of research questions and dissemination of findings
2. Increased collaboration among sociologists and researchers in the field of mental retardation to develop multivariant theoretical models and methodologies for studying the complexities and heterogeneity of family life from a systems perspective
3. Use of control groups comprised of families with nonhandicapped children to determine the differential impact of retardation on the family system
4. Increased emphasis on rigorous instrument development
5. Increased emphasis on family strengths, rather than deficits, as a guide to intervention development
6. Development of a predictive taxonomic key of intervention to assist practitioners

in tailoring intervention strategies to the critical dimensions of family hetereogeneity

7. Longitudinal research programs to study the impact of interventions on families across the life cycle

REFERENCES

Altman, K., & Mira,M. (1983). Training parents of developmentally disabled children. In J. G. Matson & R. Andrasik (Eds.), *Treatment issues and innovations in mental retardation* (pp. 303–371). New York: Plenum Publishing Corp.

Avis, D. W. (1985). Deinstitutionalization jet lag. In A. P. Turnbull & H. R. Turnbull (Eds.), *Parents speak out* (pp. 181–191). Columbus, OH: Charles E. Merrill Publishing Co.

Baker, B. L. (1983). Parents as teachers: Issues in training. In J. A. Mulick & S. M. Pueschel (Eds.), *Parent professional partnerships in developmental disability services* (pp. 55–74). Cambridge, MA: The Ware Press.

Barnard, R. N., & Kelly, J. F. (1980). Infant intervention: Parental considerations. In *Guidelines for early intervention programs* (pp. 33–55). Salt Lake City: University of Utah College of Nursing.

Benson, H., & Turnbull, A. P. (1986). Approaching families from an individualized perspective. In R. H. Horner, L. H. Meyers, & H. D. Fredericks (Eds.), *Education of learners with severe handicaps: Exemplary service strategies*. Baltimore: Paul H. Brookes Publishing Co.

Berardo, F. M. (1980). Decade review: Some trends and directions for family research and theory in the 1980's. *Journal of Marriage and the Family, 42*(4), 723–728.

Birenbaum, A. (1971). The mentally retarded child in the home and the family cycle. *Journal of Health and Social Behavior, 12,* 55–65.

Boggs, E. M. (1979). Allocation of resources for family care. In R. H. Bruininks, & G. C. Krantz (Eds.), *Family care of developmentally disabled members: Conference proceedings* (pp. 47–62). Minneapolis: University of Minnesota.

Breslau, N. (1982). Siblings of disabled children: Birth order and age-spacing effects. *Journal of Abnormal Child Psychology, 10*(1), 85–96.

Bristol, M. M., & Schopler, E. (1983). Stress and coping in families of autistic adolescents. In E. Schopler & G. B. Mesibov (Eds.), *Autism in adolescents and adults* (pp. 251–278). New York: Plenum Publishing Corp.

Broderick, C. B. (1971). Beyond the five conceptual frameworks: A decade of development in family theory. In C. B. Broderick (Ed.), *A decade of family research and action* (pp. 3–23). Minneapolis: National Council on Family Relations.

Caplan, G. (1976). The family as a support system. In G. Caplan & M. Killilea (Eds.), *Support systems and mutual help* (pp. 19–36). New York: Grune & Stratton.

Carter, E., & McGoldrick, M. (1980). The family life cycle and family therapy: An overview. In E. Carter & M. McGoldrick (Eds.), *The family life cycle: A framework for family therapy* (pp. 3–21). New York: Gardner Press.

Colon, F. (1980). The family life cycle of the multi-problem poor family. In E. Carter and M. McGoldrick (Eds.), *The family life cycle: A framework for family therapy* (pp. 343–382). New York: Gardner Press.

Conroy, J. W., & Latib, A. (1982). *Family impacts: Pre-post attitudes of 65 families of clients deinstitutionalized June 1980 to May 1982.* Unpublished manuscript, Temple University Developmental Disabilities Center, Philadelphia.

Dean, A., & Lin, N. (1977). The stress buffering role of social support. *Journal of Nervous and Mental Disease, 165,* 403–416.

Diamond, S. (1981). Growing up with parents of a handicapped child: A handicapped persons's perspective. In J. L. Paul (Ed.), *Understanding and working with parents of children with special needs* (pp. 23–50). New York: Holt, Rinehart & Winston.

Dunlap, W. R., & Hollingsworth, J. S. (1977). How does a handicapped child affect the family? Implications for practitioners. *The Family Coordinator, 26*(3), 286–293.

Duvall, E. (1957). *Family development.* Philadelphia: J. B. Lippincott Co.

Falicov, C. J., & Karrer, B. M. (1980). Cultural variations in the family life cycle: The Mexican-American family. In E. Carter & M. McGoldrick (Eds.), *The family life cycle: A framework for family therapy* (pp. 383–426). New York: Gardner Press.

Farber, B. (1962). Effects of a severely mentally retarded child on the family. In E. P. Trapp & P. Himeleston (Eds.), *Readings on the exceptional child* (pp. 227–246). New York: Appleton-Century-Crofts.

Farber, B., & Ryckman, D. B. (1965). Effects of severely mentally retarded children on family relationships. *Mental Retardation Abstracts, 2,* 1–17.

Fotheringham, J. B., & Creal, D. (1974). Handicapped children and handicapped families. *International Review of Education, 20*(3), 353–371.

Friedman, E. H. (1980). Systems and ceremonies: A family view of rites of passage. In E. A. Carter & M. McGoldrick (Eds.), *The family life cycle: A framework for family therapy* (pp. 429–460). New York: Gardner Press.

Friedrich, W. N. (1979). Predictors of coping behavior of mothers of handicapped children. *Journal of Consulting and Clinical Psychology, 47*(6), 1140–1141.

Gallagher, J. J., Cross, A., & Scharfman, W. (1981). Parental adaptation to a young handicapped child: The father's role. *Journal of the Division for Early Childhood, 3,* 3–14.

Grossman, F. K. (1972). *Brothers and sisters of retarded children: An exploratory study.* Syracuse, NY: Syracuse University Press.

Haley, J. (1973). *Uncommon therapy.* New York: W. W. Norton & Co.

Hareven, T. K. (1982). American families in transition, historial perspectives on change. In F. Walsh (Ed.),

Normal family processes (pp. 446–466). New York: The Gilford Press.

Hill, R. (1949). *Families under stress.* New York: Harper & Row.

Hill, R. (1964). Methodological issues in family development research. *Family Process, 3*(1), 186–206.

Hill, R. (1970). *Family development in three generations.* Cambridge, MA: Schenkman Publishing Co.

Hill, R., & Rodgers, R. H. (1969). The developmental approach. In H. T. Christensen (Ed.), *Handbook of marriage and the family* (pp. 171–211). Chicago: Rand McNally & Co.

Holman, T. B., & Burr, W. R. (1980). Beyond the beyond: The growth of family theories in the 1970s. *Journal of Marriage and the Family, 42*(4), 729–741.

Holroyd, J., & McArthur, D. (1976). Mental retardation and stress on the parents: A contrast between Down's syndrome and childhood autism. *American Journal of Mental Deficiency, 80,* 431–436.

Hubbell, R. (1981a). *Field coordinator's guide: Theoretical framework.* Washington, DC: Institute for Educational Leadership, Family Impact Seminar, George Washington University.

Hubbell, R. (1981b). The family impact seminar: A new approach to policy analysis. In H. C. Wallach (Ed.), *Approaches to child and family policy* (pp. 35–46). Boulder, CO: AAAS, Westview Press.

Hughes, S. F., Berger, M., & Wright, L. (1978). The family life cycle and clinical interventions. *Journal of Marriage and Family Counseling, 4*(4), 33–40.

Kantor, D., & Lehr, W. (1975). *Inside the family.* San Francisco: Jossey-Bass.

Keating, D. J., Conroy, J. W., & Walker, S. (1980). *Longitudinal study of the court-ordered deinstitutionalization of Pennhurst: Family impacts of residents of Pennhurst* (Contract #130-79-3). Unpublished manuscript, Temple University Developmental Disabilities Center, Philadelphia.

Kerckhoff, A., & Campbell, R. (1977). Black-white differences in the educational attainment process. *Sociology of education, 50*(1), 15–27.

Klaber, M. M. (1969). The retarded and institutions for the retarded: A preliminary research report. In S. B. Sarason & J. Doris (Eds.), *Psychological problems in mental deficiency* (pp. 148–185). New York: Harper & Row.

Korn, S. J., Chess, S., & Fernandez, P. (1978). The impact of children's physical handicaps on marital and family interaction. In R. M. Lerner & G. B. Spanier (Eds.), *Child influence on marital and family interaction—A life-span perspective* (pp. 229–326). New York: Academic Press.

Lee, G. R. (1982). *Family structure and interaction: A comparative analysis.* Minneapolis: University of Minnesota Press.

Leslie, G. R. (1976). *The family in social context* (4th ed.). New York: Oxford University Press.

McAndrew, I. (1976). Children with a handicap and their families. *Child Care, Health and Development, 2,* 213–237.

McCubbin, H. (1979). Integrating coping behavior in family stress theory. *Journal of Marriage and the Family, 41*(1,2), 237–244.

McCubbin, H. I., Joy, C. B., Cauble, A. E., Comeau, J. K., Patterson, J. M., & Needle, R. H. (1980). Family stress and coping: A decade review. *Journal of Marriage and the Family, 42*(4), 855–871.

McCubbin, H. I., & Patterson, J. M. (1981). *Systematic assessment of family stress, resources and coping: Tools for research, education and clinical intervention.* St. Paul: University of Minnesota, Department of Family Social Science, Family Stress and Coping Project.

McGoldrick, M., & Carter, E. (1982). The family life cycle. In F. Walsh (Ed.), *Normal family processes* (pp. 167–195). New York: The Gilford Press.

McGoldrick, M., Pearce, J. K., & Giordano, J. (1982). *Ethnicity and family therapy.* New York: The Guilford Press.

Meyer, R. J. (1980). Attitudes of parents of institutionalized mentally retarded individuals toward deinstitutionalization. *American Journal of Mental Deficiency, 85*(2), 184–187.

Minde, K., Hackett, J. D., Killou, D., & Silver, S. (1972). How they grow up: 41 physically handicapped children and their families. *American Journal of Psychiatry, 128*(12), 1554–1560.

Minuchin, S. (1974). *Families and family therapy.* Cambridge, MA: Harvard University Press.

Moroney, R. M. (1981). Public social policy: Impact on families with handicapped children. In J. L. Paul (Ed.), *Understanding and working with parents of children with special needs* (pp. 180–204). New York: Holt, Rinehart & Winston.

Neugarten, B. (1976). Adaptations and the life cycle. *The Counseling Psychologist, 6*(1), 16–20.

Neugarten, B., & Hagestad, G. (1977). Age and the life course. In R. H. Binstock & E. Shanas (Eds.), *Handbook on aging and the social sciences* (pp. 35–55). New York: Van Nostrand Reinhold Co.

Nevin, R., & McCubbin, H. (1979, August). *Parental coping with physical handicaps: Social policy consideration.* Paper presented at the National Council of Family Relations' Annual Meeting, Boston, MA.

Olson, D. H., McCubbin, H. I., Barnes, H., Larsen, A., Muxen, M., & Wilson, M. (1984). *One thousand families: A national survey.* Beverly Hills: Sage Publications.

Olson, D. H., Russell, C. S., & Sprenkle, D. H. (1980a). Circumplex model of marital and family systems. II: Empirical studies and clinical intervention. In J. P. Vincent (Ed.), *Advances in family intervention assessment and theory* (Vol. 1, pp. 129–179). Greenwich, CT: JAI Press.

Olson, D. H., Russell, C. S., & Sprenkle, D. H. (1980b). Marital and family therapy: A decade review. *Journal of Marriage and the Family, 42*(4), 973–993.

Olson, D. H., Sprenkle, D. H., & Russell, C. (1979). Circumplex model of marital and family systems. I: Cohesion and adaptability dimension, family types and clinical applications. *Family Process, 18,* 3–28.

Payne, J. E. (1976). The deinstitutional backlash. *Mental Retardation, 3,* 43–45.

Pearlin, L. I., & Schooler, C. (1978). The structure of coping. *Journal of Health and Social Behavior, 19,* 2–21.

Rodgers, R. (1960, August). *Proposed modifications of Duvall's family life cycle stages.* Paper presented at the American Sociological Association Meeting, New York, NY.

Rubin, L. B. (1976). *Worlds of pain: Life in the working-class family.* New York: Basic Books.

Sager, C. J., Brown, H. S., Crohn, H., Engel, T., Rodstein, E., & Walker, L. (1983). *Treating the remarried family.* New York: Brunner/Mazel.

Sailor, W., & Guess, D. (1983). *Severely handicapped students: An instructional design.* Boston: Houghton Mifflin Co.

Skrtic, T. M., Summers, J. A., Brotherson, M. J., & Turnbull, A. P. (1984). Severely handicapped children and their brothers and sisters. In J. Blacher (Ed.), *Young severely handicapped children and their families: Research in review* (pp. 215–246). New York: Academic Press.

Suelzle, M., & Keenan, V. (1981). Changes in family support networks over the life cycle of mentally retarded persons. *American Journal of Mental Deficiency, 86,* 267–274.

Terkelsen, K. G. (1980). Toward a theory of the family life cycle. In E. Carter & M. McGoldrick (Eds.), *The family life cycle: A framework of family therapy* (pp. 21–52). New York: Gardner Press.

Turnbull, A. P., Brotherson, M. J., & Summers, J. A. (1985). The impact of deinstitutionalization on families: A family systems approach. In R. H. Bruininks & K. C. Lakin (Eds.). *Living and learning in the least restrictive environment* (pp. 115–140). Baltimore: Paul H. Brookes Publishing Co.

Turnbull, A. P., Summers, J. A., & Brotherson, M. J. (1984). *Working with families with disabled members: A family systems approach.* Lawrence: Kansas University Affiliated Facility, University of Kansas.

Turnbull, H. R., III. (1981). Two legal analysis techniques and public policy analysis. In R. Haskins & J. Gallagher (Eds.), *Models for analysis of social policy: An introduction* (pp. 153–173). Norwood, NJ: Ablex Publishing Corp.

Von Bertalanffy, L. (1968). *General systems theory.* New York: George Braziller.

Wadsworth, H. G., & Wadsworth, J. B. (1971). A problem of involvement with parents of mildly retarded children. *The Family Coordinator, 28,* 141–147.

Weeks, G. R., & Wright, L. (1979). Dialectics of the family life cycle. *American Journal of Family Therapy, 1*(7), 85–91.

Wikler, L. (1981). Chronic stresses of families of mentally retarded children. *Family Relations, 30*(2), 281–288.

Wikler, L., Wasow, M., & Hatfield, E. (1981). Chronic sorrow revisited: Attitude of parents and professionals about adjustment to mental retardation. *American Journal of Orthopsychiatry, 51,* 63–70.

Wilcox, B., & Bellamy, G. T. (1982). *Design of high school programs for severely handicapped students.* Baltimore: Paul H. Brookes Publishing Co.

Wolfensberger, W. (1970). Counseling the parents of the retarded. In A. A. Baumeister (Ed.), *Mental retardation: Appraisal, education, and rehabilitation* (pp. 329–400). Chicago: Aldine Publishing Co.

Chapter

4

Siblings of Handicapped Children

Rune J. Simeonsson and Donald B. Bailey, Jr.

THE LIFE EXPERIENCES of handicapped children have changed dramatically in the last decade as a result of advocacy and public policy efforts. Models attempting to explain the variables that influence the developmental outcome of handicapped children have also changed in this period, reflecting the impact of theory and research from a variety of disciplines. Drawing on Sameroff's (1975) conceptualizations of developmental outcome, both the nativist and nurturist explanations embodied in the main effect model have been recognized as too simplistic. In its most dogmatic expression, the nativist position assumed that organic deficits inevitably resulted in a fixed outcome, such as severe mental retardation. Conversely, the nurturist position maintained that an ideal environment could essentially eradicate the effects of such deficits, yielding normal or near normal functioning. The dogmatism of the main effect model gradually gave way to a model in which interaction of the organism and environment was assumed to result in a mediated outcome, in which the severity of a condition was reduced.

Although the premise of the interactive model has been sound, there has been a growing recognition in recent years that organismic and environmental variables operate in a dynamic fashion over time to determine developmental outcome. The transactional model maintains that the interaction between child and environment changes from one occasion to the next as a function of such transactions. Central to an analysis of these transactions has been a recognition of the ongoing, pervasive, and complex influence of the family on child outcome. This recognition has been evident programmatically in requirements for family involvement at all levels of intervention for their handicapped offspring. In theoretical and empirical domains, there has been a corresponding growth of interest in defining and documenting the role of the family in child outcome (Farber, 1983).

The purpose of this chapter is to examine one particular element of family transactions; namely, the sibling relationships of handicapped children. In so doing it is recognized that the family is a system evolving over time

The preparation of this paper was supported in part by the Special Education Program, U.S. Department of Education, Contract No. 300-82-0366. The opinions expressed do not necessarily reflect the position or policy of the U.S. Department of Education, and no official endorsement by the U.S. Department of Education should be inferred.

and that any analysis of a subsystem such as sibling relationships, must take both developmental stages and the complexity of the overall system into account.

The manner in which the family is conceptualized clearly influences efforts to analyze and synthesize findings on the family. Trends in recent contributions to the literature on the family of the handicapped child have been to view the family system as being characterized by developmental, structural, and/or functional components. In a previous review on this topic, various perspectives on functions of the family were considered (Simeonsson & Simeonsson, 1981). Developmental approaches were identified, such as Havighurst's (1972) notion of developmental tasks for child and family and Solomon's (1973) notion of developmental stages for the family unit. Along a similar line, Cerreto and Miller (1981) have drawn on Erikson's and Havighurst's concepts of stages and tasks to review the family's role in socialization of mentally retarded children. Turnbull and her colleagues (1983) have drawn on the framework of Minuchin (1974) and proposed a representation of the family involving four variations, nine family functions, and eight family life-cycle stages.

A model that has had heuristic value for the authors in a consideration of the family and sibling relationships of handicapped children is the triaxial model proposed by Tseng and McDermott (1979). In this model, the first axis is longitudinal in nature and considers the family's development. The second axis is cross-sectional and focuses on the structural relationships of individual family members. The third axis is also cross-sectional and structural in nature, but views the family in terms of subgroups and subsystems. The value of the model is that from an analytic point of view an independent consideration can be made of the family in terms of its development, its structure, and its function. The functioning of a family may, for example, be maladaptive on the developmental axis but not on a structural axis. Pathology should thus not be automatically inferred for all dimensions if maladaption is evident on one dimension. Of the classifications

described by Tseng and McDermott (1979), those pertaining to parent-child subsystems, sibling subsystems, and coping dysfunctions may be of particular relevance to an analysis of sibling relationships of handicapped children.

The authors acknowledge at the outset that the definition of the "normal" or "ideal" family both in terms of structure and function is currently debated. However, it is assumed that the fundamental goal of applied research with families should be the identification of conditions that optimize family functioning. In the context of this chapter, the authors propose that there are three basic characteristics of an optimal or ideal family:

1. The ideal family is one that supports the role and development of each family member, both as individuals as well as members of the family unit.
2. The ideal family has the resources to cope with internal and external sources of stress.
3. The ideal family engages in within-family interactions that are mutually satisfactory.

Three specific questions are explored in this chapter: 1) What are the general effects attributable to sibling relationships of handicapped children? 2) to what extent are these effects a function of the context and role of sibling relationships?, and 3) what are the implications of findings for research and clinical service? In carrying out the review and analysis of the literature several qualifications need to be stated. For the sake of practicality, as in the previous review (Simeonsson & McHale, 1981), the word "sibling" is used only to refer to the nonhandicapped sister(s) and/or brother(s) of the handicapped child. This is done to reduce the confusion that is likely to occur if the word sibling is alternatively used for both handicapped and nonhandicapped children in the family. The word "handicapped child" is used in a broad sense encompassing children who are mentally retarded, as well as those having various chronic conditions and impairments influencing developmental outcome. Although type and severity of impairment may be variables of interest in their own right, the choice of a general, rather than specific, approach was adopted for two reasons. First, from a conceptual standpoint, many issues in sibling relationships are likely to be generic in regard to children with developmental problems. Second, from a practical standpoint, a larger literature can be reviewed when a broad definition of handicap or disability is used. The literature review is selective, however, in order to complement an increasing number of publications on this topic (Cerreto and Miller, 1981; Lobato, 1983; McKeever, 1983; Murphy, 1982; Siemon, 1984). These published reviews provide a background for the synthesis and interpretation of findings examined in this chapter.

A REVIEW OF CURRENT LITERATURE

In an earlier review of research on the sibling relationships in families with a handicapped child (Simeonsson & McHale, 1981), the authors found that a number of factors, either singly or in combination, influenced sibling adjustment. These factors reflected both direct and indirect influences on the nature of the relationship and adjustment of siblings and are summarized in Table 1. The nature of the evidence was such that the identification of a factor as associated with good adjustment did not

Table 1. Factors associated with adjustment of siblings of handicapped children

Positive adjustment	Negative adjustment
Small family	Large family
Sibling younger than handicapped child	Sibling older than handicapped child
Male handicapped child	Female handicapped child
Silbling and handicapped child same gender	Sibling and handicapped child different gender
Handicapped child older than sibling	Handicapped child younger than sibling
Severe level of impairment	Mild level of impairment
Impairment of undefined, ambiguous nature (e.g., mental retardation)	Impairment, visible, clearly defined (e.g., blind)

imply that its reciprocal was associated with poor adjustment. Furthermore, inadequacies of design and analysis limited the possibility of generalizing a finding to siblings as a group. The synthesis of that evidence, however, led to a schematic represention of the nature of family and sibling relationships. Although somewhat simplistic in format, it summarized agent-recipient roles of the principals in terms of the sibling-handicapped child, the sibling-parent, and the handicapped child-parent relationships. Each of these relationships are likely to influence the adjustment of individual family members and of the family as a unit.

In this chapter, the literature is examined with a focus on the two relationships in which the sibling has a direct agent and recipient role; namely, the sibling-parent and sibling-handicapped child relationships. The handicapped child-parent relationship undoubtedly has an indirect impact on the siblings, but is a topic beyond the scope of this review.

In a search of the literature to update the previous review (Simeonsson & McHale, 1981), 19 studies were found that dealt with some aspect of the sibling relationships of handicapped children. The conceptual framework, issues, methodology, and experimental rigor varied widely across these studies. Included among these studies are clinical research reports, single-subject intervention designs, and comparative studies of siblings of handicapped and nonhandicapped children. To facilitate interpretation, the findings of each study were reviewed and coded in terms of the context in which the relationship occurred (sibling-parent versus sibling-handicapped child), the role of the relationship (agent versus recipient), and the valence of observed effects (positive versus negative). If all the effects reflected only one role and were only of one valence, then a single entry was made. However, if the findings were variable, several entries were made as appropriate. A summary of this review process is presented in Table 2, which provides an overall picture of the patterns of effects.

As Table 2 reveals, a variable pattern is evident in terms of the context, direction, and val-

Table 2. Sibling relationship effects (summary of findings)

		Handicapped child characteristics			Sibling characteristics			Order	
Investigators	Type	CA	M	F	CA	M	F	O	Y
Blackard & Barsh, 1982	MR	3–18	29	14	—	—	—	—	
McHale, Simeonsson, & Sloan, 1983	AUT/MR	6–15	30	30	6–15	15	15		
Breslau, Weitzman, & Messenger, 1981	CI, CP MH	3–18			6–18	105	134		
Breslau, 1982	CI, CP MH	3–18			6–18	—	—	—	
Miller & Cantwell, 1976	DD/MR	4,11	1	1	15–20	5	3	8	
Cash & Evans, 1975	MR	1–3	2	1	3–6		3	3	
Schreibman, O'Neill, & Koegel, 1983	AUT	5,8,8	2	1	8,11,13	1	2	3	
Chinitz, 1981	CP, MR MH	3–11	—	—	7–14	—	—	—	—
Colletti & Harris, 1977	AUT/DD	9,9	1	1	10,11 12	2	1	3	
Taylor, 1980	CI	—	—	—	7–12	14	11	25	
Lavigne & Ryan, 1979	CI	—	—	—	3–13	—	—	—	—
Gayton, Friedman, Tavormina, & Tucker, 1977	CI	5–18	—	—	5–18	—	—	—	—
Wellen & Broen, 1982	Lang. delayed	3½–4	3	1	6–9	1	3	4	
Mates, 1982	AUT	4–17	—	—	6–17	18	15	25	8
Caradang, Folins, Hines, & Steward, 1979	CI	—	—	—	6–15	—	—	—	—
Harder & Bowditch, 1982	CI	—	—	—	7–16	7	12	19	
Breslau, 1983	CI,CP MH	3–18	—	—		—	—	—	—
Ferrari, 1984	AUT/DD CI				6–13	16	16	16	16
Harvey & Greenway, 1984	CP,OI	9–11	20	13	7–15	16	17	16	17

CA = chronological age; M = male; F = female; O = older; Y = younger.
MR = mentally retarded; AUT = autistic; CI = chronically ill; CP = cerebral palsied; MH = mentally handicapped; DD = developmentally disabled; OI = orthopaedically impaired.

Table 2. (*continued*)

Dependent variables	Sibling-parent Agent +	Agent −	Recipient +	Recipient −	Sibling-handicapped child Agent +	Agent −	Recipient +	Recipient −
Parent vs. professional perception				X				
Interview sibling, family, peer relationships rating scale				X	X	X		
Psychiatric screening inventory			X	X				
Psychiatric screening inventory			X	X				
Behavior modification			X		X			
Behavior modification					X			
Behavior modification					X		X	
Counselling group				X	X		X	X
Behavior modification					X			
Interview	X		X	X	X	X		X
Louisville Behavior Checklist								X
Self-concept, locus of control, etc.							X	
Dialogue interruption						X		
Behavior rating scales, achievement, self-concept			X					
Understanding of illness								X
Interview	X		X	X				X
Psychiatric screening, inventory				X				X
Self-concept, Child Behavior Checklist, adjustment rating							X	X
Self-concept								X

ence of effects. On the basis of this review, it is interesting to note that there were only two effects that appeared to relate to the agent role in sibling-parent relationships, whereas entries occurred in all the other possible categories. Furthermore, in about one-half of the studies (9), a single category accounted for reported effects, whereas for the remaining 10 studies, variable effects were found for contexts, role, and/or valence.

In terms of the sibling-parent relationship, most of the effects seemed to pertain to a recipient role of siblings; that is, effects reflecting responses and reactions of siblings to parent and/or family characteristics. There were an equal number of studies that reported positive and negative effects; sometimes both effects were found in the same study.

Positive effects generally encompassed sibling acceptance of family adjustment to the presence of a handicapped child. Breslau, Weitzman, and Messenger (1981) found no differences on total scores on the Psychiatric Screening Inventory between siblings of disabled children and reference groups, but differences were obtained on selected components of the Psychiatric Screening Inventory. Along a similar line, Mates (1982) found that the scores of male and female siblings of autistic children on measures of home and school adjustment, school achievement, and self-concept did not differ significantly from normative values. In an interview study of siblings of chronically ill children, Taylor (1980) reported positive agent roles for siblings in terms of supporting the family. In a recipient role, siblings were also reported to have developed empathy and understanding. Harder and Bowditch (1982) found variable effects associated with the impact of cystic fibrosis children on the sibling-parent relationship. A final study reporting on positive effects was that of Miller and Cantwell (1976), in which the use of successful behavioral techniques by older siblings of a moderately retarded boy resulted in decreasing family arguments.

Negative results found in sibling-parent relationships were similar to those that have been reported frequently in earlier research on sib-

ling adjustment. The issue of reduced parental time for siblings of chronically ill (Taylor, 1980), as well as for siblings of autistic and mentally retarded children (McHale, Simeonsson, & Sloan, 1983) was a frequent finding. Feelings of being left out (Blackard & Barsh, 1982), being excluded from the parent-special child dyad (Taylor, 1980), having more expected of them (Blackard & Barsh, 1982; Harder & Bowditch, 1982), and resenting such additional responsibilities (Chinitz, 1981) were concerns common to siblings of multi-handicapped, chronically ill, and mentally retarded children. Siblings also reported the receipt of "bribes" to compensate for inadequacies in the sibling-parent relationships (Chinitz, 1981). On formal inventories of psychological functioning, siblings of disabled children were also found to have significantly higher scores on subscales reflecting inappropriate behaviors, such as fighting and delinquency (Breslau, 1982; Breslau et al., 1981).

In a consideration of the sibling-handicapped child relationship, seven studies reported positive effects for the agent role, and two studies reported negative effects. In terms of positive effects, McHale et al. (1983) found that mothers rated siblings of autistic and mentally retarded children as more supporting and less hostile than siblings of nonhandicapped children. Taylor (1980) reported that siblings assisted in the care of chronically ill children by administering treatments and medications and providing encouragement to them. In five studies siblings were identified as teachers/trainers of handicapped children. In the context of a counseling group, siblings expressed satisfaction in their role as teachers for mentally retarded and multihandicapped children (Chinitz, 1981). Positive effects in the form of behavior change in handicapped children through sibling involvement were reported by Miller and Cantwell (1976) and Colletti and Harris (1977). In a study of behavioral training, 8- to 13-year-old siblings of autistic children demonstrated the ability to apply behavioral procedures effectively and to serve as behavior change agents (Schreibman,

O'Neill, and Koegel, 1983). Positive effects of siblings as behavior change agents have even been reported for preschool siblings of very young handicapped children (Cash & Evans, 1975) providing evidence for the significant role that siblings can play in contributing to the management and training of handicapped children.

One of the studies coded as reporting a negative effect for siblings in the agent role was a study of language-delayed preschoolers (Wellen & Broen, 1982). In a somewhat novel experiment, language-delayed preschoolers were asked questions about a story in the presence of older siblings. In a comparative study, siblings of language-impaired children were found to interrupt the question-answer interaction at a rate similar to that of siblings of younger, non-language-impaired children. This rate was much higher (75%) than that of age-matched siblings of older non-language-impaired children. Furthermore, at a qualitative level, siblings of language-impaired children tended to provide the answer, whereas siblings of non-language-impaired children tended to rephrase questions and/or provide hints. In the second study in this category with chronically ill children (Taylor, 1980), siblings reported that they said or did things that were cruel or angry.

In the recipient role of the sibling-handicapped child relationship, positive effects were coded for five studies, and negative effects were coded for eight studies. In a study of chronically ill children, Gayton, Friedman, Tavormina, and Tucker (1977) found that both the chronically ill children and their siblings performed within normal limits on a battery of personality tests. Ferrari (1984) found siblings of autistic and diabetic children to have higher social competence scores than siblings of healthy children. McHale's et al. (1983) study of siblings of autistic and mentally retarded children revealed that they were more accepting than siblings of nonhandicapped children. Interestingly, there were no differences in embarrassment between siblings of handicapped and nonhandicapped groups. Chinitz (1981) reported that siblings were pleased by the accomplishments of their handicapped family members. Along a similar line, siblings were found to express positive sentiments after they were successful in the application of behavior modification procedures with autistic children (Schreibman et al., 1983).

Negative effects of the recipient role for siblings have been reported in eight studies of chronically ill children and/or handicapped children. In Taylor's (1980) study of chronically ill children, siblings reported feelings of inferiority and guilt, as well as entertaining death wishes for their handicapped brothers and sisters. Breslau (1983) found that chronically ill children and their siblings had higher scores on conflict with parents and on regressive-anxious behavior, whereas Harder and Bowditch (1982) reported siblings to be worried about the death of their brother or sister with cystic fibrosis. In another study of chronic illness, siblings of children with different types of chronic illnesses had scores symptomatic of irritability and social withdrawal (Lavigne & Ryan, 1979). Caradang, Folins, Hines, and Steward (1979) found lower levels of understanding of illness in siblings of diabetic children. In some personal domains, Chinitz (1981) found that siblings of multihandicapped children expressed anger over damage to personal belongings and restrictions on family activities attributable to handicapped brothers or sisters. Finally, the presence of a chronically ill or handicapped child also appears to result in poorer self-concepts of siblings (Ferrari, 1984; Harvey & Greenway, 1984).

CONCLUSIONS

The preceding review has indicated that the effects of sibling relationships in families of handicapped children do not conform to a consistent pattern. Clearly, the variability in type and quality of investigations contribute to the difficulty of summarizing and interpreting findings. As has been found in the authors' own research, comparative analyses of siblings of handicapped and nonhandicapped children may be confounded by scaling dimensions of instruments and the effects of averaging variable performance (McHale et al., 1983).

Despite these limitations, however, some tentative conclusions can be drawn. Consistent with the summary of earlier research findings (Simeonsson & McHale, 1981), a number of the studies reviewed here have reported differential age and/or sex effects for adjustment of siblings of handicapped children. Young siblings of chronically ill children, for example, have been found to have higher psychopathology scores (Lavigne & Ryan, 1979). Closeness in age of sibling to handicapped child may also contribute to poorer adjustment (Taylor, 1980). Male gender is another factor associated with poorer adjustment, as found by Lavigne & Ryan (1979) in siblings of chronically ill children, although same-sex effects may be attributable to sample characteristics (Ferrari, 1984). Age and gender may in fact be interactive as reported by Breslau et al. (1981) in that male siblings who were younger than the handicapped child had higher impairment scores on a psychological inventory. The reverse was true for female siblings. In a subsequent report, Breslau (1982) indicated that a third variable—age spacing—influenced measures of psychological functioning; younger male siblings whose age spacing was close to that of the disabled child had higher impairment scores. Given these and earlier findings, it seems reasonable to assume that the adjustment of siblings who are younger and closer in age to a handicapped child is likely to be more demanding than that of older siblings with greater age spacing. Male gender may also be a factor, although it is likely to be confounded by age as well as the gender of the handicapped child (Simeonsson & McHale, 1981).

An important finding is that siblings of handicapped children are often not unilaterally characterized by maladjustment, but do in fact have positive, constructive reactions to the presence of a disabled or handicapped brother or sister. The growing literature on siblings as behavioral change agents is encouraging in that it not only demonstrates that siblings can take an active role in the teaching/training of handicapped children but also that secondary gains are obtained in the sense of competence and self worth provided for the sibling. As indicated in Table 2, 7 of 17 studies pertained to the agent role in sibling-handicapped child relationships. The identification of means whereby the agent role of siblings can be increased in this relationship would seem a desirable goal in research and practice. This suggestion is made cautiously, however, in light of previous research indicating that siblings of handicapped children either have, or perceive themselves as having, greater caregiving responsibilities than children whose siblings are not handicapped. Winton and Turnbull (1981) found that parents of handicapped children often preferred not to be teachers of their children. This finding may also pertain to siblings of handicapped children, particularly if training responsibilities are time-consuming and long-term in nature. Because all the studies of siblings as tutors have been short-term studies, further investigations of sibling perceptions of such responsibility should be conducted. Furthermore, it may be appropriate to consider activities that take alternate forms of teaching to promote the agent role of siblings in their relationship with handicapped brothers or sisters. Categories, such as manager, helper, and so forth, described by Brody and Stoneman (1983) may be particularly germane.

In reviewing the findings, several themes have emerged: 1) Regardless of the specific chronic and/or handicapping condition, siblings demonstrate similar personal and social reactions, 2) younger and closer age-spaced siblings seem to have more difficulty adjusting; and 3) the handicapping condition per se does not appear to determine whether the sibling reaction will be positive or negative. It may be useful to conceptualize these themes in terms of three dimensions that mediate the adjustment of siblings of special children (see Figure 1). In regard to the commonality of sibling reactions across chronic and handicapping conditions, the authors propose that there are child variables influencing the sibling reaction that transcend the particulars of the im-

	Adjustment		Maladjustment
1. **Synchrony of Development**	Recognizes and accepts asynchrony of development of handicapped child		Failure to recognize or accept asynchrony of development of handicapped child
2. **Personal Comparison**	Accepts/resolves discrepancy between self and handicapped child		Unable to accept or resolve discrepancy between self and handicapped child
3. **Personal Evaluation**	Sense of real or perceived competence by sibling relative to handicapped child		Sense of real or perceived incompetence by sibling relative to handicapped child

Figure 1. Siblings of handicapped children: dimensions of adjustment.

pairment or disability. In other words, the re-action of siblings is likely to be mediated by individual differences of the handicapped child in the form of traits, temperament, and functional behavior as much as it is by the nature of the handicapping condition itself. This interpretation would account for the fact that there are wide differences in sibling reaction to children with the same handicapping condition. The systematic exploration of individual differences in sibling adjustment to handicapped children may be a fruitful area for research.

The synchrony dimension as shown in Figure 1 is proposed as an explanation for the generic reaction of siblings to children with various chronic conditions or impairments. The developmental progression of handicapped children is often attenuated or fixated relative to the continued progression of the family and siblings through developmental stages. To the extent that there is perceived or real asynchrony between the progress of the handicapped child and that of the family, sibling maladjustment may result. It is proposed that siblings who can recognize and accept this asynchrony of development are more likely to make the necessary personal and familial adjustments than those who are unable to do so.

Second, the authors propose that the poorer adjustment of younger and closer age-spaced siblings is due to difficulty in resolving discrepancies between themselves and their handi-capped brother or sister. Younger children are accustomed to seeing older children perform in a more mature and competent fashion than themselves. The discrepancy between expectation and reality for the younger sibling of a handicapped child is likely to be difficult to resolve cognitively and affectively. When age spacing is close, personal comparison may make the discrepancy particularly obvious. In the search for developmentally appropriate ways to help young siblings resolve such discrepancies, knowledge about the development of reasoning in children may be a useful reference source.

Finally, the authors propose that an important variable determining adjustment of siblings is the extent to which they are and/or perceive themselves to be competent relative to the handicapped child. The finding that adjustment of older siblings (adolescents, adults) is often better than that of younger siblings may very well be a reflection of the fact that older individuals are more competent than younger ones. The studies of siblings as teachers/trainers provide support for this proposal in their findings of direct effects on behavior change in handicapped children and the indirect effects on siblings in terms of a sense of personal competence. The study by Cash and Evans (1975) is particularly germane in that it demonstrates that even preschool-age siblings can be trained to be effective change agents for handicapped brothers and sisters. Research that extends these applications may serve not only to enhance sibling adjustment but, equal- ly important, also to promote the development of the handicapped child.

REFERENCES

Blackard, M. K., & Barsh, E. T. (1982). Parent's and professional's perceptions of the handicapped child's impact on the family. *TASH Journal, 7,* 62–70.

Breslau, N. (1982). Siblings of disabled children: Birth order and age-spacing effects. *Journal of Abnormal Child Psychology, 10,* 85–96.

Breslau, N. (1983). The psychological study of chron- ically ill and disabled children: Are healthy siblings ap- propriate controls? *Journal of Abnormal Child Psychol- ogy, 11,* 379–391.

Breslau, N. Weitzman, M., & Messenger, K. (1981). Psychologic functioning of siblings of disabled chil- dren. *Pediatrics, 67* (3), 344–353.

Brody, G. H. & Stoneman, Z. (1983). Children with atypical siblings: Socialization outcomes and clinical participation. In B. B. Lakey & A. Kazdin (Eds.), *Ad- vances in Clinical Child Psychology, Vol. 6,* New York: Plenum.

Caradang, J. L. A., Folins, C. H., Hines, P. A., & Stew- ard, M. S. (1979). The role of cognitive level and sib- ling illness in children's conceptualizations of illness. *American Journal of Orthopsychiatry, 49,* 474–481.

Cash, W. M., & Evans, I. M. (1975). Training pre- school children to modify their retarded siblings' be- havior. *Journal of Behavioral Therapy and Experimen- tal Psychiatry, 6,* 13–16.

Cerreto, M. C., & Miller, N. B. (1981). Siblings of hand- icapped children. Unpublished manuscript, University of Texas Medical Branch, Galveston, Texas.

Chinitz, S. P. (1981). A sibling group for brothers and sisters of handicapped children. *Children Today,* 21– 23.

Colletti, G., & Harris, S. L. (1977). Behavior modifica- tion in the home: Siblings as behavior modifiers, par- ents as observers. *Journal of Abnormal Child Psychol- ogy, 5,* 21–30.

Farber, B. (1983, September). *Historical contexts of re- search on families with mentally retarded persons.* Pa- per presented at the NICHHD Conference on Research on Families with Retarded Children, Quail Roost, NC.

Ferrari, M. (1984). Chronic illness: Psychosocial effects on siblings—I. Chronically ill boys. *Journal of Child Psychology and Psychiatry, 25,* 459–476.

Gayton, W. F., Friedman, S. B., Tavormina, J. F., & Tucker, F. (1977). Children with cystic fibrosis: 1. Psychological test findings of patients, siblings, and parents. *Pediatrics, 59* (6), 888–894.

Harder, L., & Bowditch, B. (1982). Siblings of children with cystic fibrosis perceptions of the impact of dis- ease. *Chidren's Health Care, 10,* 116–120.

Harvey, D. H. P., & Greenway, A. P. (1984). The self concept of physically handicapped children and their non-handicapped siblings: An empirical investigation. *Journal of Child Psychology and Psychiatry, 25,* 273– 284.

Havighurst, R. J. (1972). *Developmental tasks and edu- cation* (3rd ed.). New York: McKay.

Lavigne, J. V., & Ryan, M. (1979). Psychologic adjust- ment of siblings of children with chronic illness. *Pedi- atrics, 63* (4), 616–622.

Lobato, D. (1983). Siblings of handicapped children: A review. *Journal of Autism and Developmental Disor- ders, 13,* 347–364.

Mates, T. E. (1982). Siblings of autistic children: Their adjustment and performance at home and in school as a function of their sex and family size. Unpublished doc- toral dissertation, University of North Carolina at Chapel Hill.

McHale, S. M., Simeonsson, R. J., & Sloan, J. (1983). Children with handicapped brothers and sisters. In E. Schopler and G. Mesibov (Eds.), *Issues in autism: Vol. 2. The effects of autism on the family* (pp. 327–342). New York: Plenum.

McKeever, P. (1983). Siblings of chronically ill children: A literature review with implications for research and practice. *American Journal of Orthopsychiatry, 53,* 209–218.

Miller, N. B., & Cantwell, D. P. (1976). Siblings as ther- apists: A behavioral approach. *American Journal of Psychiatry, 133,* 447–450.

Minuchin, S. (1974). *Families and family therapy.* Cambridge, MA: Harvard University Press.

Murphy, M. A. (1982). The family with a handicapped child: A review of the literature. *Developmental and Behavioral Pediatrics, 3,* 73–82.

Sameroff, A. J. (1975). Early influences on development: Fact or fancy. *Merrill-Palmer Quarterly, 21,* 267–294.

Schreibman, L., O'Neill, R. E., & Koegel, R. L. (1983). Behavioral training for siblings of autistic children. *Journal of Applied Behavior Analysis, 16,* 129–138.

Siemon, M. (1984). Siblings of the chronically ill or dis- abled child. *Nursing Clinics of North America, 19,* 295–307.

Simeonsson, R. J., & McHale, S. M. (1981). Review: Research on handicapped children: Sibling rela- tionships. *Child: Care, Health and Development, 7,* 153–171.

Simeonsson, R. J., & Simeonsson, N. E. (1981). Parent- ing handicapped children: Psychological aspects. In J. Paul (Ed.), *Understanding and working with parents of children with special needs* (pp. 51–58). New York: Holt, Rinehart & Winston.

Skritic, T. M., Summers, J. A., Brotherson, M. J., & Turnbull, A. P. (1984). Severely handicapped children and their brothers and sisters. In J. Blacker (Ed.), *Young severely handicapped children and their fami- lies: Research in review,* New York: Academic Press.

Solomon, M. A. (1973). A developmental conceptual premise for family therapy. *Family Process, 12,* 179– 188.

Taylor, S. C. (1980). The effect of chronic childhood ill- nesses upon well siblings. *Maternal-Child Nursing Journal, 9,* 109–116.

Tseng, W. & McDermott, J. F. (1979). Triaxial family classification: A proposal. *Journal of the American Academy of Child Psychiatry, 18* (1), 22–43.

Turnbull, A. P., Summers, J. A., & Brotherson, M. J. (1983, September). *Family life cycle: Theoretical and empirical implications and future directions for families with mentally retarded members.* Paper presented at NICHHD Conference on Research on Families with Retarded Children, Quail Roost, NC.

Wellen, C., & Broen, P. (1982). The interruption of young children's responses by older siblings. *Journal of Speech and Hearing Disorders, 47,* 204–210.

Winton, P. J., & Turnbull, A. P. (1981). Parent involvement as viewed by parents of preschool handicapped children. *Topics in Early Childhood Special Education, 1* (3), 11–19.

PARENTING OF HANDICAPPED CHILDREN

Chapter

5

Research on Fathers of Young Handicapped Children

Evolution, Review, and Some Future Directions

Marie M. Bristol and James J. Gallagher

ALTHOUGH THE LITERATURE on normal child development often appears independent of the literature on atypical child development, the purpose of this chapter is to illustrate how concepts of normal child development have influenced and continue to influence research on fathers of disabled children. This chapter examines how the research questions asked and the answers found regarding fathers of developmentally disabled children have been guided, and sometimes limited, by prevailing psychological concepts of family influence and normal child development. It also points out gaps in research on atypical development when viewed from the perspective of emerging concepts of family influence. Tracing this path should also serve to illustrate the growing rapprochement between psycho-

logical and sociological research with these families. Finally, suggestions for future research and services for fathers of developmentally disabled children are offered.

SOCIAL POLICY AND PATERNAL INVOLVEMENT

Before beginning to assess the role of fathers in both child development and family adaptation to disabled children, it is important to allude briefly to three social policy issues: deinstitutionalization, mandated early intervention programs, and discussions of a major initiative to extend early intervention programs to fathers, as well as mothers.

As a result of a national commitment to a policy of deinstitutionalization, increasing

The preparation of this chapter was supported in part by the Special Education program, Special Education and Rehabilitative Services, U.S. Department of Education, Contract No. 300-82-0366. The opinions expressed do not necessarily reflect the position or policy of the U.S. Department of Education, and no official endorsement by the U.S. Department of Education should be inferred.

numbers of even the most severely and profoundly handicapped children now spend all or most of their lives at home with their families. The reality of the situation, then, is that fathers, as well as other family members, both affect and are affected by the presence of the developmentally disabled child in the home.

A major social policy response to dealing with this phenomenon has been the development of intervention programs designed to give parents the necessary skills and support to cope with the often difficult and atypical behaviors of their young developmentally disabled children. Although parental training is only a small part of an adequate service ecology for these families, there is convincing evidence that such training facilitates the progress of the developmentally disabled child. It has been shown to be superior to direct child intervention alone in maintaining and generalizing gains in appropriate child behavior and decreases in bizarre or inappropriate behavior (Koegel, Schreibman, Britten, Burke, & O'Neill, 1981). Even with severely disabled children, such as autistic children, parent training coupled with parent support services has been shown to be effective in improving parental teaching skills, reducing children's inappropriate behaviors, and increasing children's functional skills (Marcus, Lansing, Andrews, & Schopler, 1978; Short, 1984), and it appears to be related to reduced maternal stress and the prevention of unnecessary institutionalization (Bristol & Schopler, 1983; Schopler, Mesibov, & Baker, 1982; Short, 1984).

In the vast majority of programs, however, "parents" in reality equal mothers. Although some early intervention programs offer specific activities for fathers, most programs operate during hours when fathers are unavailable, and most are frankly puzzled about whether or how to involve fathers (Bristol & Gallagher, 1982).

The confusion or lack of information about fathers extends not only to their roles in programs but to their roles in families as well. In a recent study, Gallagher, Cross, and Scharfman (1981) found that both mothers and fathers of handicapped children thought fathers should take a more active role in the family, but neither group appeared to know just what form this involvement should take.

What role(s), then, for which fathers in which families will help promote successful family adaptation while facilitating the development of the developmentally disabled child? The answer to such a question is of more than academic interest because there are an increasing number of early intervention programs that involve fathers, as well as mothers. It is timely then to reflect on what is known from psychological research on the contribution of fathers to child progress and successful family adaptation to developmentally disabled children.

REASONS FOR NEGLECT OF FATHERS

The relative paucity of studies that address the issue of fathers and the progress of their developmentally disabled offspring is readily apparent. This neglect of fathers in psychological research is not unique to the field of handicapped individuals. Until recently, such paternal neglect had been a hallmark of most psychological theories and research programs in the study of nonhandicapped children as well. In fact, if the role of the father in child development was originally addressed at all, it was usually in terms of father absence through death or divorce (Belsky, 1981; Hetherington, Cox, & Cox, 1978).

Reasons for this neglect of fathers include the following:

The difficulty of gaining access to fathers for research studies or clinical interventions

Research paradigms and data analysis strategies that were more suited to the study of dyadic, rather than triadic or larger social systems

A focus on a narrow range of child development gains as the outcome measure of successful early intervention (Karnes & Teska, 1975) that stems from a failure to conceive of intervention in the broader context of the entire family

Theoretical biases that stressed the uniqueness of mothers in promoting child socialization and education in a dyadic or two-person context (Bowlby, 1951, 1969; Freud, 1948; Maccoby & Masters, 1976).

EVOLUTION OF PSYCHOLOGICAL CONCEPTS OF THE FATHER'S ROLE IN CHILD DEVELOPMENT

The evolution of the father's role in child development from a vague figure on the periphery of the "unique" dyad of mother and child to an equal partner in an ecological model of the family has occurred in a relatively short time. This evolution is traced briefly in Figure 1. Examples from both the child development literature and the literature on developmentally disabled children are included to illustrate how psychological concepts of the fathers' role affect research designs and findings. (Note that this sequence reflects the development of psychological research strategies. Sociologists have traditionally begun with the larger family concept, but, with few exceptions [Farber, Jenne, & Toigo, 1960], have paid less attention to the child development focus.)

The various models of developmental influence presented are not considered to be mutually exclusive, and chronologically earlier models are often legitimate and necessary subparts of later, more complex models. Seeds of more complex models are often also apparent in chronologically earlier studies. The categorization of a particular research study within a particular model was based on whether the chapter authors judged that the research illustrated a specific type of family concept and not on any statement of intent by the original author.

For the most part, examples in this chapter are also limited to empirical research studies and are meant to be illustrative, rather than exhaustive. Although much important research on fathers has been generated by studies of father-absent families (see Herzog & Sudia, 1973; Hetherington, 1981; or Shinn, 1978, for reviews of results on studies of single-parent families), this review is limited to studies of fathers in intact families.

THE UNIDIRECTIONAL DYAD: PRIMACY OF MOTHERS

Normal Child Development

Traditionally, the role of the father, especially in infancy, had been deemphasized. In discussing the concept of attachment or of prevailing psychodynamic theories of child development, virtually all theorists focused on the importance of the mother-child relationship to the exclusion of the father (Bowlby, 1951, 1958, 1969; Freud, 1948; Maccoby & Masters, 1970). Initially, then, the father is pictured as an outside person, with influence on socialization essentially passing from mother to child (Bowlby, 1951) (Figure 1, I).

Research with Developmentally Disabled Children

In this conceptualization of child socialization, the mother was primarily responsible for either the success or the failure of the child's development. Research in the area of developmentally disabled children sought to demonstrate, in a unidirectional way, how parents, usually mothers, may have *caused* various handicaps in their children or how they at least evidenced overcontrolling, punitive, or otherwise abnormal parenting practices (Kogan, Wimberger, & Bobbitt, 1969) when compared with parents of normal children. The use of normal control groups, of course, failed to take into account the fact that the developmentally disabled child's behaviors were different from those of normal children and elicited different responses from parents. Because fathers were seen as peripheral in this process, they were seldom subjects of this research.

The effect of this conceptualization of family influence is strikingly evident in early (pre-1965) research on families of autistic children. These early studies of parents of autistic children relied on indirect measures of parental personality and attitudes and compared parents of autistic children with parents of normal children. As a result of such studies, parents of autistic children were purported to be "cold," "mechanical," "insensitive to the needs of the child," "overprotective," or "cynical,

The father in child development	Concept of family influence	Implications for family research with normal children (illustrative examples)	Implications for family research with handicapped children (illustrative examples)
F M → C (I)	*Unidirectional dyad* Mother responsible for socialization (or failure of socialization) of young children. Father unimportant.	Studies focus on effect of mother on child (Bowlby, 1951). Failure to acknowledge contribution of child to interaction. Fathers generally excluded from studies.	Studies focus on how parents of handicapped children "cause" handicaps (e.g., Down syndrome blamed on alcoholism of mother [Hayden & Haring, 1974]; autism on parental rejection [Eisenberg, 1957]). Emphasis on pathogenic mothers.
F M ↔ C (II)	*Interactive dyad* Contribution of child characteristics to M-C interactions acknowledged. Father still peripheral.	Reciprocity of mother-child interaction over time studied. Growing literature on "child effects" on caregiver (Bell, 1968; Lewis & Rosenblum, 1974; Thomas & Chess, 1977). Father-infant relationships still "insignificant and essentially redundant" (Ainsworth, in Lamb, 1978a).	Beginning and slow acknowledgment of impact of handicapped child characteristics on mothers in interaction (Beckman, 1983; Bristol, 1979; Cummings, Bayley & Rie, 1966; Fraiberg, 1974; Rondal, 1978; Stone & Chesney, 1978). Fathers still largely ignored.
C M ← → F (III)	*Multiple dyads* Family essentially conceived as multiple pairs of dyads. Both mother and father directly affect child development.	Direct interactions of mothers and infants, and fathers and infants studied. Little acknowledgement of significance of M-F relationship to child development (Lamb, 1977).	Increased interest in impact on fathers (Cummings, 1976) but, in general, mothers and fathers still studied separately, if fathers included at all. Comparative studies of mothers and fathers (Tallman, 1965; Tavormina, Boll, Dunn, Luscomb, & Taylor, 1981).
Marital relationships Child behavior and development Parenting (IV)	*Family system* Effect of either parent on child may be direct or mediated not only by other parent, but by relationship between those parents.	Studies of both direct and indirect effects of father on child (Weinraub, 1978). Mother-father relationships may affect maternal behavior (Parke & O'Leary, 1976), father-child relationships (Pedersen, Anderson, & Cain, 1977), or	Studies of impact of handicapped child on marriage (Farber, 1959; Love, 1973); family functioning (Fotheringham, Shelton, & Hoddinott, 1972; Holroyd & McArthur, 1976); siblings (Gath, 1972); family task allocation (Gallagher, Scharfman, & Bristol,

Figure 1.   The evolution of the father's role in psychological research on normal and atypical child development. (From Bristol, 1983; reprinted by permission. Copyright © 1983 by Marie M. Bristol.)

		child outcome (Biller, 1970) or, in turn, be affected by any of these (Belsky, 1981).	1984).
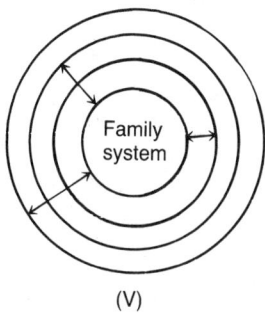(V)	*Family ecological system* The entire family seen as *one* of an interactive, interdependent *set* of systems "nested" within each other. Child affects and is affected by family system as well as by other systems of which family is a part.	Child, mother, father reciprocally affect each other and are affected by larger informal and formal systems in which they are "nested." (Bronfenbrenner 1977; Crnic, Greenberg, Ragozin, Robinson, & Basham, 1983; Garbarino, 1977).	The development of the handicapped child depends upon factors both within and beyond family. (Bristol, 1979; Bristol, 1985; Friedrich & Friedrich, 1981; Holroyd, 1974; Nihira, Meyers, & Mink, 1980; Turnbull & Winton, 1984).

Figure 1.   (*continued*)

obsessive, and passive." Parents who asked questions, gave directions, and structured situations were said to be "intrusive." Those who did not were said to be "perplexed."

Because of the predominant Freudian orientation of the times, most of the responsibility for child pathology was attributed to the mother. In fact, Eisenberg (1957) referred to the father as "the forgotten man." When the father was included, however, it was to illustrate his share of the "blame" for the child's disorder. In his study of 100 fathers of autistic children, Eisenberg (1957) concluded that the majority of fathers suffered from "serious personality difficulties that markedly impaired the fulfillment of a normal paternal role and that seriously influence the pattern of family living." He suggested that the mother alone is not the culprit, but that father and mother together caused the psychopathology in the autistic child. Similar findings regarding fathers were reported by Donnelly (1960), and Lennard, Beaulieu, and Embrey (1966).

As evidence of a biological basis for autism emerged, the injustice of these early charges became clear. Schopler (1978) reviewed the results of over 100 research studies of families of autistic children and found a statistically significant effect for time of publication. The majority of studies that emphasized parental causation of autism in their children were published before 1965. Using mainly clinical impressions, they tended to confirm the prevail-

ing psychoanalytic, unidirectional parent-cause model of child development.

The particular conceptualization of family influence therefore shaped the question to be asked—"How did these parents cause their child's handicap?"—and the methodology to be used. Because the influence was thought to be unidirectional, the contribution of child characteristics to parental responses was ignored. The major focus of research was a dyadic one, largely excluding fathers from research. When fathers were included, it was mainly to share the blame for the child's handicap.

THE INTERACTIVE DYAD

Normal Child Development

Some researchers (Gallagher, 1956; Sears, Maccoby, & Levin, 1957) had openly questioned the adequacy of the unidirectional model of child development in the 1950s. However, it was not until the publication of Bell's classic papers (Bell, 1968, 1971) on the reinterpretation of the direction of effect in correlational studies of child socialization that serious attention was paid to the contribution of child characteristics to parent-child interaction and subsequent child development. On the basis of his review, Bell concluded that both the social response and control behaviors of parents are organized in hierarchical caregiving repertoires. Differences in congenital child characteristics, such as impaired sensorimotor abilities, differential responsiveness to parents, and differences in activity levels, elicit and reinforce different levels and intensities of parent caregiving responses (Figure 1, II). Sameroff's (1975) concept of a transactional model in which parent and child mutually modify each other over time is a further extension of this conceptualization.

This change in conceptualization of family influence led to increased research in normal development on child differences detectable in early infancy and their effects on caregivers, usually mothers (Lewis & Rosenblum, 1974). As more sophisticated technology for data collection became available, it was also possible to measure at least some aspects of the reciprocity of these relationships (Bakemann, 1977; Parke, 1978; Sackett, in press) and to develop observational systems to measure limited aspects of the reciprocal nature of the more complex behaviors of young children beyond infancy (Farran & Haskins, 1980).

Research with Developmentally Disabled Children

There is considerable evidence that developmentally disabled children are generally different from birth and are deficient in many of the areas that Bell has indicated as instrumental in affecting parent caregiving and social response behaviors. (See Ramey, Beckman-Bell, & Gowen, 1981, for an extensive review of this topic.) It is therefore reasonable to expect that child differences could explain many of the parental differences found earlier in comparisons of parents of handicapped and non-handicapped children. (See Bristol & Schopler, 1984, for a reinterpretation of the direction of effect in research on parents of autistic children.) An interactive conceptualization of family influence then led to investigation not only of the possible impact of the parent on the handicapped child but also to investigations of the impact of the handicapped child on the parent.

In research with families of developmentally disabled children, the literature assessing the impact of different handicaps (Bristol & Schopler, 1984; Cummings, Bayley, & Rie, 1966; Holroyd & McArthur, 1976; Stone & Chesney, 1978) and different specific characteristics of handicapped children (Beckman, 1983; Bristol, 1979; Fraiberg, 1974; Kogan & Tyler, 1973; Rondal, 1978) on mothers reflects a recognition of the contribution of child characteristics. Because studies focused mainly on the impact of the child on the caregiver, and caregivers were generally mothers, fathers were still largely ignored.

MULTIPLE DYADS

Normal Child Development

In this conceptualization of family influence, the father's role is seen simply as the addition of an individual who increases the opportunities for the number of possible dyadic or two-person relationships (Figure 1, III). Using this model, the usual research paradigm in normal development is to have the father take the role previously taken by mothers—for example, in Ainsworth's (1978) stranger paradigm—and look for similarities and differences in maternal and paternal behaviors and infants' responses to them. Even in the initial work done in this area, the importance of the father's role in normal child development was clear.

Differences in Father/Child, Mother/Child Interaction In affecting child outcomes, Lamb (1978a) stresses the importance of regarding the father not as a replacement for, but as an addition to the mother. (This contrasts significantly with Ainsworth's [1978] comment that father-infant relationships are "insignificant and essentially redundant.") Although the relationships between mother and child and father and child are similar in many ways, they are also qualitatively different, with fathers (usually noncaregivers) more likely to engage their infants in physically stimulating and idiosyncratic play while mothers' contact more often revolves around caregiving activities. In his review of this research, Lamb (1978a) concludes that fathers of nonhandicapped children provide different experiences for their children and therefore make different contributions to their children's development.

Pedersen, Anderson, and Cain (1980a) also caution that virtually all the major comparisons of maternal and paternal behavior in the infancy period included samples heavily weighted in favor of traditional couples in which the wife was the caregiver and the father was the only breadwinner. When Pedersen (1975) used a sample of working mothers who were themselves away from the child most of the day, the mothers engaged in many of the behaviors thought to be gender-specific to fathers. It is at this point that closer attention to more "sociological" concepts, such as family structure and task and role allocation, became necessary in order to avoid overgeneralizing because of sample selection bias.

Fathers and Child Outcome In addition to comparisons of the direct interactions of normal children with both mothers and fathers, the multiple dyad conceptualization of family influence helped focus research efforts on the possible effects that fathers had on longer-term outcomes for their children.

Reviewing research using such paradigms in normal child development, Lamb (1976) suggests that many fathers are accessible and responsive to their infants and are important figures in their infants' lives. He reviews evidence of an attachment bond between fathers and infants and concludes that, during the first year, there is no demonstrable preference by infants for either parent in the home or the laboratory, except in limited stress situations when they show some preference for their mothers. Apparently, physical caregiving is not necessary for attachments to form, although fathers appear to be as "sensitive" to infant signals as mothers (Parke & Sawin, 1976) and are capable of competent caregiving (Parke, 1978).

Because there is empirical evidence that the amount of time spent together is a poor predictor of the quality of the infant's relationships with either father or mother (Pedersen & Robson, 1969), the time spent between father and child, although limited, has important implications for child development. In fact, fathers'

relative scarcity and the differences in their behaviors compared to mothers may give fathers a special salience or novelty value for the child. Little contact under these circumstances can have a substantial impact. Lamb (1978) notes that, among his many roles, the father may serve as the medium through which the values and role demands of the social system are interpreted to the child. (Belsky [1981] warns, however, that many such commonly held ideas about fathers are merely untested hypotheses.) On the basis of data showing that father absence is more acute for young children and that sex-role assignment may be made before 18 months of age, Lamb (1978) concludes that, although the influence of the father is felt throughout the lifespan of the child, it is particularly critical in infancy. Results of this and similar research lead to the conclusion that fathers affect the gender role identity (Lamb, 1978), achievement motivation (Baruch & Barnett, 1978; Radin, 1981), and cognitive development (Biller, 1974; Busse, 1969) of their normal offspring.

This multiple dyad conceptualization of family influence on child development, then, allows for multiple influences on child outcome. Because the focus still remains on individual family members, however, only direct effects of one family member on another are considered.

Research with Developmentally Disabled Children

The potential research questions growing out of this multiple dyad conceptualization are the following: How do mothers and handicapped children affect each other?, how do fathers and handicapped children affect each other?, and how are these influences the same or different for mothers and fathers?

This conceptualization of family influence has had an impact on research on fathers of developmentally disabled children. However, the direction of effect is almost universally the effect of the child on the father, and observational studies comparing contingent interactions of handicapped children with both mothers and fathers are almost nonexistent. (See

Stoneman & Brody [1982] below). The focus of most comparative studies has been on the differential effects of developmentally disabled children on fathers and mothers. Results of studies assessing whether mothers or fathers are more adversely affected by their disabled child are mixed. Also, unlike research on normal children, few studies have assessed the effect of fathers on outcomes for their developmentally disabled children.

Differences in Father/Child, Mother / Child Impact   Cummings (1976) found in his study of 240 fathers of mentally retarded, chronically ill, neurotic, and healthy children that fathers reported more stress than a sample of mothers of similar children. He found that fathers of mentally retarded children may undergo long-term personality changes of a neurotic type and have few constructive outlets for such stress. Fathers reported awareness of the negative aspects of the child's care, but were involved in few of the rehabilitative aspects. Only half of the mothers and fathers in the study, however, were couples, so such comparisons can only be suggestive, and no data are presented on the effects of either parent on the children.

These results contrast with those of Tavormina, Boll, Dunn, Luscomb, and Taylor (1981) who found that 133 mothers of diabetic, asthmatic, cystic fibrotic, and hearing impaired children reported both more problems and more involvement than fathers with their chronically ill children. The stress was clearly taking a toll on both parents, whose functioning fell between that reported for either "normal" or poorly adjusted parents on measures of personality styles, attitudes, perspectives, and coping strategies. Type of child illness affected parental scores, reflecting a differential impact according to type of handicap. The indirect effects of one parent on another were not studied, nor were parental variables related to child outcome. In both of these studies, however, the effect of child characteristics is controlled by use of comparison groups of parents of children with differing handicapping conditions.

Studies by Gumz and Gubrium (1972), Hersch (1970), and Love (1973) also con-cluded that the impact on a father of having a handicapped child is different from that on mothers. Fathers appeared to accept the diagnosis with less emotion, to be more objective, less emotionally involved, and more future-oriented, worrying particularly about the long-term economic support of the handicapped child. However, this objectivity is not universal as Kanner (1954), Meyerowitz and Farber (1966), and Wadsworth and Wadsworth (1971) note. A prolonged period of denying the reality of the handicap appears to be common among minimally involved fathers who do not interact with the children often enough to be forced to recognize the severity of the problem.

These studies therefore parallel in some ways the comparative mother/father normal child development studies, but they reveal some significant differences. First, the effects of the child on the family are almost always assumed to be negative and, with few exceptions (Schaefer & Edgerton, 1981; Stoneman & Brody, 1982), the chosen research instruments generally do not allow for documentation of any positive effects. Second, a search for systematic studies of families of developmentally disabled children that assessed either the reciprocal or even the unidirectional effect of fathers on outcomes for their developmentally disabled children yielded few studies.

In a review of over 60 research studies of parental involvement in early education programs for young developmentally disabled children (Wiegerink, Hocutt, Posante-Loro, & Bristol, 1980), none were found that assessed the effects of fathers' attitudes, attributes, or behaviors on developmentally disabled children's outcomes. Few "parent outcome" studies can be found that assess either effects of the father on the developmentally disabled child or the effect of the early intervention program on fathers or the rest of the family. A study by Stoneman and Brody (1982) discussed below did assess the extent to which children complied with fathers' requests, but did not relate this behavior to later child outcome. Only one study (Tallman, 1965) was found that assessed the direct effects of the father on later child outcome.

Direct Effects of Fathers on Handicapped Children In his study of 80 mothers and 69 fathers of moderately to severely retarded children age 6–12, Tallman (1965) found that fathers were less skillful (adaptable) than mothers in providing responses to 15 problematic parent–retarded child situations, more affected by the more visibly handicapped Down syndrome children than by non–Down retarded children, and experienced an extreme reaction of involvement or withdrawal to the birth of a retarded son. The ways in which one parent mediated the effect of the child on the other were not determined.

When Tallman examined the differential relationship of mother and father variables to developmentally disabled child outcome, he did not find any significant relationships between paternal problem-solving ability and child competence over a 1- and 2-year period. The mother's problem-solving ability, however, was significantly associated with subsequent child competence. No attempt was made to test whether paternal coping indirectly influenced the child's subsequent functioning by directly affecting maternal coping, because only direct effects of both mother and father on the child were tested. The study is significant, however, because it is one of the few studies of handicapped children that specifically measured both maternal *and* paternal influence on child outcome as suggested by the multiple dyad concept of family influence.

THE FAMILY SYSTEM

Normal Child Development

In the course of the studies of mother-infant and father-infant dyads of nonhandicapped disabled children, it was noted that, when both mothers and fathers were present, the level of interaction with the children was reduced because mother and father spent time interacting with each other instead of solely with the child (Belsky, 1979, Parke & O'Leary, 1976; Pedersen, Anderson, & Cain, 1977). Fathers not only *directly* influence their children when alone with them, but also *indirectly* influence them by distracting maternal attention or by affecting their wives' parenting styles or attitudes (Lewis & Weinraub, 1976). This recognition of the indirect effects of fathers on child development was consistent with an emerging recognition of the family as an interactive system, rather than merely a collection of individuals or dyads (Figure 1, IV). Although psychological research continued to focus on child development to a greater extent perhaps than sociologists were wont to do, the rapprochement between the two fields at the present time may be discerned from the number of writers from both disciplines addressing the topic of family systems. It is noteworthy, however, that such sociologists as Farber had taken this approach as early as 1959 (Farber, 1959).

Indirect or "Second Order" Effects Some authors (Clarke-Stewart, 1977; Lewis & Weinraub, 1976) contend that the primary way that fathers of nonhandicapped children influence their children (infants, in these cases) is through their wives. Because fathers generally spend very little time interacting with their children—estimates range from less than a minute (Rebelsky & Hanks, 1971) to more than an hour per day (Pedersen & Robson, 1969)—this indirect influence through the mothers may be their primary mode of influence. Weinraub (1978) summarizes data that suggest the strength of these indirect effects on children's ability to cope with father absence. Children's emotional adjustment shows little relationship to any direct measures of father's absence, such as duration or age of onset. Instead, the child's emotional adjustment appears to depend on the mother's perceptions of her ability to cope, her attitude toward her husband, and her attitude toward the child.

There is also evidence that the mother's perception of support from the father affects her responsivity and feeding behavior to her infant (Feiring & Lewis, 1978) and her display of positive affect toward the child (Parke & O'Leary, 1976). Some evidence (Pedersen, Anderson, & Cain, 1980b) also suggests that the mother's relationship to the father affects the father-child relationship. Paternal support has also been shown to be related to successful adaptation to pregnancy (Shereshefsky & Yarrow, 1973), maternal distress during labor (Anderson & Standley, 1977), and the practice of breast feeding (Switzky, Vietze, & Switzky, 1979).

Because the father's direct interactions with the young child are generally very limited, it appears that the father's most powerful influence on his children may be indirect (i.e., the father may affect the mother's ability to cope or her attitudes or behaviors toward the child). A family systems model provides for both discussion and measurement of such indirect as well as direct family influences.

Research with Developmentally Disabled Children

This broader family systems conceptualization can be seen in studies of the effects of developmentally disabled children on mother-father relationships and sibling adjustment, in studies of the indirect effects of paternal support, and in naturalistic observational studies of the family.

Effects on Mother-Father Relationships A family systems perspective suggests that the study of child development should include not only the direct and indirect effects of individuals in the family on one another but also the effect of roles or relationships on one another (Belsky, 1981).

Results of studies examining the impact of parenting developmentally disabled children on marital relationships are mixed. In addition to general limitations in social activities, parents of retarded children report high levels of desertion (Reed & Reed, 1965). Love (1973) reports that the divorce rate among parents of mentally retarded children may be triple the national average, whereas suicide may be double the national average. Adequate data are not presented in these studies to support these claims, a criticism that can also be leveled at many of the studies that conclude that marital separation and divorce rates are not higher for families of disabled children. (See Darling & Darling, 1982, for a review of these studies.) Research with more adequate comparison samples is needed in this area.

If they remain married, fathers of retarded children are reported to show greater marital strain than mothers (Schonnell & Watts, 1956), and both Farber (1959) and Fowle (1968) report marital tension in families of retarded children. Farber (1959) reports from a cross-sectional study that marital tension increases with the age of the retarded child, and Fowle's work (1968) suggests that marital role tension is the same whether the mentally retarded child remains at home or is institutionalized. Farber's study of 240 intact families of severely retarded children (IQ<50) with at least one additional sibling notes the effect of marital adjustment on sibling communication and adjustment (Farber & Jenne, 1963), one of the few examples of effects of relationships on child development (Farber, 1959; 1960). Holt (1958) reports extensive marital disruption and subsequent negative effects on siblings, with a greater effect noted in the lower socioeconomic classes. Lonsdale (1978) and Schipper (1959) also report an adverse effect of retardation on marital integration, although Kramm (1963) does not report such an effect. A more recent study (Bristol, 1984a) of young autistic and communication-impaired children finds that the majority of parents who remained married scored in the average or above average range on a test of marital adjustment.

It may be that group averages obscure the bimodal distributions of data on marital satisfaction. In a study of marital happiness of families of children with a variety of handicaps (Krause-Eheart, 1981), approximately one-half of the mothers reported that the handicapped child did not affect their marriages. The remaining half of the mothers were divided into two approximately equal groups, one of which felt that the children had adversely affected their marriages and the other that felt that having a developmentally disabled child had actually strengthened theirs.

In terms of the effects of marriage on child outcome, studies have indicated that single-parent families with developmentally disabled children experience more stress (Beckman, 1983; Holroyd, 1974) and that single parents are judged in interviewer ratings as having more difficulty in accepting and adapting to their disabled child (Bristol, 1985) than two-parent families. In all three of these studies, however, groups were not matched on social class, so the effect may relate less to marriage and more to mother's education, financial status, or other variables. In fact, in the Bristol study, when the effect of maternal education was statistically corrected, differences in mean ratings between single- and two-parent families disappeared. Marital satisfaction in two-parent families, however, is one of the best predictors of coping with the child (Friedrich, 1977). A family systems perspective encourages investigation of such indirect effects.

Indirect Effects of Paternal Support A recent study (Gallagher, Scharfman, & Bristol, 1984) indicates that, despite the increased demands posed by the developmentally disabled child, fathers of young developmentally disabled children do not help mothers with family tasks any more than do comparable fathers of nonhandicapped children. Lack of such instrumental support may be important to child and family outcomes, but at the present time, such indirect effects on child outcome have not been documented.

In his study of 201 families of severely retarded children in England, Holt (1958) noted that many fathers and siblings were adversely affected by the retarded children, not directly, but indirectly because of the mother's exhaustion and subsequent neglect. This is an anecdotal comment, however, rather than a research finding, and the relationship of these observations to child functioning is unknown.

Work by Gallagher et al. (1981) and McNeil and Chabassol (1981) demonstrates that both mothers and fathers of developmentally disabled children believe that it is appropriate for fathers to be involved in the problems of their handicapped children. The Gallagher study suggests that fathers appear to be willing to take a more active role, although both parents are unsure of what that role should be. Mothers

and fathers of the hearing-impaired children in the McNeil and Chabassol study considered the role of the father in the life of a hearing-impaired child to be as important as the role of the mother. Fathers also indicated as great a willingness as mothers to participate in a parent education activity.

The form that additional involvement should take is not known, but a study by Stoneman and Brody (1982) indicates that, in their homes, fathers were only half as likely as mothers to take the role of teacher, a common goal for mothers in early intervention training programs. Whether this is "good" or "bad" has not yet been determined, but it suggests that training fathers to be teachers of their children would certainly change, if not cause conflict with, existing family roles.

An understanding of how much time fathers actually spend with their developmentally disabled children would help one evaluate the relative likelihood of direct and indirect paternal effects on child outcomes. At the present time, however, no accurate estimates are available of the amount of time that fathers typically spend with their handicapped children or with the child's siblings, either alone or with others. In addition, it is not known whether the amount or distribution of this time is related to child progress or successful family adaptation to the developmentally disabled child. In an ongoing study of fathers of handicapped children, the authors are studying relationships between the amount and distribution of both emotional and instrumental support and subsequent (6 months and 18 months later) child progress and family adaptation.

The competency of fathers when they do interact with their disabled children is also not known. Parke & O'Leary's (1976) work with fathers of very young, nonhandicapped children suggests that fathers can be as competent and sensitive as mothers in caring for their infants. There is some indication that fathers may be more effective than mothers in getting compliance from their handicapped youngsters (Stoneman & Brody, 1982). Tallman's (1965) work, however, suggests that fathers of retarded children may be less competent than mothers in solving problems related to their retarded children, but he found that relative paternal competence was not related to later child progress. In fact, probably the most glaring omission in the literature on fathers of developmentally disabled children at the present time is the lack of consistent evidence that anything that fathers do affects long-term outcomes for their handicapped children.

Indirect Effects on Maintenance of the Disabled Child in the Home   One of the few specific tests of the effect of the father on the family's acceptance or rejection of the retarded child is provided in a pilot study by Peck and Stephens (1960). This early study is remarkable for using not only parent report measures but also including inhome ratings (Fels Behavior Scale). It appears on the basis of this limited study ($N = 10$) that the father, not the mother, sets the pattern for family acceptance or rejection of the developmentally disabled child. The correlation between paternal acceptance or rejection and the amount of family acceptance or rejection observed in the home was .81. The comparable maternal acceptance-family acceptance correlation for mothers was .09. This is an interesting finding that, if replicated with a larger sample, would be an important demonstration of an indirect paternal effect that might have relevance to preventing institutionalization of severely developmentally disabled children.

A study by Bristol (1984a) appears to corroborate this finding. Maternal perception of adequacy of paternal support in 45 families of autistic and communication-impaired children was found to be significantly related not only to maternal depression and maternal marital satisfaction but also to an interviewer rating of acceptance of the child and quality of parenting in these homes. These results suggest that fathers do affect their children by indirectly affecting the mother's ability to cope with the care that the children require. The relationship of such acceptance/rejection to child functioning was not tested in either study. A family systems approach, however, does allow for examination of both direct and indirect effects within the family.

Naturalistic Observational Studies of the Family   Another example of research on a family system is the series of family observational studies by Stoneman and Brody (1982). The studies present an interesting and unique picture of functional role relationships in 15 families with handicapped children and 8 contrast families with young, nonhandicapped children. Frequencies of occurrence of specific behaviors and roles were recorded, as well as sequential coding of contingent responsiveness. Observations took place in the home, first during a selected task and then during an unstructured naturalistic observation. Parents of Down syndrome children assumed the manager role more frequently, emitted more positive verbal and physical behaviors toward their children, and touched their offspring more frequently than did parents of nonhandicapped children, whereas these parents interacted with their children as playmates more often. Mothers of Down syndrome children assumed the role of teacher almost twice as often as any other group. Down syndrome children were also differentially responsive to mothers and fathers and responded to a lower proportion of managing, teaching, and information-seeking attempts than did the nonhandicapped children.

As predicted from the normal child development literature, parents decreased the amount of interaction with their children when their spouse was present, and both families with and without handicapped children let the mother "manage" the parent-child interactions. The effects of these interactions on any subsequent behavior or outcomes were not assessed, but the studies provide a vivid view of how conceiving of the family as a system allows for the assessment of both direct and indirect effects.

FAMILY ECOLOGICAL SYSTEMS PERSPECTIVE

Normal Child Development

The issue of family functioning is a complex one that does not yield easily to simple unidirectional, bidirectional, or even tridirectional research models. Including fathers in the understanding of family functioning is an important addition, but the fathers, as well as all the other family members, are affected by and, in turn, affect the larger formal and informal systems with which the family interacts. A developmental ecological systems approach (Figure 1, V) (Bronfenbrenner, 1977; Garbarino, 1977) places the family system (above) in a larger extrafamilial context.

A family ecological systems perspective offers the promise of providing a framework in which to assess the relative contribution of various internal and external influences on the child and on family adaptation to the developmentally disabled child. It focuses on the contextual nature of human development and suggests that understanding and lasting interventions are possible only when the personal, interpersonal, social, demographic, and ideological contexts of the individual are examined. Because the model is developmental, it also encompasses a dynamic lifespan perspective that includes both the concepts of child development and family development, two linked concepts that were previously the separate domains of psychologists and sociologists, respectively. (A discussion of a complete family developmental/ecological systems approach is beyond the scope of this chapter. The reader is referred to papers by Belsky, 1981; Feiring & Lewis, 1978; Tseng & McDermott, 1979; Turnbull, Brotherson, & Summers, 1985; and Von Bertalanffy, 1968, for a more detailed discussion.)

Investigations using this conceptualization of family influence have been fruitful in studying child abuse (Garbarino, 1977) and social support (Wahler, 1980) in families of nonhandicapped children. Although the terminology may differ somewhat as both psychologists and sociologists use this approach, the best skills of both disciplines are required to do justice to this type of model. For example, in addition to the usual psychological constructs, such as cognitive and emotional development or paternal self-esteem, development in this context involves life stages, boundary permeability, roles, family structure and functions, and other sociological constructs.

Research with Developmentally Disabled Children

Although it is not possible in a single study to do a completely exhaustive ecological evaluation, various aspects of the ecology can be observed. One aspect that has been studied is extrafamilial support and its relationship to mother-child interaction (Crnic, Greenberg, Ragozin, Robinson, & Basham, 1983). In a study of 40 mothers of autistic children, Bristol (1979) found that one of the variables that distinguished high-stress from low-stress mothers of autistic children was the perceived adequacy of an informal social support group consisting of family, extended family, friends, neighbors, and other parents of developmentally disabled children. In a subsequent study (Bristol, 1984b), such social support was also significantly positively correlated with marital satisfaction, inversely correlated with maternal reports of symptoms of depression within the past week, and positively correlated with an interviewer rating of family adaptation to the developmentally disabled child. A developmental/ecological systems perspective allows for and encourages such investigations of both intra- and extrafamilial influences on parent-child interaction and subsequent child development.

An understanding of the complexity of child development, thus, encompasses not only the influence of mothers, fathers, and other immediate and extended family members, but also the mutual effects of outside agencies and services.

Indirect Effects of Early Intervention on the Family Since the 1960s, government sponsored programs have worked directly with families to improve the development of young children. The efficacy of involving mothers in these efforts has since been demonstrated for both nonhandicapped (Lazar & Darlington, 1978) and handicapped children (Koegel et al., 1981, Marcus et al., 1978; Short, 1984). Because the concept of influence was originally one of mother to child, it seemed sufficient, at first, to focus only on mother and child and to measure the success of the intervention in terms of a narrow focus on cognitive gains in the child. (The controversy that followed in analyzing the outcome of the Head Start program is well known.)

Maternal involvement in programs for developmentally disabled children is now an established aspect of most effective programs. Outcome, however, continues to be measured mainly in terms of child progress. There are few studies of the impact of the program on the mother herself and even fewer that attempt to assess the impact of the child's intervention on the larger family.

In the study discussed above (Bristol, 1984a), low-stress mothers of autistic children were compared with high-stress mothers of autistic children comparable in social class, mother's age, number of children in the family, child IQ, and percent of severely autistic children. In addition to characteristics of the child and the adequacy of informal social support that differentiated the groups, low-stress mothers reported more adequate activities and services for their autistic children. A post hoc analysis (Bristol, 1985) revealed that the vast majority of mothers in the low-stress group had children receiving services from TEACCH, a program that, in addition to providing direct services for children, provided training and support services for parents. The majority of the highest-stress group were receiving services in local nonTEACCH special education programs that generally did not provide parent support services. (Mothers were categorized as high or low stress on the basis of the reported number of parental and family coping problems.) This study suggests that intervention that includes maternal training and parent support services may have a beneficial effect on the family, at least as seen from the mother's perspective.

Indirect Effects of Intervention on the Nonparticipating Spouse In a study by Fewell (1983), fathers who participated for 1 year in an early intervention program experienced less stress, less sadness, and fewer problems than they had evidenced when newly enrolled in the program. Their wives who had not been directly involved in the program themselves also appeared to benefit from the intervention, showing a significant decrement

in stress in dealing with child problems over that time. The study is remarkable first, for involving fathers rather than mothers in an early intervention program and then, for assessing the impact of the intervention on the nonparticipating family member.

All indirect effects, however, are not desirable. In evaluating the outcome of a training program for mothers of developmentally disabled children 2–6 years of age, Sandler, Coren, and Thurman (1983) assessed paternal as well as maternal change in families in which only the mother was enrolled in the program. They found that both maternal and paternal changes in attitudes toward themselves, their special child, their other children, and their spouses were correlated with child progress. As children improved, mothers tended to express more positive attitudes. However, child improvement tended to be associated with negative attitude change in the father. (No significance levels are given, and the word "tended" suggests something less than a robust finding, but the study is noteworthy for empirically raising the issue of possible negative effects.) The authors suggest that

> The time a mother spent teaching her handicapped child in the present study may have been related to greater progress by the child, but at the expense of time which might otherwise have been spent with other family members. This may have caused a negative attitude shift in the father. (Sandler et al., 1983, p. 358)

The authors conclude that the error is not in teaching the mothers, but rather in excluding the fathers when their wives are receiving intervention and gaining new knowledge and skills. Such a conclusion is strictly conjecture, but constitutes a testable hypothesis. Certainly, programs that make such excessive demands on mothers that they are forced to neglect other important family functions would do well to monitor the unintended family consequences of such interventions.

A family ecological systems conceptualization would both predict some internal reverberations from outside intervention and would result in the selection of a research design that would assess such indirect and, often unintended, effects of an extrafamilial influence.

Advances in multivariate data analysis strategies have made the consideration of such complex schemes more feasible in recent years.

CONCLUSIONS AND
IMPLICATIONS FOR FUTURE RESEARCH

Emerging concepts of normal family influence thus have shaped to some extent the questions asked and answers found regarding fathers of disabled children. Showing the conceptualizations of family influence as a progression is not meant to disparage earlier or simpler models. Instead, so little is presently known regarding fathers of developmentally disabled children that information at all levels is needed. At the simplest level, it is not yet known how much time fathers spend in contact with their handicapped children or how they spend that time. More importantly, it is not known to what extent such paternal contact makes a difference in the disabled child's development.

Regardless of the complexity of the paradigm used, it is clear that little is presently known about either the direct or indirect effects of fathers on their disabled children. More observational studies of contingent interaction are needed, as well as studies that assess the direct and indirect effects of paternal roles, attributes, attitudes, and behaviors on long-term child and family outcomes. The limited data presently available suggest that two of the father's most critical roles may be supplying support to the child's mother and communicating to the family that their burden of care is worthwhile.

Fathers then are seen as potent sources of support for their wives and families (Bristol, 1984b). Pedersen, Rubenstein, and Yarrow (1979) point out, however, that there are virtually no systematic studies of the type, amount, or sources of support that fathers themselves need to adapt successfully to having a handicapped child. Studies of this topic are also clearly needed.

Research instruments should also be designed or chosen so that positive as well as negative effects of developmentally disabled children on fathers can be measured, and assumptions of pathology should be superseded by studies of factors relating to successful adaptation by fathers and families. Recently, models have been tested predicting successful adaptation in mothers of disabled children (Bristol, 1984a; Bristol, in press). The applicability of such models to fathers should also be assessed.

With few exceptions (Fotheringham, Shelton, & Hoddinott, 1972; Tallman, 1965), data regarding fathers were also collected at a single point in time. Longitudinal research on fathers and families is needed. Although such studies are costly, they are critical to an understanding of the dynamic changes that occur not only in the development of the child and the father but also in the development of the family and the community.

Review of the current research on families also reveals studies that do not specify the race or social class of the parents, the sex of the children, or the percentage of response from families contacted. Others do not specify methods of subject recruitment, and few indicate the amount or adequacy of services that the child's parent is presently receiving. Greater specification of subject variables is needed if results are to be interpreted accurately.

It is also clear that the data that will answer the question raised in this chapter's introduction—what roles for which fathers in which families will help promote successful family adaptation while facilitating the development of the disabled child—are not yet available.

Because so little is known about the optimum role of fathers in facilitating the development of their handicapped children, caution is advised in devising intervention programs that may place fathers in conflict with existing family roles and responsibilities. Respect for family cultural values and beliefs requires the encouragement of types and levels of paternal involvement with the child and the child's program that meet the families' real needs, rather than the convenience or bias of the intervention staff. Before beginning to involve fathers programatically, both mothers' and fa-

96

thers' perceptions of appropriate program roles need to be ascertained. For example, parents who believe that their child's improvement depends on professionals rather than on parents may be unlikely to participate actively in a parent training program (De Vellis et al., 1985). At the very least, the broader impact on the family of any intervention program should be monitored in such a way as to detect both desirable and undesirable intended and unintended consequences of the intervention on other family members.

Finally, the complexity of the family and the limitations of methodologies require that research not be limited to a single methodology or even a single operationalization of family influence. There is no one best research method for studying fathers or families. The choice of a method depends on the stage of the research, the purpose for which the data are being collected, the question asked, and the population being studied. Researchers, however, should be aware of the concept of family influence implied by their choice of paradigm and, at least in interpreting their results, should acknowledge the larger context of the family ecology that may limit or clarify their findings.

REFERENCES

Ainsworth, M. D. (1978). Personal communication cited in Lamb, M. The father's role in the infant's social world. In J. H. Stevens & M. Mathews (Eds.), *Mother/child, father/child relationships* (pp. 87–108). Washington, DC: National Association for the Education of Young Children.

Anderson, B. J., & Standley, K. (1977). Manual for naturalistic observation of the childbirth environment. *JSAS Catalogue of Selected Documents in Psychology, 8,* 6 (MS No. 1413).

Andrews, G. (1968). Determinants of Negro family decisions in management of retardation. *Journal of Marriage and the Family, 30,* 612–617.

Bakemann, R. (1977). Untangling streams of behavior: Sequential analyses of observation data. In G. Sackett (Ed.), *Observing behavior: Data collection and analysis methods* (pp. 63–78). Baltimore: University Park Press.

Baruch, G. D., & Barnett, R. (1978). *The competent woman.* New York: Arvington.

Beckman, P. B. (1983). Characteristics of handicapped infants: A study of the relationship between child characteristics and stress as reported by mothers. *American Journal of Mental Deficiency, 88,* 150–156.

Bell, R. Q. (1968). A reinterpretation of the direction of effects in studies of socialization. *Psychological Review, 75*(2), 81–95.

Bell, R. Q. (1971). Stimulus control of parent or caretaker behavior by offspring. *Developmental Psychology, 4,* 63–72.

Bell, R. Q. (1978). A reinterpretation of the direction of effects in studies of socialization. *Psychological Review, 75,* 81–95.

Belsky, J. (1979). The interrelation of parental and spousal behavior during infancy in traditional nuclear families: An exploratory analysis. *Journal of Marriage and the Family, 41,* 749–755.

Belsky, J. (1980). A family analysis of parental influences on infant exploratory competence. In F. Pedersen (Ed.), *The father infant relationship: Observational studies in a family context* (pp. 87–110). New York: Praeger Special Studies.

Belsky, J. (1981). Early human experience: A family perspective. *Developmental Psychology, 17*(1), 3–23.

Bettleheim, B. (1967). *The empty fortress—Infantile autism and the birth of the self.* New York: The Free Press.

Biller, H. B. (1970). Father absence and the personality development of the male child. *Developmental Psychology, 2,* 181–201.

Biller, H. B. (1974). *Paternal deprivation: Family, school, sexuality and society.* Lexington, MA: D. C. Heath & Co.

Bowlby, J. (1951). *Maternal care and mental health.* Geneva: World Health Organization.

Bowlby, J. (1958). The nature of the child's tie to his mother. *International Journal of Psychoanalysis, 39,* 350–373.

Bowlby, J. (1969). *Attachment and loss. Vol. 1.* New York: Basic Books.

Bristol, M. M. (1979). *Maternal coping with autistic children: The effect of child characteristics and interpersonal support.* Unpublished doctoral dissertation, University of North Carolina at Chapel Hill.

Bristol, M. M. (1983, April). *Stress in families of handicapped children: Focus on fathers.* Invited paper presented at the Special Education for the 80's Conference, Louisiana State Department of Education, Baton Rouge.

Bristol, M. M. (1984a). Family resources and successful adaptation to autistic children. In E. Schopler & G. Mesibov (Eds.), *The effects of autism on the family* (pp. 289–311). New York: Plenum Publishing Corp.

Bristol, M. M. (1984b, October). *Families of developmentally disabled children: Healthy adaptation and the double ABCX model.* Paper presented at the Family Systems and Health Pre-conference workshop, National Council on Family Relations, San Francisco, CA.

Bristol, M. M. (1985). Designing programs for young developmentally disabled children: A family systems approach to autism. *Remedial and Special Education, 4*(6), 46–53.

Bristol, M. M. (in press). The home care of developmentally disabled children: Some empirical support for a conceptual model of successful coping with family stress. In P. Vietze & S. Landesman-Dwyer (Eds.), *Living with retarded people.* Washington, DC: Monographs of the American Association on Mental Deficiency.

Bristol, M. M., & Gallagher, J. J. (1982). A family focus for intervention. In C. Ramey & P. Trohanis (Eds.), *Finding and educating the high risk and handicapped infant* (pp. 137–161). Baltimore: University Park Press.

Bristol, M. M., & Schopler, E. (1983). Stress and coping in families of autistic adolescents. In E. Schopler & G. Mesibov (Eds.), *Autism in adolescents and adults* (pp. 251–278). New York: Plenum Publishing Corp.

Bristol, M. M., & Schopler, E. (1984). A developmental perspective on stress and coping in families of autistic children. In J. Blacher (Ed.), *Families of severely handicapped children* (pp. 91–141). New York: Academic Press.

Bronfenbrenner, U. (1977). Toward an experimental ecology of human development. *American Psychologist, 32*(7), 513–531.

Busse, T. V. (1969). Child-rearing antecedents of flexible thinking. *Developmental Psychology, 1,* 585–591.

Clarke-Stewart, K. A. (1977, March). *The father's impact on mother and child.* Paper presented at the meeting of the Society for Research in Child Development, New Orleans, LA.

Crnic, K. A., Greenberg, M. T., Ragozin, A. S., Robinson, N. M., & Basham, R. B. (1983). Effects of stress and social support on mothers and premature and full-term infants. *Child Development, 54,* 209–217.

Cummings, S. T. (1976). The impact of the handicapped child on the father: A study of fathers of mentally retarded and chronically ill children. *American Journal of Orthopsychiatry, 36,* 246–255.

Cummings, S. J., Bayley, H. C., & Rie, H. E. (1966). Effects of the child's deficiency on the mother: A study of mothers of mentally retarded, chronically ill and neurotic children. *American Journal of Orthopsychiatry, 36,* 595–608.

Darling, R. B., & Darling, J. (1982). *Children who are different: Meeting the challenge of birth defects in society.* St. Louis: The C. V. Mosby Company.

DeMyer, M. (1976). *Parents and children in autism.* Silver Spring, MD: V. H. Winston & Sons.

De Vellis, R.K., DeVellis, B., Revicki, D. A., Lurie, S. J., Runyan, D. K., & Bristol, M. M. (1985). Development and validation of the Child Improvement Locus of Control (CILC) Scales. *Journal of Social and Clinical Psychology, 3,* 308–325.

Donnelly, E. M. (1960). The quantitative analysis of parent behavior toward psychotic children and their siblings. *Genetic Psychology Monographs, 62,* 331–376.

Eisenberg, L. (1957). The fathers of autistic children. *American Journal of Orthopsychiatry, 27,* 715–725.

Farber, B. (1959). Effects of a severely mentally retarded child on family integration. *Monographs of the Society for Research in Child Development, 24* (2, Serial No. 71).

Farber, B. (1960). Perceptions of crisis and related variables in the impact of a retarded child on the mother. *Journal of Health and Human Behavior, 1,* 108–118.

Farber, B., & Jenne, W. C. (1963). Family organization and parent-child communication: Parents and siblings of a retarded child. *Monographs of the Society for Research in Child Development, 28,* (Whole Number 91).

Farber, B., Jenne, W. C., & Toigo, R. (1960). Family crisis and the decision to institutionalize the retarded child. *Council of Exceptional Children Research Monograph Series, Series A, 1.*

Farran, D. C., & Haskins, R. T. (1980). Reciprocal influence in the social interactions of mothers and 3-year-old children from different socioeconomic backgrounds. *Child Development, 51,* 780–791.

Feiring, C. (1976, March). *The preliminary development of a social systems model of early infant-mother attachment.* Paper presented at the Eastern Psychological Association Convention, New York, NY.

Feiring, C., & Lewis, M. (1978). The child as a member of the family system. *Behavioral Science, 23,* 225–233.

Fewell, R. R. (1983, May). *Supporting extended family members: Summary of research findings.* Paper presented at the 107th meeting of the American Association for Mental Deficiency, Dallas, TX.

Fotheringham, J. B., Shelton, M., & Hoddinott, B. A. (1972). The effects on the family of the presence of a mentally retarded child. *Canadian Psychiatric Association Journal, 17,* 283–290.

Fowle, C. M. (1968). The effect of the severely mentally retarded child on his family. *American Journal of Mental Deficiency, 73,* 468–473.

Fraiberg, S. (1974). Blind infants and their mothers: An examination of the sign system. In M. Lewis & L. A. Rosenblum (Eds.), *The effect of the infant on its caregiver* (pp. 215–232). New York: John Wiley & Sons.

Freud, S. (1948). *An outline of psychoanalysis.* New York: W. W. Norton.

Friedrich, W. (1977). Ameliorating the psychological impact of chronic physical disease on the child and family. *Journal of Pediatric Psychology, 2,* 26–31.

Friedrich, W. M., & Friedrich. W. L. (1981). Psychosocial assets of parents of handicapped and nonhandicapped children. *American Journal of Mental Deficiency, 85*(5), 551–553.

Gallagher, J. J. (1956). Rejecting parents? *Exceptional Children, 22,* 273–276.

Gallagher, J. J., Cross, A., & Scharfman, W. (1981). Parental adaptation to a young handicapped child: The father's role. *Journal of the Division for Early Childhood, 3,* 3–14.

Gallagher, J. J., Scharfman, W., & Bristol, M. M. (1984). The division of responsibilities in families with preschool handicapped and nonhandicapped children. *Journal of the Division of Early Childhood, 8,* 3–11.

Garbarino, J. (1977). Human ecology of child maltreatment: A conceptual model for research. *Journal of Marriage and the Family, 39,* 721–735.

Gath, A. (1972). The effects of mental subnormality on the family. *British Journal of Hospital Medicine, 8,* 147–150.

Gumz, E. J., & Gubrium, J. F. (1972). Comparative parental perceptions of a mentally retarded child. *American Journal of Mental Deficiency, 77,* 175–180.

Hayden, A., & Haring, N. (1974). Early intervention for high risk infants and young children: Programs for Down's Syndrome children. In T. D. Tjossem (Ed.), *Intervention strategies for high risk infants and young children* (pp. 573–607). Baltimore: University Park Press.

Hersch, A. (1970). Changes in family functioning following placement of a retarded child. *Social Work, 14*, 93–102.

Herzog, E., & Sudia, C. E. (1973). Children in fatherless families. In B. M. Caldwell & H. N. Ricciuti (Eds.), *Review of child development research* (Vol. 3, pp. 141–232). Chicago: University of Chicago Press.

Hetherington, E. M. (1981). Children and divorce. In R. Henderson (Ed.), *Parent-child interaction: Theory, research, and prospects* (pp. 33–58). New York: Academic Press.

Hetherington, E., Cox, M., & Cox, R. (1978). The development of children in mother-headed families. In H. Hoffman & D. Reiss (Eds.), *The American family: Dying or developing?* (pp. 117–145). New York: Plenum Publishing Corp.

Holroyd, J. (1974). The questionnaire on resources and stress: An instrument to measure family response to a handicapped member. *Journal of Community Psychology, 2*, 92–94.

Holroyd, J., & McArthur, D. (1976). Mental retardation and stress on the parents: A contrast between Down's Syndrome and childhood autism. *American Journal of Mental Deficiency, 80*, 431–436.

Holt, X. S. (1958). The influence of a retarded child upon family limitation. *Journal of Mental Deficiency Research, 2*, 28–34.

Hunt, J. M. (1979). Psychological development: Early experience. *Annual Review of Psychology, 30*, 103–143.

Kanner, L. (1954). To what extent is early infantile autism determined by constitutional inadequacies? *Proceedings of the Association for Research in Nervous and Mental Diseases, 33*, 378–385.

Karnes, M. B., & Teska, J. A. (1975). Children's response to intervention programs. In J. J. Gallagher (Ed.), *The application of child development research to exceptional children* (pp. 196–243). Reston, VA: Council for Exceptional Children.

Koegel, R. L., Schreibman, L., Britten, K. R., Burke, J. C., & O'Neill, R. E. (1981). A comparison of parent training to direct child treatment. In R. L. Koegel, A. Rincover, & A. L. Egel (Eds.), *Educating and understanding children* (pp. 260–279). San Diego: College Hill Press.

Kogan, K. L., & Tyler, N. (1973). Mother-child interaction in young physically handicapped children. *American Journal of Mental Deficiency, 77*, 492–497.

Kogan, K. L., Wimberger, H. C., & Bobbitt, R. A. (1969). Analysis of mother-child interaction in young mental retardates. *Child Development, 40*(3), 799–811.

Kotelchuck, M. (1976). The infant's relationship to the father: Experimental evidence. In M. E. Lamb (Ed.), *The role of the father in child development* (pp. 329–344). New York: John Wiley & Sons.

Kramm, E. R. (1963). *Families of mongoloid children.* Washington, DC: U.S. Department of Health, Education, and Welfare Administration, Children's Bureau.

Krause-Eheart, B. (1981, April). *Special needs of low-income mothers of developmentally delayed children.* Paper presented at the National Conference of the Society for Research in Child Development, Boston, MA.

Lamb, M. E. (1975). Fathers: Forgotten contributors to child development. *Human Development, 18*, 245–266.

Lamb, M. E. (1976). Effects of stress and cohort on mother- and father-infant interaction. *Developmental Psychology, 12*, 435–443.

Lamb, M. E. (1977). Father-infant and mother-infant interaction in the first year of life. *Child Development, 48*, 167–181.

Lamb, M. E. (1978a). The father's role in the infant's social world. In J. H. Stevens & M. Mathews (Eds.), *Mother/child, father/child relationships* (pp. 87–108). Washington, DC: National Association for the Education of Young Children.

Lamb, M. E. (1978b). Infant social cognition and "special order" effects. *Infant Behavior and Development, 1*, 1–10.

Lazar, I. & Darlington, R. B. (1978). Lasting effects of early education. *Monographs of the Society for Research in Child Development, 47* (No. 2–3, Serial No. 175).

Lennard, H. L., Beaulieu, M. R., & Embrey, M. G. (1966). Interaction in families with a schizophrenic child. *Archives of General Psychiatry, 12*, 166–183.

Lewis, M., & Feiring, C. (1978). The child's social world. In R. M. Lerner & G. B. Spanier (Eds.), *Child influences on marital and family interaction: A life-span perspective* (pp. 47–69). New York: Academic Press.

Lewis, M., & Rosenblum, L. A. (1974). *The effect of the infant on its caregiver.* New York: John Wiley & Sons.

Lewis, M., & Weinraub, M. (1976). The father's role in the child's social network. In M. E. Lamb (Ed.), *The role of the father in child development* (pp. 157–184). New York: John Wiley & Sons.

Lonsdale, G. (1978). Family life with a handicapped child: The parents speak. *Child: Care, Health and Development, 4*, 99–120.

Love, H. (1973). *The mentally retarded child and his family.* Springfield, IL: Charles C. Thomas Publications.

Maccoby, E. E., & Masters, J. C. (1970). Attachment and dependency. In P. H. Mussen (Eds.), *Carmichaels' manual of child psychology* (Vol. 2, 3rd ed., pp. 73–157). New York: John Wiley & Sons.

Marcus, L., Lansing, M., Andrews, C., & Schopler, E. (1978). Improvement of teaching effectiveness in parents of autistic children. *Journal of the American Academy of Child Psychiatry, 17*, 625–639.

McCubbin, H. (1979). Integrating coping behavior in family stress theory. *Journal of Marriage and the Family, 42*, 237–344.

McNeil, M., & Chabassol, D. (1981). Parents' perceptions of fathers' involvement with hearing-impaired children. *Psychological Reports, 49*, 803–806.

Meyerowtiz, H. D., & Farber, B. (1966). Family background of educable mentally retarded children. In B. Farber (Ed.), *Kinship and family organization* (pp. 388–398). New York: John Wiley & Sons.

Nihira, K., Meyers, C. E., & Mink, A. (1980). Home environment, family adjustment, and the development of mentally retarded children. *Applied Research in Mental Retardation, 1*, 5–24.

Parke, R. D. (1978). Parent infant interaction: Progress, paradigms, and problems. In G. P. Sackett & H. C. Haywood (Eds.), *Application of observations: Ethological methods to the study of mental retardation* (pp. 69–93). Baltimore: University Park Press.

Parke, R. D., & O'Leary, S. (1976). Father-mother-infant interaction in the newborn period: Some findings, some observations, and some unresolved issues. In K. Riegel & J. Meacham (Eds.), *The developing individual in a changing world: Vol. 2. Social and environmental issues* (pp. 653–663). The Hague: Mouton & Company.

Parke, R. D., & Sawin, D. B. (1976). The father's role in infancy: A re-evaluation. *The Family Coordinator, 25,* 365–371.

Peck, J. R., & Stephens, W. B. (1960). A study of the relationships between the attitudes and behaviors of parents and that of their mentally defective child. *American Journal of Mental Deficiency, 64,* 839–844.

Pedersen, F. A. (1975, August). *Mother, father and infant as an interaction system.* Paper presented at the annual convention of the American Psychological Association, Chicago, IL.

Pedersen, F. A., Anderson, B. J., & Cain, R. L. (1977, March). *An approach to understanding linkages between the parent-infant and spouse relationships.* Paper presented at the meeting of the Society for Research in Child Development, New Orleans, LA.

Pedersen, F., Anderson, B., & Cain, R. (1980a). Conceptualization of father influences in the infancy period. In M. Lewis & L. Rosenblum (Eds.), *The social network of the developing infant* (pp. 45–66). New York: Plenum Press.

Pedersen, F. A., Anderson, B. J., & Cain, R. L. (1980b). Parent-infant and husband-wife interactions observed at age five months. In F. Pederson (Ed.), *The father-infant relationship: Observational studies in a family setting* (pp. 71–86). New York: Praeger Publishers.

Pedersen, F. A., & Robson, K. S. (1969). Father participation in infancy. *American Journal of Orthopsychiatry, 39,* 466–472.

Pedersen, F. A., Rubenstein, J. L., & Yarrow, L. J. (1979). Infant development in father-absent families. *The Journal of Genetic Psychology, 135,* 51–61.

Radin, N. (1981). The role of the father in academic, cognitive and intellectual development. In M. E. Lamb (Ed.), *The role of the father in child development* (rev. ed.) (pp. 379–427). New York: John Wiley & Sons.

Ramey, C. T., Beckman-Bell, P., & Gowen, J. W. (1981). Infant characteristics and infant-caregiver interactions: Implications from research for educating handicapped infants. In J. J. Gallagher (Ed.), *New directions in exceptional children* (pp. 59–83). San Francisco: Jossey-Bass.

Rebelsky, F., & Hanks, C. (1971). Fathers' verbal interaction with infants in the first three months of life. *Child Development, 42,* 63–68.

Reed, E. W., & Reed, S. C. (1965). *Mental retardation: A family study.* Philadelphia: W. B. Saunders Co.

Rondal, J. A. (1978). Maternal speech to normal and Down's Syndrome children matched for mean length of utterance. *American Association on Mental Deficiency Monographs, 3.*

Sackett, G. (in press). Analysis of sequential social interaction data: Some issues, recent developments, and a causal inference model. In J. Osofsky (Ed.), *Handbook of infant development* (2nd ed.). New York: John Wiley & Sons.

Sameroff, A. J. (1975). Early influences on development: Fact or fancy? *Merrill Palmer Quarterly, 21,* 267–294.

Sandler, A., Coren, A., & Thurman, S. K. (1983). A training program for parents of handicapped preschool children: Effects upon mother, father, and child. *Exceptional Children, 49*(4), 355–358.

Schaefer, E. S., & Edgerton, M. (1981, April). *Parental modernity in childrearing and educational attitudes and beliefs.* Paper presented at the meeting of the Society for Research in Child Development, Boston, MA.

Schaffer, H. R., & Emerson, P. E. (1964). The development of social attachments in infancy. *Monographs of the Society for Research in Child Development, 29*(Serial No. 94).

Schipper, M. T. (1959). The child with mongolism in the home. *Pediatrics, 24,* 132–144.

Schonnell, F. J., & Watts, E. H. (1956). A first survey or the effects of a subnormal child on the family unit. *American Journal of Mental Deficiency, 51,* 210–219.

Schopler, E. (1971). Parents of psychotic children as scapegoats. *Journal of Contemporary Psychotherapy, 4,* 17–22.

Schopler, E. (1978). Limits of methodological differences between family studies. In M. Rutter & E. Schopler (Eds.), *Autism: A reappraisal of concepts and treatment* (pp. 297–302). New York: Plenum Publishing Corp.

Schopler, E. Mesibov, G., & Baker, A. (1982). Evaluation of treatment for autistic children and their parents. *Journal of the American Academy of Child Psychiatry, 21,* 262–267.

Sears, R. R., Maccoby, E. E., & Levin, H. (1957). *Patterns of child rearing.* New York: Harper & Row.

Shereshefsky, P. M., & Yarrow, L. J. (1973). *Psychological aspects of a first pregnancy and early postnatal adaptation.* New York: Raven Press.

Shinn, M. (1978). Father-absence and children's cognitive development. *Psychological Bulletin, 85,* 295–324.

Short, A. (1984). Short-term treatment outcome using parents as co-therapists for their own autistic children. *Journal of Child Psychology and Psychiatry and Allied Disciplines, 25,* 443–458.

Stone, N. W., & Chesney, B. H. (1978). Attachment behaviors in handicapped infants. *Mental Retardation, 16,* 8–12.

Stoneman, Z., & Brody, G. H. (August, 1982). *Observational research on retarded children, their parents, and their siblings.* Paper presented at the NICHHD Lake Wilderness Conference, University of Washington, Seattle, WA.

Switzky, L. T., Vietze, P., & Switzky, H. (1979). Attitudinal and demographic predictors of breast-feeding and bottle-feeding behavior of mothers of six-week-old infants. *Psychological Reports, 45,* 3–14.

Tallman, I. (1965). Spousal role differentiation and the socialization of severely retarded children. *Journal of Marriage and the Family, 27,* 37–42.

Tavormina, J. B., Boll, T. J., Dunn, N. J., Luscomb, R. L., & Taylor, J. R. (1981). Psychosocial effects on parents of raising a physically handicapped child. *Journal of Abnormal Child Psychology, 9*(1), 121–131.

Thomas, A., & Chess, S. (1977). *Temperament and development.* New York: Brunner/Mazel.

Tseng, W., & McDermott, J. F. (1979). Triaxial family classification: A proposal. *Journal of the American Academy of Child Psychiatry, 18*(1), 22–43.

Turnbull, A. P., Brotherson, M. J. & Summers, J. A. (1985). The impact of deinstitutionalization on families: A family systems approach. In R. H. Bruininks & K. C. Lakin (Eds.), *Living and learning in the least restrictive environment* (pp. 115–140). Baltimore: Paul H. Brookes Publishing Co.

Turnbull, A. P., & Winton, P. J. (1984). Parent involvement policy and practice: Current research and implications for families of young severely handicapped children. In J. Blacher (Ed.), *Severely handicapped children and their families: Research in review.* (pp. 367–395). New York: Academic Press.

Von Bertalanffy, L. (1968). *General systems theory.* New York: George Braziller.

Wadsworth, H. G., & Wadsworth, J. B. (1971). A problem of involvement with parents of mildly retarded children. *The Family Coordinator, 20,* 141–147.

Wahler, R. G. (1980). The insular mother: Her problems in parent-child treatment. *Journal of Applied Behavior Analysis, 13,* 207–219.

Weinraub, M. (1978). Fatherhood: The myth of the second-class parent. In J. H. Stephens & M. Mathews (Eds.), *Mother/child, father/child relationships* (pp. 109–135). Washington, DC: National Association for the Education of Young Children.

Wiegerink, R., Hocutt, A., Posante-Loro, R., & Bristol, M. (1980). Parent involvement in early education programs for handicapped children. *New Directions for Exceptional Children, 1,* 67–85.

Chapter

6

Fathers, Families, and Support Systems

Their Role in the Development of At-Risk and Retarded Infants and Children

Ross D. Parke

A NARROW CONCEPTUALIZATION of the family unit has been common in theories concerning families of both retarded and non-retarded individuals. The premise of this chapter is that the theoretical and empirical conceptualization of the environment needs to be expanded beyond the traditional view of the mother-child dyad to include both father-child and mother-father-child relationships and a wider range of socializing agents and contexts. Recognition of the embeddedness of the family in its ecological context is needed in order to understand how families function on a daily basis and cope with stressful events. To illustrate the value of this expanded view of the family, the impact of the birth of a premature infant on family functioning is discussed. In addition, the impact of a handicapped infant on families is examined in order to evaluate how

the severity of the stressful event can modify family adaptation.

IMPACT OF PRETERM AND HANDICAPPED INFANTS ON THE MOTHER-CHILD RELATIONSHIP

The birth of a premature infant is often a stressful event, as evidenced by descriptions portraying parents with infants in at-risk nurseries as shocked, angry, and otherwise emotionally distraught (Kennedy, 1973; Kopf & McFadden, 1974; Slade, Redl, & Manguten, 1977). Likewise, parents of handicapped infants express a similar emotional sequence of disappointment, denial, anger, and guilt (Holt, 1957; Klaus & Kennell, 1982; Legeay & Keogh, 1966; Marion, 1981). Yet reactions to the birth of a premature infant are likely to differ

Preparation of this chapter was supported by NICHD Grant No. PO1 HD05951, NICHD Training Grant No. HD07205, and the National Foundation March of Dimes.
Thanks to Karen McGuire and Wilma Hardin for their assistance in the preparation of this manuscript.

across families. The degree of stress associated with this event is determined, in part, by the parents' subjective perceptions of the event. In turn, it is assumed that their perceptions will influence their interactions with their infants. This cognitive-mediational approach suggests that parental knowledge, expectations, and labeling must be considered in order to understand the degree of stress, as well as the parents' treatment of their infant (Leiderman, 1982; Parke, 1978; Sameroff, 1982).

The survival rate of the low birth weight infant has increased greatly in recent years due to advances in medical care and technology (Klaus & Fanaroff, 1979; Kopp, 1983). Many of these "new" survivors often have serious medical difficulties, as well as a higher rate of short-term and long-term developmental problems than normal infants. Caputo and Mandell (1970) point out a number of outcomes that may make the low birth weight infant "at risk" for possible parental maltreatment. Some of the outcomes may alter the parent-child relationship in the early postpartum months, whereas others may not affect the parent-child dyad until the child is beyond infancy.

In addition to the disruption of family harmony caused by the birth of any infant (e.g., additional tasks associated with caregiving, modifications of schedules and activities, readjustment of the marital relationship [Cowan & Cowan, 1984; Entwisle & Doering, 1981]), the birth of a premature infant further increases familial stress in a number of ways. First, the immature development of the infant may require special medical support procedures, which in turn may lead to separation of the mother from her infant. Although early separation may cause short-term stress on the family, follow-up studies indicate no long-term impact (i.e., 2 years) of this type of separation on the development of these infants (Leiderman, 1981, 1982).

Second, the low birth weight premature infant violates many parental expectations. In addition to arriving early, often before parental preparations for birth are completed, these infants differ from full-term infants in their appearance, cries, feeding needs, interaction-

al demands, and developmental progress, which, in turn, can contribute further to the stress associated with their arrival (Brooks & Hochberg, 1960; Frodi, Lamb, Leavitt, Donovan, Neff, & Sherry, 1978). For example, in their study, Frodi et al. (1978) documented that, in addition to their appearance, the high-pitched cry patterns of the premature infant are rated by parents as more disturbing, irritating, and annoying. In addition, the parents who responded found premature infants to be less pleasant and were less eager to interact with a preterm than a full-term infant. More recently, Stern and Hildebrandt (1984) found that mothers rated infants labeled premature as less physically developed, less attentive, slower, less smart, quieter, more sleepy, and more passive than the same infants labeled full-term. These studies provide support for the existence of a prematurity stereotype among adults. In turn, these biased perceptions may lead to a self-fulfilling prophecy whereby the premature infant comes to exhibit the expected negative behavior. These findings underscore the value of a cognitive-mediational approach (Parke, 1978). Violations of expectations are not restricted to preterm infants; other studies indicated that handicapped infants violate parental expectations of rearing a normal, well-functioning child as well (Canning & Pueschel, 1978).

Preterm infants place greater demands on their caregivers than term infants (Freidman & Sigman, 1981). For example, feeding disturbances are more common among low birth weight infants (Klaus & Fanaroff, 1979). Moreover, premature infants are behaviorally different than their term peers; as Goldberg (1979) reported, premature infants spend less time in an alert state, are more difficult to keep in alert states, are less responsive to sights and sounds than term infants, and provide less distinctive cues to guide parental treatment. In view of these behavioral characteristics, it is not surprising that parents have to work "harder" when interacting with a premature infant. Brown and Bakeman (1980) have documented that preterm infants are more difficult and less satisfying to feed than term infants; during feeding interactions, preterms contributed less to maintenance of the interactive flow than term infants, and the burden of maintaining the interaction fell disproportionately on the mothers of these preterms. Other observational studies of Down syndrome children (Stoneman, Brody, & Abbott, 1983), developmentally delayed infants (Vietze, Abernathy, Ashe, & Faulstich, 1978), and severely handicapped infants (Walker, 1982) report a similar pattern of reduced responsivity during social interchanges. Together, these studies confirm that children with a variety of limiting conditions are less responsive during parent-child interaction.

Not only does the preterm infant modify caregiver behavior but expectations concerning developmental timetables may be altered as well. Recently, Smith, Leiderman, Selz, MacPherson, and Bingham (1981) found that mothers of preterm infants rated developmental milestones for their own child differently than for a typical child. In rating their own children, they predicted substantial lags for their own child until approximately 2 years of age. Beyond 2 years, they expected more rapid development in social, psychomotor, and cognitive development than the rate of progress expected by the mothers of full-term infants. These data suggest that parents of preterm infants may have unrealistic expectations for their young children, which, in turn, may be a contributing factor in later dysfunctional parent-child relationships, such as child abuse (Egeland & Brunnquell, 1979).

The remainder of this chapter argues that an expanded characterization of the social context of the premature infant, as well as the handicapped and retarded infant, is necessary to understand better the nature of the environment in which these infants and children develop.

FATHERS AND TRIADS: EXPANDING THE CONTEXT OF DEVELOPMENT

The Father-Infant Relationship

In recent years, the father's role in infancy has been increasingly recognized (Lamb, 1981; Parke, 1981; Parke & Tinsley, 1984). Fathers are active and interested contributors in early infancy, and competent in their execution of early caregiving tasks, such as feeding and diapering (Parke & Sawin, 1976; 1980). Until recently, the focus was nearly exclusively on fathers of term infants, but researchers have begun to explore the special role of fathers in families with preterm infants, as well as handicapped and retarded infants. The role of fathers in caregiving and play with normal full-term infants, as well as with special infants, such as premature and handicapped infants, is examined in this discussion.

The birth of a premature infant elicits greater father involvement in caregiving; this heightened involvement may, in part, be due to the additional time, energy, and skill required to care for preterm infants. A recent investigation by Yogman (1984) illustrates this finding. Twenty preterm and 20 full-term infants were followed longitudinally from birth to 18 months. On the basis of father reports of routine caregiving at 1, 5, and 18 months, Yogman found that fathers of the preterm infants reported engaging in more of the caregiving tasks at each age than the comparison group of fathers of full-term infants. The differences were especially marked and statistically significant by 18 months, when fathers were more likely to take the infant to a physician, to bathe the infant, and to get up at night to console their infant. In summary, the birth of a premature infant appears to elicit greater father participation in caregiving.

Does father participation increase in the case of handicapped infants and children? Although the data are neither abundant nor entirely consistent, research suggests that fathers of retarded infants and children tend *not* to show increased involvement in child care. In fact, the level of participation in caregiving of fathers of retarded children is low (Andrew, 1968; Holt, 1957). In one of the rare observational studies in this area, Stoneman et al. (1983) found that mothers of handicapped infants assumed the role of teacher more frequently in a structured interaction situation than did fathers. Mothers and fathers did not differ in their level of teaching in families of nonhandicapped children. Unfortunately, the level of father involvement in routine caregiving activities of handicapped children was not assessed in this investigation. Lamb (1984) suggests that

> this reflects the fact that fathers obtain less satisfaction from retarded than normal children (Cummings, 1976) and the fact that paternal involvement—unlike maternal involvement—is discretionary. The paternal role is defined in such a way that fathers can increase or decrease their involvement depending on their preferences and satisfactions whereas traditionally mothers are expected to show equivalent commitment to all their children—regardless of personal preferences or the individual characteristics of their children. (pp. 16–17)

However, not all investigators find this pattern of low involvement. In an early study, Tallman (1965) found that fathers of handicapped children became highly involved in child care, but only with boys. This heightened involvement of fathers with their sons is consistent with earlier studies of nonretarded infants (Parke & Sawin, 1976, 1980). Others find no differences in the level of father involvement with handicapped and nonhandicapped children. In a more recent investigation of the division of role responsibilities in families of handicapped and nonhandicapped children by Gallagher, Scharfman, and Bristol (1984), there was no difference in the roles of mothers and fathers in the families of handicapped and nonhandicapped children. However, the involvement of the children in national demonstration programs for preschool handicapped children may have reduced the necessity for role realignments in these families. More attention to this issue is needed with a wider range of samples. The application of observational and time-diary strategies would help clarify the inconsistencies in this area.

Play patterns, as well as levels of involvement in caregiving, may be different for fathers of premature infants than for fathers of term infants. In a comparative observational investigation of the interaction patterns of fathers with premature and term infants in the high-risk nursery and at home shortly after the infant's discharge, styles of father-infant play with the preterm and full-term infants differed (Tinsley, Johnson, Szczypka, & Parke, 1982). Fathers exhibited their characteristic higher rate of physical play (bounce-stretch) than mothers, but only when the infant was born at term. When the infant was born prematurely, there was no mother-father difference in play style. The differences were particularly marked by 3 weeks; in the high-risk nursery, there were no differences between mothers and fathers in their treatment of either term or premature infants.

Other evidence is consistent with these findings. Yogman (1982) studied fathers of preterm and full-term infants during a 3-minute episode of face-to-face play in the laboratory. The games were categorized as arousing if they involved proximal activities (e.g., tactile and limb movement games), or as nonarousing if they were assumed to maintain rather than arouse the infant's attention (e.g., verbal and visual games). Fathers of preterm infants played fewer and shorter games and fewer arousing games than did fathers of full-term infants. Fathers were less able to engage their preterm infants directly in play compared to the full-term infants. Possibly, fathers assume that the premature infant is fragile and unable to withstand robust physical stimulation; this assumption, in turn, leads to an inhibition of fathers' usual play style. Moreover, because preterm infants have more difficulty with motor activity and tone and with state regulation and hypersensitivity, vigorous stimulation may stress and disorganize an already vulnerable infant. In view of this feedback, fathers may not only shift their play style to a less stressful mode, but may interact less.

Studies of how fathers with infants with varying types of handicapping conditions modify their play patterns would be worthwhile. Observational studies by Walker (1982) of the social interactions between mothers and handicapped infants suggest that the handicapped infant is less reinforcing, less interesting, and more difficult as a social partner. In her studies, mothers accounted for a large share of the playful stimulation, whereas the infant contribution was severely limited. Parallel work with fathers using an observational strategy would help further illuminate the father's role in the early development of handicapped infants.

The Family Triad: Mother-Father-Infant

Models that limit examination of the effects of interaction patterns to only the father-infant and mother-infant dyads and the direct effects of one individual on another are inadequate for understanding the impact of social interaction patterns in families, especially in families with preterm infants or handicapped infants (Lewis & Feiring, 1981; Parke, Power, & Gottman, 1979; Parke & Tinsley, 1982).

Triadic contexts in which mother, father, and infant interact together merit further examination. Similarly, indirect as well as direct paths of mutual influence within families are important. A parent may influence a child through the mediation of another family member's impact (e.g., a mother may contribute to the father's positive affect toward his child by praising his caregiving skill). Another way in which one parent may indirectly influence the child's treatment by other agents is by modifying the infant's behavior. Child behavior patterns that develop as a result of parent-child interaction may, in turn, affect the child's treatment by other social agents. For example, irritable infant patterns induced by an insensitive and impatient mother may, in turn, make the infant more difficult for the father to handle and pacify. Thus, patterns developed in interaction with one parent may alter interaction patterns with another caregiver. In larger families, siblings can play a similar mediating role.

The triadic setting can modify the nature of parent-infant interaction patterns. Parents have been shown to behave differently when alone with their infant than when interacting with the infant in the presence of the other parent. In the author's earlier studies (Parke, Grossman, & Tinsley, 1981; Parke & O'Leary, 1976), the presence of the other parent significantly altered the behavior of the partner. Although there was an overall reduction in the level of interaction in the presence of a spouse, not all behaviors decreased. Specifically, each parent expressed more positive affect (smiling) toward their infant and showed a higher level of exploration when the other parent was present. In studies of premature infants and their parents, similar patterns were found (Tinsley et al., 1982). The family context appeared to elicit greater affective and exploratory behavior on the part of both parents. These results indicate that parent-infant interaction with either premature or term infants cannot be understood by focusing solely on parent-infant dyads.

Moreover, recent research with Down syndrome infants and their parents underscores the importance of examining the family triad (Stoneman et al., 1983). These investigators found that the interactive behavior of mothers and fathers decreased when the other parent was present. However, fathers were more affected than mothers. Although mothers remained involved with their children in both the dyadic and triadic contexts, fathers tended to play a less active role when the mother was present. "This is consistent with research suggesting that mothers continue to assume a managing, parenting role across family groupings; whereas in mother-father-child triads fathers tend to defer to mothers decreasing their interaction time with children" (Stoneman et al., 1983, p. 599). However, there were no differences across families of retarded and nonretarded children.

Of even greater importance is the impact of spousal support on parental competence. In a recent study of 4- to 8-month-old infants and their parents, Dickie and Matheson (1984) examined the relationships between parental competence and spousal support. Parental competence was based on home observations and involved a variety of components, such as emotional consistency, contingent responding, and warmth and pleasure in parenting. Emotional support—a measure of affection, respect, and satisfaction in the husband-wife relationship—and cognitive support, an index of husband-wife agreement in child care, were positively related to maternal competence. Just as paternal support relates positively to maternal competence, there is evidence that maternal support is similarly linked to father's parenting competence. These same investigators found that maternal emotional support and cognitive support were related to paternal competence. In fact, spousal support was a more important correlate of competence in fathers than mothers. The level of emotional and cognitive support successfully discriminated high- and low-competency fathers, but failed to do so in the case of mothers. In short, successful paternal parenting may be particularly dependent on a supportive intrafamilial environment.

Nor is the importance of spousal support restricted to families of healthy infants. A supportive spousal relationship can serve to buffer or diminish the negative impact of giving birth to a handicapped or retarded infant. Support for this hypothesis comes from a study of maternal adjustment to having a handicapped child (Friedrich, 1979). Marital satisfaction was found to be the best predictor of maternal coping behavior.

Unfortunately, stressful events, such as the birth of a premature or retarded infant, may often have a disruptive impact on the marital relationship. In turn, this disruption may reduce the level of mutual support that spouses provide to each other in stressful circumstances. Of relevance to this issue is the work of Leiderman (1981) and Leiderman and Seashore (1975). These investigators examined the relationship of prematurity to marital stability. In the 2-year period following hospital discharge, marital discord, often leading to separation or divorce, was higher for the families of preterm infants who were initially separated from their mothers. As Leiderman and Seashore suggest, "separation in the newborn period does have an effect, albeit non-specific, by acting through the family as a stress that creates disequilibrium in the nuclear family structure" (Leiderman & Seashore, 1975, pp. 229–230). Although the Leiderman work provides further support for considering the family unit, the specific ways in which the birth of a preterm infant affects relationships among family members remain unclear.

Just as in the case of preterm infants, the birth of a retarded child often has a negative impact on the marital relationship. Specifical-

ly, a number of investigators have found extensive marital and family disruption as a result of the birth of a retarded or handicapped child (Farber, 1959, 1960; Holt, 1957; Lonsdale, 1978; Tew, Lawrence, Payne, & Rawnsley, 1977). Moreover, nonretarded siblings tend to be negatively affected (Farber, 1960; Holt, 1957), and further childbearing tends to cease (Carver & Carver, 1972).

The importance of these findings is clear: In order to understand either the mother-infant or father-infant relationship, the total set of relationships among the members of the family needs to be assessed. Although interviews are helpful, they are not sufficient; rather, direct observations of both mother *and* father alone with their infants, as well as the mother, father, and infant together, are necessary to understand the effects of the birth of either a premature or handicapped infant.

Beyond the Nuclear Family: The Role of Extrafamilial Support Systems

A further extension of this theoretical framework—from the dyad to the triad to the family in its ecological context—is needed to understand the environment and the development of either the at-risk or retarded infant. Families do not exist as units independent of other social organizations within society. Thus, families need to be viewed within their social context, and recognition of the role of the community as a modifier of family modes of interaction is necessary for an adequate theory of early development (Cochran & Brassard, 1979; Parke & Tinsley, 1982).

To understand the specific functions that extrafamilial support systems play in modulating interaction patterns in families of premature and/or handicapped or retarded infants, an appreciation of the problems associated with the care of these types of infants is necessary. Infants who are born prematurely or with a handicapping condition may be at risk as a result of: 1) limited knowledge of development on the part of parents, 2) inappropriate infant care skill, and/or 3) the stress associated with the care and rearing of a preterm infant. Extrafamilial support systems can alleviate these problems by: 1) providing accurate timetables for the development of infants with special problems, 2) monitoring current infant care practices and providing corrective feedback in order to improve infant care skills, and 3) providing relief from stress associated with the birth and care of the preterm and/or handicapped infant.

There are a variety of support systems of special relevance to at-risk infants and families. Two kinds of support systems operate: formal (e.g., health care facilities, social service agencies, recreational facilities), and informal (e.g., extended families, neighbors, and co-workers). These programs serve the educational functions of providing child care information, as well as alleviating stress associated with premature or ill infants. Support systems that serve an educational function include hospital-based courses in child care and child-rearing, visiting nurse programs, well-baby clinics, follow-up programs, and parent discussion groups. Some other supportive programs that offer stress relief are family and group day care facilities, baby-sitting services, mother's helpers, homemaker and housekeeping services, drop-off centers, crisis nurseries, and hotlines.

Evidence upholding the role of formal and informal support systems in regulating family ability to cope with at-risk infants is limited. In the next section, some illustrative studies of the role of support systems in modifying family management of infant care and development are reviewed. Although some recent studies involve informal social support systems, many of the studies have primarily involved modification of the formal support systems available to families. Finally, in some cases, formal and informal support are provided together, underscoring the interconnectedness of these two levels of social support for families.

The Impact of Informal Support Systems on Families A number of studies have suggested that there is a positive relationship between informal social networks and a family's adaptation to stressful events, such as divorce (Hetherington, Cox, & Cox, 1982) and job loss (Bronfenbrenner & Crouter, 1982). Of particu-

lar relevance are recent investigations concerning the relationship between social networks and mother-child interaction.

Unger (1979) examined the influence of social networks on mother-infant interaction in a small sample of white, low-income mothers and their young infants (under 6 months). Using the HOME Scale (Elardo, Bradley, & Caldwell, 1975) to assess interaction, Unger found that mothers who experienced high levels of stress were found to be more actively involved with their infants when they had weekly contact with friends than when they had infrequent contact. Parents also appeared more responsive to their infants if they were receiving material resources from their network members. In a related study that also employed the HOME Scale, Pascoe, Loda, Jeffries, and Earp (1981) found a positive relationship between the level of maternal social support and selected subscales from the HOME Scale in a group of families with 3-year-old children. Unfortunately, Pascoe et al. did not examine both intrafamilial (i.e., spouse support) and extrafamilial social support separately, therefore hindering an evaluation of the relative importance of differing sources of support. However, studies by Pascoe et al. (1981) and Unger and Powell (1980) are important in view of the previously established positive relationship between the HOME Scale and mental test performance (Bradley & Caldwell, 1976). More recently, Crnic, Greenberg, Ragozin, Robinson, & Basham (1983), using samples of both preterm and full-term infants, reported positive relationships between informal social support and the quality of mother-infant interaction. These investigations suggest that social support may affect infant and child developmental outcomes indirectly through modifying the nature of parent-child interaction patterns.

Moreover, Crockenberg (1981) found that the extent to which mothers utilized social support networks was related to the infant's pattern of attachment to its mother. Especially in the case of irritable infants (a characteristic common in many premature infants), utilization of social support was associated with secure attachment. This study provides an excellent illustration of the interplay of individual characteristics (temperament) and the role of the social environment (social support networks) on later patterns of infant-mother attachment. In view of the evidence that the quality of early attachment is associated with later peer social competence (Pastor, 1981), this finding is of particular importance.

Unfortunately, little evidence is available concerning the utilization and impact of social support systems on families of preterm infants. It is assumed that social networks will be particularly important in the families of preterm infants who are under greater initial stress than families of term infants. Although many of the children in the Pascoe et al. (1981) study were either born prematurely or were ill as infants, no assessments were made of the social networks of these families when their children were infants. More recent evidence (Parke, Tinsley, & Volling, 1982) indicates that parents are more likely to use social support systems when their infants were born prematurely than when their infants are born at term. However, mothers are more likely to utilize informal support networks than fathers, whereas fathers are more likely to use formal agencies for information. This suggests the importance of distinguishing formal and informal support systems and underscores the necessity of providing formal support systems for families including fathers.

In the case of families with retarded children, social networks are particularly important aids to successful coping and adaptation. However, a number of studies have documented that these families are socially isolated (Birenbaum, 1970; Carver & Carver, 1972; Illingworth, 1967). In a recent study, McDowell and Gabel (1981) found significantly smaller social networks for parents of mentally retarded infants as compared to a contrast group of parents of normally developing infants; the difference was due to reduced extended kinship networks. There are many reasons for this isolation. First, the families may be too emotionally and physically exhausted to maintain ties with friends and relatives. Second, the assumed stigma of a retarded child in the family

may lead parents to avoid outside social contacts. Third, others may ostracize the family of a retarded person due to lack of acceptance and understanding. Fourth, such relatives as grandparents may be less able to provide emotional support in the case of the birth of a retarded or handicapped infant, due, in part, to their own grief over the discovery that their grandchild is handicapped (Berns, 1980; Solnit & Stark, 1961). Moreover, the grandparents themselves may need support and may become an additional burden for the parents (Gabel & Kotsch, 1981). Finally, many potential social support agents in the informal network, such as friends or relatives, may be less capable of providing assistance in child care when the child is handicapped due to the need for specialized arrangements for these kinds of children (Gabel & Kotsch, 1981). In view of the heavy reliance on professional assistance in the case of retarded and handicapped children, the role of formal support systems is examined next.

The Impact of Formal Support Systems on Families   In recent years, a number of investigators have recognized the hospital as a provider of social support for parents and, in particular, the postpartum period as a convenient time point for initiating supportive services for parents of infants. Parents are accessible at this point, and motivation for learning about infant development and caregiving skills is often high during this time.

The value of hospital-based programs for mothers is illustrated in the work of Badger, Burns, and Vietze (1981). Teenage mothers who were assumed to be at risk for later parenting problems were recruited in the hospital during the postpartum period and given a series of weekly classes that included instruction in stimulating their infant's social and cognitive skills and information about infant nutrition, family planning, and health care. Results indicated that young teenage mothers (16 years or younger) and their infants profit from this intervention effort. Specifically, the infants of high-risk mothers who attended classes had normal Bayley scores at 1 year, in contrast to a comparison group who had significantly lower Bayley mental scores, emphasizing that social support can indirectly as well as directly affect family members. Furthermore, the mothers who attended the classes were more physically and emotionally responsive to their infants than mothers in the comparison samples. Unfortunately, the relative contribution of the components that may account for the observed differences in infant functioning are unclear.

This early postpartum period can be used effectively to provide support for fathers as well. This is demonstrated by a recent hospital-based study (Parke, Hymel, Power, & Tinsley, 1980). During the mother's postpartum hospitalization, one group of fathers was shown a short videotape that modeled positive father-infant interaction and caregiving involvement with young infants. In comparison to a control group of fathers who did not see the videotape, fathers who viewed the film in the hospital increased their knowledge about infant perceptual abilities, believed more strongly that infants need stimulation, and were more responsive to their infants during feeding and play. Based on diary reports of caregiving activities in the home at 3 months, fathers of boys who saw the film were more likely to diaper and feed their infants than fathers in the no-film control group. In summary, the film intervention significantly modified selected aspects of father behavior and attitudes both in the hospital and through the first 3 months of their infants' lives.

Further evidence of the effectiveness of a film intervention during the postpartum period comes from a recent study by Arbuckle (1983). In this project, Arbuckle used a film intervention developed by Parke et al. (1980). Entitled *Becoming a Family,* the film demonstrated the same behaviors, such as feeding and diapering, playing, and infant capabilities, as were included in the Parke et al. (1980) film intervention. In contrast to the earlier film, this film depicted *both* mothers and fathers actively engaged in caregiving and game playing. Assessment of the impact of the film 4–6 weeks later indicated that first-time fathers who saw the film, in comparison to a no-film control group of fathers, had greater knowledge of infant sensory and cognitive capabilities and were higher

in their perception of the importance of providing infant affection and stimulation. Moreover, the fathers who saw the film reported higher levels of involvement in the daily caregiving of their babies 4–6 weeks after the intervention. No sex of infant differences were reported. Despite the limitation of this study because of its reliance on self-report measures, the similarity of the findings across these two film intervention studies underscores the potential value of this approach for modifying paternal behavior. Further work is clearly justified; particularly important would be studies that isolate the effective components of these film intervention programs.

In a recent study, Dickie and Carnahan (1980) provided training to mothers and fathers of 4- to 12-month-old infants in order to increase parents' competence. Utilizing Goldberg's notion of competence as paternal ability to assess, predict, elicit, and provide contingent response experiences for their infants, these investigators provided eight 2-hour weekly training sessions. Training emphasized individual infant variation, knowledge of the infant's temperament and cues, provision of contingent experiences, and awareness of the infant's effect on the parents. Fathers who had participated in the training sessions, in contrast to fathers who had not participated, increased their interactions with their infants; specifically, they talked, touched, held, attended more, and gave more contingent responses to infant smiles and vocalizations. The infants of the trained fathers sought interaction more than infants of fathers in the control group. However, mothers in the trained group decreased their interactions. In view of this fact that training did increase the judgments of the spouse's competence, it is possible that the wives of the trained fathers encouraged their competent husbands to assume a greater share of the infant care and interactional responsibilities. Interestingly, this finding underlines the reciprocal nature of the mother-father relationship and provides further support for viewing the family as a social system in which the activities of one member have an impact on the behavior of other family members.

Another set of studies illustrates the potential role of health care providers, such as pediatricians, in playing a supportive role for parents of young children. Chamberlin (1979) reports that mothers who participated in an educational program concerning child development during pediatric well-baby visits increased their knowledge of child development and perceptions of being supported in the caregiving role. A second study (Whitt & Casey, 1982) suggests that mothers who were provided with an office-based pediatric intervention program which emphasized physical and preventive child care, developmental norms, and information on infant communication abilities during well-baby exams, demonstrated a more positive relationship with their infants. Again, given the problematic medical status of many premature infants, utilization of pediatric visits as support mechanisms for families of premature infants appears to be a promising form of supportive intervention. Together, these intervention studies illustrate the ways in which such formal institutions as hospitals and other health care facilities can potentially affect infants through the modification of the skills of mothers, fathers, or both parents.

There are many intervention programs for retarded and handicapped infants and children. However, few of these programs are specifically designed to either enlist or assist fathers. In view of this lack of specific attention to fathers, it is not surprising that father participation in programs is very low (Meyer, Vadasy, Fewell, & Schell, 1982). Because of the difficulties that fathers, in particular, have in adjusting to and accepting the birth of a retarded child, it is important to include fathers in future intervention efforts.

Recently, several programs have finally targeted fathers for participation. For example, the University of Washington's Supporting Extended Family Members (SEFAM) is specifically organized to assist fathers of handicapped infants (Meyer et al., 1982; Vadasy, Fewell, Meyer, Schell, & Greenberg, 1984). In a weekly program in which fathers and children meet with male teachers, "fathers learn activities and games that they can enjoy with their

children, share their concerns with other fathers, and learn how to help their family cope effectively with the responsibilities of caring for and educating a child with special needs" (Vadasy et al., 1984, p. 14). A small sample of fathers of handicapped children who had participated in a pilot program for 1–3 years was compared with fathers who had just entered the program. Fathers who had been in the pilot program were less depressed, had more positive feelings about their interactions with their children, and had greater access to social supports than the newly enrolled fathers.

Finally, informal and formal social support systems can often be combined to aid families. Links between formal and informal support systems can assume a variety of forms, such as: 1) strengthening the informal network through formal intervention (Powell, 1979), 2) mobilizing existing social networks in times of stress (Rueveni, 1979), and 3) using informal network members to help individuals utilize formal support services (Olds, 1981).

A number of innovative projects aimed at assisting families of handicapped children have begun to include extended family members in the design of their intervention programs. The Family, Infant, and Toddler Project (Gabel & Kotsch, 1981), which includes bimonthly evening clinics for extended families, has found that parents report that their kin are more understanding and helpful after attending the family clinics. Other programs are beginning to be developed that are aimed at aiding the extended family network in supporting handicapped children and their parents (Berger & Fowlkes, 1980; Olds, 1981). These intervention efforts are consistent with the ecological framework outlined in this chapter. However, the details of the puzzle are only partially clear, and the specific direct and indirect ways in which different types of informal and formal supportive interventions alter families of handicapped and nonhandicapped infants and children are not yet well understood. Descriptive studies of how families spontaneously use and profit from available formal and informal network resources, as well as experimental interventions in which the contributions of specific parts of the network are manipulated, are both useful strategies for future research.

CONCLUSION

As argued in this chapter, in order to understand the development of at-risk infants and children, as well as retarded and handicapped individuals, it is necessary to expand the conceptualization of the "environment." The restrictive use of environment to mean only the mother-infant dyad is no longer adequate. Instead, the father-child relationship as well as the family triad of mother, father, and child merit further examination. In addition, the family is embedded in a set of informal and formal social support systems that can signifi-

cantly modify the interaction of family members and thereby often affect the developing infant and child. A single research strategy aimed at clarifying these issues is insufficient, but a continuing commitment to observational strategies will help increase the quality of research findings in this domain. Although there are similarities in the impact of such different kinds of infants as preterm, handicapped, and retarded on family adaptation, there are differences as well; future research should be carefully designed to assess the differential impact of various types of infants and children on families. In the final analysis, better understanding will lead to more effective strategies for helping at-risk and retarded children and their families.

REFERENCES

Andrew, G. (1968). Determinants of Negro family decisions in management of retardation. *Journal of Marriage and the Family, 30,* 612–617.

Arbuckle, M. B. (1983). *The effects of educational intervention on fathers' relationships with their infants.* Unpublished doctoral dissertation, University of North Carolina, Greensboro.

Badger, E., Burns, D., & Vietze, P. (1981). Maternal risk factors as predictors of developmental outcome in early childhood. *Infant Mental Health Journal, 2,* 33–43.

Berger, M., & Fowlkes, M. A. (1980). Family intervention project: A family network model for serving young handicapped children. *Young Children, 35,* 22–32.

Berns, J. H. (1980). Grandparents of handicapped children. *Social Work, 25,* 238–239.

Birenbaum, A. (1970). On managing a courtesy stigma. *Journal of Health and Social Behavior, 11,* 196–206.

Bradley, R. H., & Caldwell, B. M. (1976). Early home environment and changes in mental test performance in children from 6 to 36 months. *Developmental Psychology, 12,* 93–97.

Bronfenbrenner, U., & Crouter, A. C. (1982). Work and family through time and space. In S. B. Kamerman and C. D. Hayes (Eds.), *Families that work: Children in a changing world.* Washington, DC: National Academy Press.

Brooks, V., & Hochberg, J. (1960). A psychological study of "cuteness." *Perceptual and Motor Skills, 11,* 205.

Brown, J. V., & Bakeman, R. (1980). Relationships of human mothers with their infants during the first year of life: Effects of prematurity. In R. W. Bell & W. P. Smotherman (Eds.), *Maternal influences and early behavior.* Holliswood, NY: Spectrum.

Canning, C. D., & Pueschel, S. M. (1978). An overview of developmental expectations. In S. M. Pueschel (Ed.), *Down Syndrome children: Growing and learning.* Fairway, KS: Andrews & McMeel.

Caputo, D. V., & Mandell, W. (1970). Consequences of

low birth weight. *Developmental Psychology, 3,* 363–383.

Carver, N., & Carver, J. (1972). *The family of the retarded child.* Syracuse:NY: Syracuse University Press.

Chamberlin, R. W. (1979, August). *Effects of educating mothers about child development in physicians' offices on mother and child functioning over time.* Paper presented at the American Psychological Association, New York, NY.

Cochran, M. M., & Brassard, J. A. (1979). Child development and personal social networks. *Child Development, 50,* 601–616.

Cowan, P., & Cowan, C. (1984, August). *The process of family formation.* Paper presented at the Meeting of the American Psychological Association, Toronto, Canada.

Crnic, K. A., Greenberg, M. T., Ragozin, A. S., Robinson, N. M., & Basham, R. B. (1983). Effects of stress and social support on mothers and premature and full-term infants. *Child Development, 54,* 209–217.

Crockenberg, S. B. (1981). Infant irritability, mother responsiveness, and social support influences on the security of infant-mother attachment. *Child Development, 52,* 857–865.

Cummings, S. T. (1976). The impact of the child's deficiency on the father: A study of fathers of mentally retarded and of chronically ill children. *American Journal of Orthopsychiatry, 46,* 246–255.

Dickie, J. R., & Carnanan, S. (1980). Training in social competence: The effects on mothers, fathers and infants. *Child Development, 51,* 1248–1251.

Dickie, J. R., & Matheson, P. (1984). *Mother-father-infant: Who needs support?* Paper presented at the Annual Meeting of the American Psychological Association, Toronto, Canada.

Egeland, B., & Brunnquell, D. (1979). An at-risk approach to the study of child abuse: Some preliminary findings. *Journal of the American Academy of Psychiatry, 18,* 219–235.

Elardo, R., Bradley, R., & Caldwell, B. (1975). The relations of infants' home environments to mental test performance from 6 to 36 months: A longitudinal analysis. *Child Development, 46*, 71–76.

Entwisle, D., & Doering, S.G. (1981). *The first birth*. Baltimore: Johns Hopkins University Press.

Farber, B. (1959). Effects of a severely mentally retarded child on family integration. *Monographs of the Society for Research in Child Development, 24* (Whole No. 71).

Farber, B. (1960). Family organization and crisis: Maintenance of integration in families with a severely mentally retarded child. *Monographs of the Society for Research in Child Development, 25* (Whole No. 75).

Freidman, S. L., & Sigman, M. (Eds.). (1981). *Preterm birth and psychological development*. New York: Academic Press.

Friedrich, W. N. (1979). Predictors of the coping behavior of mothers of handicapped children. *Journal of Consulting and Clinical Psychology, 47*, 1140–1141.

Frodi, A. M., Lamb, M. E., Leavitt, L. A., Donovan, W. L., Neff, C., & Sherry, D. (1978). Fathers' and mothers' responses to the faces and cries of normal and premature infants. *Developmental Psychology, 14*, 490–498.

Gabel, H., & Kotsch, L. S. (1981). Extended families and young handicapped children. *Topics in Early Childhood Special Education, 1*, 29–36.

Gallagher, J. J., Scharfman, W., & Bristol, M. (1984). The division of responsibilities in families with preschool handicapped and nonhandicapped children. *Journal of the Division of Early Childhood, 8*, 3–12.

Goldberg, S. (1979). Premature birth: Consequences for the parent-infant relationship. *American Scientist, 67*, 214–220.

Hetherington, E. M., Cox, M., & Cox, R. (1982). Effects of development on parents and children. In M. E. Lamb (Ed.), *Non-traditional families*. Hillsdale, NJ: Erlbaum.

Holt, K. S. (1957). *The impact of mentally retarded children upon their families*. Unpublished doctoral dissertation, University of Sheffield, England.

Illingworth, R. S. (1967). Counseling the parents of the mentally handicapped child. *Clinical Pediatrics, 6*, 340–348.

Kennedy, J. (1973). The high risk maternal infant acquaintance process. *Nursing Clinics of North America, 8*, 549–556.

Klaus, M. H., & Fanaroff, A. A. (1979). *Care of the high-risk neonate* (2nd ed.). Philadelphia: W. B. Saunders Co.

Klaus, M. H., & Kennell, J. H. (1982). *Parent-infant bonding*. St. Louis, MO: C. V. Mosby Co.

Kopf, R. C., & McFadden, E. L. (1974). Nursing intervention in the crisis of newborn illness. *Journal of Nursing Midwifery, 16*, 629–636.

Kopp, C. (1983). Risk factors in development. In P. H. Mussen (Ed.), *Handbook of child psychology* (Vol. 2). New York: John Wiley & Sons.

Lamb, M. E. (1981). *The role of the father in child development* (2nd ed.). New York: John Wiley & Sons.

Lamb, M.E. (1984). Fathers of exceptional children. In M. Seligman (Ed.), *A comprehensive guide to understanding and treating the family with a handicapped child*. New York: Grune & Stratton.

Legeay, C., & Keogh, B. (1966). Impact of mental retardation on family life. *American Journal of Nursing, 66*, 1062–1065.

Leiderman, P. H. (1981). Human mother-infant social bonding: Is there a sensitive phase? In K. Immelman, G. W. Barlow, L. Petrinovich, & M. Main (Eds.), *Behavioral development*. New York: Cambridge University Press.

Leiderman, P. H. (1982). Social ecology and childbirth: The newborn nursery as environmental stressor. In N. Garmezy & M. Rutter (Eds.), *Stress, coping, and adaptation*. New York: McGraw-Hill.

Leiderman, P. H., & Seashore, M. J. (1975). Mother-infant separation: Some delayed consequences. *Parent-infant interaction*. (CIBA Foundation Symposium 33). Amsterdam: Elsevier.

Lewis, M., & Feiring, C. (1981). Direct and indirect interactions in social relationships. In L. Lipsitt (Ed.), *Advances in infancy research* (Vol. 1). New York: Ablex Publishing Corporation.

Lonsdale, G. (1978). Family life with a handicapped child: The parents speak. *Child: Care, Health, and Development, 4*, 99–120.

Marion, R. L. (1981). *Education, parents, and exceptional children*. Rockville, MD: Aspen Systems Corporation.

McDowell, J., & Gabel, H. (1981). *Social support among mothers of retarded infants*. Unpublished manuscript, George Peabody College, Nashville.

Meyer, D. J., Vadasy, P. F., Fewell, R. R., & Schell, G. (1982). Involving fathers of handicapped infants: Translating research into program goals. *Journal of the Division for Early Childhood, 5*, 64–72.

Old, D. L. (1981). The prenatal/early infancy project: An ecological approach to prevention. In J. Belsky (Ed.), *In the beginning: Readings in infancy*. New York: Columbia University Press.

Parke, R. D. (1978). Parent-infant interaction: Progress, paradigms, and problems. In G. P. Sackett (Ed.), *Observing behavior: Theory and applications in mental retardation*. Baltimore: University Park Press.

Parke, R. D. (1981). *Fathers*. Cambridge, MA: Harvard University Press.

Parke, R. D., Grossman, K., & Tinsley, B. R. (1981). Father-mother-infant interaction in the newborn period: A German-American comparison. In T. M. Field, A. M. Sostek, P. Vietze, & P. H. Leiderman (Eds.), *Culture and early interactions*. Hillsdale, NJ: Lawrence Erlbaum Associates.

Parke, R. D., Hymel, S., Power, T. G., & Tinsley, B. R. (1980). Fathers and risk: A hospital-based model of intervention. In D. B. Sawin, R. C. Hawkins, L. O. Walker, & J. H. Penticuff (Eds.), *Psychosocial risks in infant-environment transactions*. New York: Brunner/Mazel.

Parke, R. D., & O'Leary, S. E. (1976). Father-mother-infant interaction in the newborn period: Some findings, some observations, and some unresolved issues. In K. Riegel & J. Meacham (Eds.), *The developing individual in a changing world: (Vol 2). Social and environmental issues*. The Hague: Mouton.

Parke, R. D., Power, T. G., & Gottman, J. M. (1979). Conceptualizing and quantifying influence patterns in the family triad. In M. E. Lamb, S. T. Suomi, & G. R. Stephenson (Eds.), *Social interaction analyses: Meth-*

odological issues. Madison: The University of Wisconsin Press.

Parke, R. D., & Sawin, D. B. (1976). The father's role in infancy: A re-evaluation. *The Family Coordinator, 25,* 365–371.

Parke, R. D., & Sawin, D. B. (1980). The family in early infancy: Social interactional and attitudinal analyses. In F. A. Pedersen (Ed.), *The father-infant relationship.* New York: Praeger Publishers.

Parke, R. D., & Tinsley, B. R. (1982). The early environment of the at-risk infant: Expanding the social context. In D. Bricker (Ed.), *Intervention with at-risk and handicapped infants: From research to application.* Baltimore: University Park Press.

Parke, R. D., & Tinsley, B. R. (1984). Historical and contemporary perspectives on fathering. In K. A. McCluskey & H. W. Reese (Eds.), *Life-span developmental psychology: Historical and generational effects.* New York: Academic Press.

Parke, R. D., Tinsley, B. R., & Volling, B. (1982). *The development of the preterm infant and social support utilization.* Unpublished manuscript, University of Illinois, Champaign-Urbana.

Pascoe, J. M., Loda, F. A., Jeffries, V., & Earp, J. A. (1981). The association between mothers' social support and provision of stimulation to their children. *Developmental and Behavioral Pediatrics, 2,* 15–19.

Pastor, D. L. (1981). The quality of mother-infant attachment and its relationship to toddlers' initial sociability with peers. *Developmental Psychology, 17,* 326–335.

Powell, D. R. (1979). Family-environment relations and early child-rearing: The role of social networks and neighborhoods. *Journal of Research and Development in Education, 13,* 1–11.

Rueveni, U. (1979). *Networking families in crisis.* New York: Human Services Press.

Sameroff, A. (1982). The environmental context of developmental disabilities. In D. Bricker (Ed.), *Intervention with at-risk and handicapped infants.* Baltimore: University Park Press.

Slade, C. I., Redl, O. J., & Manguten, H. H. (1977). Working with parents of high-risk newborns. *Journal of Obstetric and Gynecologic Nursing, 6,* 21–26.

Smith, C., Leiderman, P. H., Selz, L., MacPherson, L., & Bingham, E. (1981). *Maternal expectations and developmental milestones in physically handicapped infants.* Paper presented at the Biennial Meeting of the Society for Research in Child Development, Boston, MA.

Solnit, A. J., & Stark, M. H. (1961). Mourning and the birth of a defective child. *Psychoanalytic Study of the Child, 16,* 523–537.

Stern, M., & Hildebrandt, K. A. (1984). Prematurity stereotype: Effects of labeling on adults' perceptions of infants. *Developmental Psychology, 20,* 360–362.

Stoneman, Z., Brody, G. H., & Abbott, D. (1983). In-home observations of young Down Syndrome children with their mothers and fathers. *American Journal of Mental Deficiency, 87,* 591–600.

Tallman, I. (1965). Spousal role differentiation and the socialization of severely retarded children. *Journal of Marriage and the Family, 27,* 37–42.

Tew, B. J., Lawrence, K. M., Payne, H., & Rawnsley, K. (1977). Marital stability following the birth of a child with spina bifida. *British Journal of Psychiatry, 131,* 79–82.

Tinsley, B. R., Johnson, P., Szczypka, D., & Parke, R. D. (1982, March). *Reconceptualizing the social environment of the high-risk infant: Fathers and settings.* Paper presented at the International Conference on Infant Studies, Austin, TX.

Unger, D. G. (1979). *An ecological approach to the family: The role of social networks, social stress and mother-child interaction.* Unpublished master's thesis, Merrill-Palmer Institute, Detroit, MI.

Unger, D. G., & Powell, D. R. (1980). Supporting families under stress: The role of social networks. *Family Relations, 29,* 566–574.

Vadasy, P. F., Fewell, R. R., Meyer, D. T., Schell, G., & Greenberg, M. T. (1984). Involved parents: Characteristics and resources of fathers and mothers of young handicapped children. *Journal of the Division for Early Childhood, 8,* 13–25.

Vietze, P. M., Abernathy, S. R., Ashe, M. L., & Faulstich, G. (1978). Contingent interaction between mothers and their developmentally delayed infants. In G. P. Sackett (Ed.), *Observing behavior: Theory and applications in mental retardation.* Baltimore: University Park Press.

Walker, J. A. (1982). Social interactions of handicapped infants. In D. Bricker (Ed.), *Intervention with at-risk and handicapped infants.* Baltimore: University Park Press.

Whitt, J. K., & Casey, P. H. (1982). The mother-infant relationship and infant development: The effect of pediatric intervention. *Child Development, 53,* 948–956.

Yogman, M. W. (1982). Development of the father-infant relationship. In H. Fitzgerald, B. Lester, & M. W. Yogman (Eds.), *Theory and research in behavioral pediatrics* (Vol. 1). New York: Plenum Publishing Corp.

Yogman, M. W. (1984, May). *Fathers and preterm infants.* Paper presented at the Conference on Transitions to Fatherhood, Washington, DC.

Chapter

7

Research on
Mentally Retarded Parents

Stephen Greenspan and Karen Schlueter Budd

A CHAPTER DEALING WITH mentally re-
tarded parents appears, on its face, to have little
place in a volume dealing mainly with families
whose children are mentally retarded. A case
can be made, however, for including such a
chapter if one considers that the most salient
characteristic of the offspring raised by both
sets of parents is that they are "at risk." That
is, children in both types of families have a
less-than-average chance of developing into
fully competent adults. In fact, the children of
mentally retarded parents are equally, if not
more, "handicapped" in their long-run development than are all but the most severely neu-
rologically or mentally impaired youngsters.
Investigators dealing with both types of parents
are, therefore, equally engaged in the task of
identifying factors that may contribute to favorable or unfavorable outcomes for children
whose chances of successful adaptation to life
are jeopardized by some environmentally or
intrinsically based handicap. Furthermore, researchers dealing with both types of parents are
equally motivated by a desire to understand
more adequately how to give the parents of
such at-risk children the supports and skills
needed to cope with the responsibilities of par-

enthood in the face of greater-than-average
challenges and stresses. A second link between
the topic of mentally retarded parents and the
topic of families with children who are mentally retarded comes from the increasing likelihood (due to deinstitutionalization) that those
children will grow up to become sexually active adults. Thus, many mentally retarded children will some day be mentally retarded parents. Researchers and clinicians working with
the parents of these children will need to address this issue at some point.

The study of mentally retarded parents is, in
one respect, a very new issue and, in another
respect, a very old one. It is a new issue in that
only recently, with the advent of the deinstitutionalization movement, are mentally retarded
adults beginning to engage in the "nor-
malized" activity of raising a family. It is an
old issue, however, in that an initial motivation for constructing those same institutions
from which mildly retarded adults are now
being deinstitutionalized was the fear over the
genetic and societal consequences of allowing
people considered mentally deficient to pro-
create (Wolfensberger, 1975). The life histories of mentally retarded individuals (es-

pecially females) in this century is, thus, largely one of living in the community during the childhood years, being institutionalized after attainment of puberty and the first signs of sexual activity, and deinstitutionalization after the attainment of menopause or, in many cases, after sterilization has been carried out.

Ironically, one of the functions formerly performed by institutionalized mentally retarded women was to care for the young children who had been placed in those same settings. In one of the most famous natural experiments in the field of child development research, Skeels and Dye (1939) reported that mentally retarded women in a state institution served as surrogate parents for infants who were later placed in adoptive homes. This study, in which these children turned out to have normal developmental outcomes when compared to infants raised in institutions for children, is typically cited to indicate the deleterious effects of orphanages. However, relatively little note has been made of the study's other lesson; namely, that mentally retarded women are often capable, at least in the infancy period, of functioning adequately as child caregivers.

ADEQUACY OF
MENTALLY RETARDED PARENTS

Concern over the adequacy of caregiving provided by mentally retarded parents has undoubtedly been the central issue addressed in research and policy studies. In line with mental retardation research in general (Baumeister, 1967), the majority of studies have utilized a comparative paradigm in which mentally retarded parents are compared with average-IQ parents on one or more indices of parental adequacy (cf. Schilling, Schinke, Blythe, & Barth, 1982). Not surprisingly, these studies have tended to find that mentally retarded parents are, as a group, less adequate than nonretarded parents on a variety of outcomes, including observed adequacy of parenting behaviors, development of their children, or the actions taken by protective agencies. As pointed out, however, in reviews by Budd and Greenspan (1984), Fotheringham (1980), and Mira and

Roddy (1980), virtually all studies have found a sizeable percentage of mentally retarded parents to be functioning either within, or close to, normal limits, especially when compared to parents with similar demographic characteristics. Furthermore, studies have also found, contrary to stereotypes held by many professionals, that many mentally retarded parents are capable of benefiting from therapeutic and educational interventions intended to increase their child-rearing adequacy (Budd & Greenspan, in press).

Based on the finding that mentally retarded parents do not constitute a homogeneous class of equally incompetent individuals, the authors argue that researchers should lessen their heavy reliance on a comparative paradigm and instead should make greater use of correlational methods that examine sources of variance within the population of mentally retarded parents. This latter approach, which seeks to define the factors that contribute to competence or incompetence in mentally retarded parents, is more likely to enhance practical intervention efforts than is research that only measures the competency of mentally retarded parents.

Underlying much of the earlier research (and legal statutes) involving mentally retarded parents was, undoubtedly, a concern over the genetic transmission of intellectual inferiority. Such a concern is less socially acceptable today than it was 20 or 30 years ago and is, consequently, less likely to be expressed overtly. This shift in attitudes reflects, in part, greater public valuation of handicapped individuals and their rights (Wolfensberger, 1975) and, in part, greater scientific understanding of the baselessness of the eugenics movement and of the complexities involved in the inheritance of intelligence and other human behaviors (Plomin, DeFries, & McClearn, 1980).

The diminution of interest in the genetic transmission of mental retardation has also undoubtedly been influenced by a narrowing of the mental retardation construct and a consequent shrinkage in the population of parents likely to be viewed as mentally retarded. The adoption by the American Association on Mental Deficiency (AAMD), almost 25 years ago, of its dual diagnostic criteria (Heber, 1961) changed the definition of mental retardation from one based solely on IQ to one also requiring deficits in "adaptive behavior" (ability to maintain oneself independently and to engage in socially acceptable behavior). In a more recent change (Grossman, 1973), the AAMD lowered the IQ cutting score from minus one standard deviation (IQ=85) to minus two standard deviations (IQ=70). These two alterations had the effect of narrowing the mentally retarded population to only include individuals with more pervasive and severe deficits, in contrast to the broader population with which much of the existing research on mentally retarded parents was conducted.

Perhaps in part because mentally retarded parents now tend to be more globally incompetent than before, researchers now writing about the topic are most likely to emphasize the potentially negative consequences for the children. Such consequences go beyond the cultural transmission of cognitive impairment, but also include a concern about inadequate physical protection and discipline. Because of the observed heterogeneity of characteristics of mentally retarded adults (even given the dual diagnostic criteria, which are often ignored in practice), one cannot predict, on the basis of IQ, the precise pattern of strengths or deficits a mentally retarded parent will exhibit in terms of socialization skills or, for that matter, other areas of adult functioning. This problem is further exacerbated by the fact that, because of physical and social limitations associated with having an IQ below about 50, virtually all the low-IQ adults who have children or who have the option of having children are classified as "mildly retarded." Various studies (Bass, 1963; Borgman, 1969; Brandon, 1957; Sheridan, 1956) have pointed out how difficult it is to separate out, for this group, variance contributed by low intelligence from variance contributed by poverty or low socioeconomic status. There is not a sharp discontinuity in parental competence between adults whose IQs fall just above or below the 70 cutting score, just as there is not a sharp discontinuity between those parents considered "retarded"

and those considered "disadvantaged" or "neglectful."

This overlap in distributions of mentally retarded and nonretarded parents reflects, to a large extent, the fuzziness of the mental retardation construct itself and the lack of adequate, or consensually agreed on, definitional criteria. Because low IQ is associated with low socioeconomic status, and because the adaptive behavior criterion is honored more in the breach than in the observance, the decision to label a low-IQ individual as mentally retarded is a sometimes arbitrary exercise. Because many children formerly labelled "educable mentally retarded" in school are now labelled "learning disabled," it makes little sense for investigators interested in parents labelled mentally retarded to exclude from their focus parents with other diagnostic classifications.

In short, the main reason to conduct research on parents labelled mentally retarded is because there is a high likelihood that many such parents (and their children) will be at high risk. Such research (which is perhaps more appropriately conducted by investigators interested in socialization than by investigators interested in mental retardation) is useful not because it is likely to tell us anything of interest about mental retardation, but rather because it is likely to tell us something interesting about parental competence and its implications for the development of children.

A HEURISTIC MODEL LINKING CAREGIVING TO "INTELLIGENCE"

Given the desirability of adopting a multivariate assessment approach, it may be useful to discuss the dimensions of caregiver competence and to link these dimensions with aspects of intelligence in which adults labelled mentally retarded might or might not be found lacking. A model of intelligence proposed by E. L. Thorndike (1920) and used by the first author to write about personal and social competence (Greenspan, 1979, 1981) contains three components: conceptual intelligence (cognition and language), practical intelligence (mechanical and self-maintenance ability), and social intelligence (understanding of people and their behavior). These dimensions of the broad construct of intelligence can be seen as providing a base for attaining competence/incompetence in the three most widely discussed modes of child socialization: teaching, child care, and discipline.

As indicated in Figure 1, the first mode of child socialization—teaching (socialization of linguistic and cognitive development)—depends on that aspect of parental intelligence referred to as "conceptual intelligence." Because this is the aspect of intelligence most relied on in classifying an individual as mentally retarded—it is the aspect of intelligence measured by IQ tests—it is also the feature of child socialization in which mentally retarded parents, as a group, are likely to be most consistently lacking. Developmentally oriented investigators, because of their interest in cognitive development, have tended to focus on this mode of socialization when conducting research on mentally retarded parents and their children. Thus, the well-known intervention studies of Heber and Garber (1975) and Ramey and associates (Ramey, Holmberg, Sparling & Collier, 1977) have been attempts to promote normal cognitive development in young children at risk because of growing up with impoverished mothers who have low IQs.

The second mode of child socialization—child care (socialization of healthy physical development)—depends on that aspect of parental intelligence referred to as "practical intelligence." There are numerous cognitive operations involved in providing adequate child care. Mentally retarded parents, because of limitations in their reasoning processes, often commit such serious errors of judgment as providing nutrition inappropriate for young children, allowing young children to go unattended in potentially dangerous places, paying inadequate attention to children's medical needs, and so forth. Given the preoccupation that child protective agencies seem to have with the adequacy of children's physical environment and upbringing, it is not surprising that much of the research on mentally retarded parents done by social welfare and legal schol-

ars has tended to focus on this aspect of their competence/incompetence, especially in relation to the issue of termination of parental rights.

The third mode of child socialization—discipline (socialization of personality and socioemotional development)—depends on that aspect of parental intelligence referred to as "social intelligence." Because mentally retarded adults often are limited in their ability to take the perspectives of others or to understand the motives or behavior of others (Greenspan, 1979), it is not surprising that they are often quite inept at providing adequate discipline. Given their focus on children's social behavior as an outcome variable of interest, and the great deal of work that has been done in developing technologies for training parents in effective discipline, behaviorally oriented researchers, when working with mentally retarded parents, have tended to concentrate on discipline as the aspect of caregiving competence in which they are most interested (Peterson, Robinson, & Littman, 1983; Pomerantz, 1982).

The authors believe that the caregiver competence model presented above offers a potentially useful framework for addressing, both empirically and clinically, some of the issues involved in work with mentally retarded parents. One obvious benefit of the model is to point out the need to adopt a comprehensive framework in determining the caregiving adequacy of low-IQ parents. As indicated, researchers have tended to concentrate on that aspect of caregiving in which they have the most interest. The most satisfactory strategy, however, in fully understanding whether or not a parent is capable of socializing a child effectively, is to assess systematically the parent's competence in the three socialization modes of teaching, child care, and discipline.

Unfortunately, the study of child rearing is still sufficiently undeveloped so that there are neither valid measures nor, for that matter, clear-cut definitions of what constitutes minimally adequate caregiving. Only in the area of child care, because of the potential for injury and death arising from unhealthy or unsafe physical care, are professionals able to achieve

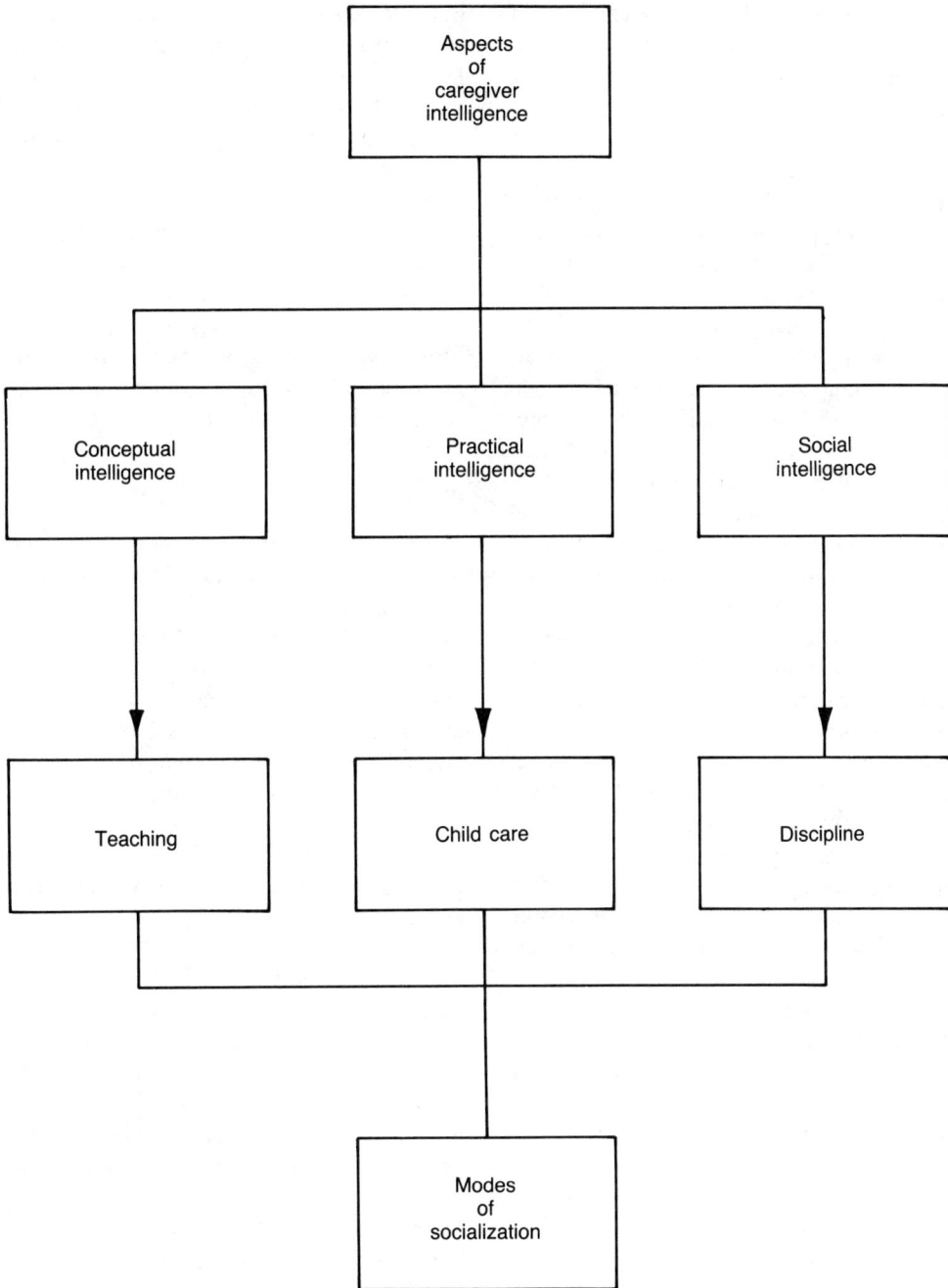

Figure 1.   A model of caregiver intelligence and socialization competence.

some degree of consensus in labelling a particular home as unsuitable. For this reason, termination of parental rights of mentally retarded parents is almost always based on failure to provide adequate physical care. This is perhaps as it should be, for it would be a serious infringement on civil liberties in this country if middle-class professionals were to threaten the parental rights of all adults whose children, in the professionals' judgment, were not being competently taught or disciplined by their parents.

Nevertheless, parents who are labelled "mentally retarded" are at a distinct disadvantage in dealing with the child protective system because many professionals have the tendency to take almost for granted that the parents will be incompetent in all aspects of child rearing. The caregiving model, and the model of intelligence underlying it, may be of use in combatting that assumption. For just as it is a fallacy to assume that low conceptual intelligence predicts low practical and social intelligence, so too is it a fallacy to assume that less than optimal ability to stimulate cognitive and linguistic development predicts inadequacy in the areas of child care and discipline. Most studies of the child-rearing adequacy of persons labelled mentally retarded, including many who were formerly institutionalized, have found a significant minority who function quite normally as parents, particularly when demographic factors are taken into account (Budd & Greenspan, 1984; Fotheringham, 1980; Mira & Roddy, 1980). These findings are usually based on global judgments or on the actions of child protective agencies. A comprehensive assessment, tapping all three socialization modes, would provide a more differentiated picture of the level and sources of variability in child-rearing competencies of adults labelled as mentally retarded.

Because mental retardation is a condition marked by deficits in thinking and problem solving (in the three modes of abstract logic, everyday living, and social behavior), mentally retarded individuals—whatever their capabilities or deficits in noncognitive aspects of personal competence—are relatively likely to exhibit poor judgment in dealing with child-rearing situations. One final implication of the cognitive model of child-rearing presented earlier, therefore, is that more effort should be made to develop assessment tools that tap cognitive operations underlying incompetent child-rearing behaviors of mentally retarded as well as nonretarded parents. Such assessment

devices, which would most likely rely on the use of hypothetical problem situations requiring a role-played solution, have been only infrequently used because of a pervasive belief that they lack the validity of in-vivo behavioral observations. Cognitive measures of parenting have, however, been found to have considerable predictive validity (cf. Greenspan, 1978), perhaps because it is possible in such measures to set up situations that occur only infrequently in real life (and only rarely in the presence of observers), but yet have special significance for determining the ability of an individual to socialize children adequately.

ISSUES IN NEED OF INVESTIGATION

The bulk of research with mentally retarded parents has been epidemiologic in nature, identifying the extent to which adults of low IQ exhibit deviant caregiving behaviors or their children experience negative developmental outcomes. As indicated earlier in this chapter, the authors believe that researchers should reorient their work toward acquiring a better understanding of why some mentally retarded parents achieve positive outcomes whereas others do not. Following are a few brief suggestions for ways in which such work might be pursued.

Parent Training Interventions

Relatively little research has been conducted into the factors contributing to successful interventions with mentally retarded parents. In a recent review of behaviorally oriented parent training programs involving mentally retarded parents (Budd & Greenspan, 1984), the authors found that some modifications of usual intervention methods are needed when working with such parents; specifically, a much broader and longer-term investment of therapist energy is needed. A survey conducted of therapists involved in interventions with mentally retarded parents revealed that nearly one-half showed moderate to extensive success with referral problems. This finding is encouraging, given the long-standing tendency of many therapists to write mentally retarded parents off as "untrainable." The same survey, however, indicated more limited impact on overall parenting competence and on transfer of acquired skills to novel situations. Much additional research is needed into the issues of designing effective training methods, enhancing generalized benefits of training, and evaluating the relative effectiveness of different modes of training.

Interactions between Retarded Parents and Protective Agencies

Mentally retarded parents often function under the close scrutiny of child protective agencies, who are quick to intervene at the first sign of problems. Although such scrutiny is often necessary and helpful, it sometimes results in the application of stricter standards of accountability toward mentally retarded parents than might be applied to "normal" parents. The problem is often exacerbated by the poor judgment shown by mentally retarded parents interacting with agencies and their frequent failure to understand the importance of making a positive impression on child protective personnel. It would be useful to learn more about the degree of understanding that mentally retarded parents have of the role of protective agencies and the degree to which they can anticipate the effect that their behavior has on the judgments and recommendations of those workers.

Role of Mentally Retarded Fathers

As is often the case in research on the socialization of at-risk children (cf. Budd & O'Brien, 1982), the study of mentally retarded parents has consisted, by and large, of the study of mentally retarded mothers. The role of fathers is, however, of obvious potential importance in determining the effectiveness of the family in coping with the demands of child rearing. Partial support for this assertion came in the authors' survey of parent training efforts, which found that mentally retarded fathers' initial competence in child rearing was predictive of positive parent training outcomes (Budd & Greenspan, in press). It appears that research on the role of mentally retarded fathers is a fruitful and largely untapped area for research activity.

Environmental Supports and Stresses

For mentally retarded parents, as for non-retarded parents, the amount of stress and the available support network that exists for coping with stress probably affect parenting competence. Such factors as marital conflict, depression, poverty, aversive extrafamilial contacts, and physical health problems have been shown to be associated with greater child-rearing difficulties and poorer responsiveness to parent training efforts in nonretarded parents (Griest & Forehand, 1982; Wahler, 1980). Mickelson's (1947) descriptive examination of families with retarded parents suggests that many of these same factors relate to the quality of care by mentally retarded parents. The number of children in the family also appears to be an important factor in some cases. Many retarded parents cope fairly adequately with one child, but are less adequate in coping with the greater responsibilities of additional children (Mickelson, 1947; Shaw & Wright, 1960).

The nature of environmental stresses and how they interact with parenting competence bears further investigation with mentally retarded parents. An important part of this research involves discovering the supports available to some families that alleviate or diminish the otherwise negative effects of stress factors. These supports may derive from community organizations (such as a local Association for Retarded Citizens), relatives, or friends and neighbors. It has been observed (Zetlin, Weisner & Gallimore, in press) in particular, that grandparents often play an especially important role in raising the children of mentally retarded children, as they do with the children of other marginal parents, such as teenagers. Edgerton (1967, p. 172) has referred to these supportive persons as "benefactors," whose involvement may play a substantial role in fostering the successful adaptation of mentally retarded adults to community life. More research is needed into the role that relatives and other benefactors can play in helping mentally retarded adults function as parents.

Developmental
Understanding of Retarded Parents

One hypothesis worthy of testing in research is the possibility that mentally retarded parents may overestimate the developmental capabilities of young children. Such an overestimation may explain the finding in the authors' survey of parent training professionals (Budd & Greenspan, 1984) that mentally retarded parents frequently treat their children in a too-old fashion, but very rarely in a too-young fashion. This phenomenon, which might be called "underprotectiveness," may be responsible for much of the behavior considered neglectful by child protective agencies. Also contributing to this underprotectiveness may be a difficulty by mentally retarded parents in foreseeing the negative consequences of potentially dangerous behaviors of young children. Because the most salient characteristic of mentally retarded parents is their inadequate understanding and judgment, it seems fruitful for researchers to pursue the possible cognitive underpinnings of much of the behavior that causes these parents to be perceived as inadequate.

The Phenomenon
of Developmental Jealousy

Reflecting the statistical phenomenon of regression to the mean, the children of mentally retarded parents tend to be significantly brighter than their parents. Thus, for many mentally retarded parents, the time will come when their children will acquire skills (such as reading) that they do not have. The authors have observed that some mentally retarded parents seem to be jealous of their child. Although this jealousy is often triggered by the attention that the child is likely to receive from other adults, it is possible that some of the parents' apparent jealousy is more existential in nature, reflecting sadness over their own failure to achieve full cognitive and social maturity. This phenomenon, which might be termed "developmental jealousy," is not limited to mentally retarded parents, but may be presumed to underlie the coolness toward children that can

sometimes be observed among various categories of disabled adults. To the authors' knowledge, no research has been conducted into this phenomenon. It would appear to be an issue worthy of investigation, especially given the possibility of making it the focus of affectively based interventions.

SOME METHODOLOGICAL
CONSIDERATIONS

The methodology of research with mentally retarded parents has tended to be relatively unsophisticated. Following are a few suggestions for how such work might be strengthened.

Appropriate Comparison Groups

Although one can question, as the authors did earlier, the use of comparative paradigms as an end in themselves in mental retardation research, there are obvious reasons why it is often useful to include a comparison group when conducting research on mentally retarded parents. Such groups help put in perspective the normative quality of the behaviors of many mentally retarded parents. It is important, however, to use comparison groups that are matched on important demographic characteristics, such as socioeconomic status. It might also be useful to compare mentally retarded parents with parents of other diagnoses, such as mental illness or learning disabilities, or whose children are at risk for other forms of disability. For example, Peterson et al. (1983) compared mentally retarded parents with both "normal" parents and parents of behavior problem children and found the inclusion of the clinical comparison group to be particularly useful.

Need to Replicate Earlier Work

One of the problems facing anyone who tries to summarize the published research literature dealing with mentally retarded parents is that most of that work was done at a time when the mentally retarded label was much more freely assigned. Therefore, it is difficult to know how relevant those earlier findings are to the current population of mentally retarded parents. It would be a positive contribution, therefore, for investigators to replicate some of the earlier research, using subjects who fit more closely the current definition of mental retardation.

Avoid Biased Samples

Most of the research with mentally retarded parents has been negatively biased by primarily using subjects who were formerly institutionalized, who were on the rolls of social service and judicial agencies, or who continued to be known in adult life as disabled. Given the fact that many individuals known in childhood or adolescence as mentally retarded cease to be identified as such in adulthood (Mercer, 1973), it is likely that there are many more low-IQ adults functioning adequately as parents than is reflected in the research literature. Investigators should, therefore, make an effort to include in their samples earlier-labelled individuals who are not currently clients of social service agencies. An ideal method for conducting such research would be through prospective longitudinal studies, although it is possible to use follow-back retrospective methods for identifying appropriate samples for current study.

Focus on Sources of Variance

A point alluded to earlier, but worthy of restatement, is that investigators should place less emphasis on questions of central tendency (i.e., how retarded parents differ from non-retarded parents) and more on questions of variability (i.e., why some retarded parents are more competent than others). The latter approach is, in the authors' opinion, more likely to result in findings that have implications for public policy and clinical practice. One way of pursuing such an approach would be to study groups of retarded parents, matched on IQ, but differing significantly in their level of adaptation to parenthood. Another way would be to utilize multivariate techniques capable of teasing out complex relationships between independent and dependent variables. Regardless of the methodology used, however, investigators should incorporate into their work an understanding of the considerable heterogeneity

in parenting competence within the class of individuals labelled mentally retarded.

Use Observational Methods

Virtually none of the research involving mentally retarded parents has used naturalistic observational methods. Instead, studies have reported demographic or historical facts about the family, measures of the physical home environment, or descriptive accounts by protective service workers as data sources about family functioning. These methods provide useful information, but they do not document empirically what mentally retarded parents actually do, or do not do, that marks them as competent or incompetent caregivers. To obtain the latter information, it would be highly useful to conduct direct observations of ongoing parent-child interactions and record specific behaviors as they occur. Sample responses of interest include parents' positive or negative attempts to control the child, appropriateness of disciplinary methods (both to the child's age and to the situation at hand), consistency of consequences for child behavior, provision of adequate care and attention to the child's safety, and so forth.

POLICY RECOMMENDATIONS

Although research on mentally retarded parents has not been voluminous, it is possible to draw some conclusions from it regarding directions for action by legislatures and social service organizations. These public policy implications are spelled out briefly below.

Avoid Automatic Termination of Parental Rights

There are still many states in which the label "mental retardation" assigned to a parent by a social service professional is sufficient grounds for terminating the custody rights of that parent (Hertz, 1979; Wald, 1975). Such a practice is, in the authors' opinion, no longer justifiable, in light of the consistent finding of considerable variability in parenting competence within the class of adults labelled mentally retarded, and the considerable amount of overlap in parenting and other forms of competence across the distributions of individuals labelled retarded and those not bearing that label. For decision-making purposes regarding legal custody, it seems as prejudicial to deny parental rights to individuals with low IQ as it would be to deny them on the basis of race, income, or any other demographic factor that might be correlated with undesirable outcomes for children.

Focus on the Welfare of the Child

The authors are not "bleeding hearts" who believe that mentally retarded parents should be allowed to retain custody of their children at all costs; indeed, the pendulum has sometimes swung too far in the direction of nonintervention-tionism. Although recent support for the rights of mentally retarded parents is a healthy development, one important criterion for judging the viability of any such arrangement should continue to be the welfare of the child. Through contacts both with parent training professionals and with mentally retarded parents, the authors have developed a deep appreciation of the great incompetence of many mentally retarded parents and of the overwhelming difficulties involved in working with them. Noting that a substantial minority of mildly retarded parents do have some competence does not gloss over the fact that a sizeable majority do not. The authors' premise, therefore, is not that all mentally retarded parents should be allowed to retain custody of their children, but that each case should be determined on its own merits and without regard to the mental retardation label. Decisions about termination of parental rights should take into account the parents' ability to provide at least adequate (although not necessarily ideal) care for the child.

Provide Counseling When Needed

Mentally retarded adults, whether parents or not, often have needs for counseling that are not being adequately met. These range from lingering feelings of sadness and anger over previous sterilization and terminations of custody, to extremely dysfunctional sexual relationships, lack of knowledge of family planning methods, and confused ideas about whether and why to have children. One obvious policy recommendation, therefore, is to make available to mentally retarded adults counseling services intended to help them deal with mental health and informational aspects of present or past parenthood.

Use Creative Approaches to Intervention

Because mentally retarded parents are likely to exhibit broad skill deficits and to have difficulty in transfering newly acquired skills, it is necessary to devise unique parent training models. These models may not be appropriate for the wider population of parents, either because of their high cost, the great amount of therapist interference in family matters, or their lack of relevance to treatment goals. A number of existing treatment models have been described in an earlier publication (Budd & Greenspan, 1984). Three approaches that might be effective are described briefly below. Only the first approach has actually been tried with mentally retarded parents.

This approach, which has been piloted in Massachusetts by Robb, Weiss, and their colleagues (Robb & Weiss, 1981), uses a day care center as a training environment for mentally retarded parents. The parents serve as day care workers and receive training in child care skills under professional supervision. This model offers the opportunity to teach a wide variety of basic child-rearing procedures to more than one parent at a time and to observe parents' acquisition of the skills in a supervised setting.

A second potentially useful approach involves a temporary live-in training program where therapists provide up to 24 hours a day of intervention to teach basic child care skills. The inspiration for this proposed approach is the "Homebuilders" program in Tacoma, Washington (Kinney, Madsen, Fleming, & Haapala, 1977), which provides up to 6 weeks of live-in crisis intervention to families of delinquent or out-of-control children in an attempt to prevent family dissolution. By living in the home of a mentally retarded parent and child, the therapist could provide moment-to-moment training and support on child management and care, as well as on related responsibilities of organizing and operating a household.

A third potential approach is a group home model, in which a small number of mentally retarded parents and their children could live together for a period of time in a supervised training setting. This approach, which derives from the same rationale as group homes for mentally retarded adults without children, would provide a protective environment for individuals in need of training and supervision while allowing for shared responsibilities and support. Although such family-style group homes have been tried with other marginal parents (primarily adolescents), it has not, to the authors' knowledge, been tried with parents identified as mentally retarded.

The virtues of all three approaches, and of other training models that might be devised, are that they all provide an opportunity for interventions that are more intense than usual and that are more ecologically valid than are interventions carried out in clinics or office settings.

Educate Protective Service Workers

Child protective service workers are legally responsible for investigating child abuse and neglect allegations, referring families for appropriate treatment, and in some cases providing training in discipline or child care. Mentally retarded parents pose special difficulties for case workers, in that their parenting inadequacies may often result from pervasive skill deficits, rather than from carelessness, lack of interest, or ill will. Child protective professionals who work with mentally retarded parents should obviously possess some understanding of mental retardation, yet it is the authors' experience that relatively few workers possess the requisite background or training. Thus, there is the ever-present danger that child protective professionals will misinterpret as "bad" (and therefore to be punished) behaviors by mentally retarded parents that are more appropriately described as "dumb" (and amenable to change, or at least more deserving of compassion).

A familiarity with mental retardation, in addition to making child protective professionals

more tolerant, might also cause them to change their intervention methods. For example, it has been noted by experienced parent therapists that intervention efforts with mentally retarded parents can benefit from the use of paraprofessionals, involvement of fathers, development of a broadly based relationship outside the teaching role, and restraint for exerting excessive control during home visits (Budd & Greenspan, in press). Although empirical evidence for the relative effectiveness of these methods is currently lacking, these approaches may provide useful guidelines for child protective workers to use when working with mentally retarded and other low-functioning clients.

CONCLUSION

This chapter may be seen as a reaction against the historic tendency to generalize about mentally retarded people as a class and to lose sight of the considerable individuality and variability within that class. Researchers, practitioners, and legal authorities have tended to act toward mentally retarded parents in terms of global stereotypes, rather than in terms of their individual characteristics. Regardless of the truth of those stereotypes, there is such widespread variability among the category of adults labelled mentally retarded that they must be viewed and treated as individuals. Virtually all these recommendations regarding methodological, conceptual and policy issues flow from this simple but fundamental point.

The issue of parenthood for mentally retarded adults is profoundly troubling for many people, including some who are sympathetic to the normalization movement. It is difficult enough for mentally retarded adults to care for their own needs, these people argue, without subjecting them to the added stress of parenthood. Furthermore, most mentally retarded parents are so unprepared for the demands of parenthood that the consequences for the development and well-being of the children involved are quite unfortunate.

The authors' response to these arguments is to say that allowing individuals labelled as mentally retarded to exercise their desire to participate in the life-giving process is the ultimate test of living in a free and humane society. Obviously, parenthood is not a good idea for many people, and there is no reason why certain individuals should not be counseled against becoming parents. People labelled mentally retarded have usually demonstrated incompetence in other situations and thus may reasonably be expected to show incompetence as parents. Yet, the same argument can be applied to a sizeable percentage of the human race. It is incumbent on us as researchers and clinicians to figure out how, if, and when we can help people with intellectual deficits to function adequately as parents, rather than to write them off as unsuitable candidates for parenthood or, for that matter, other adult social roles merely because of their deficits.

REFERENCES

Bass, M. S. (1963). Marriage, parenthood, and prevention of pregnancy. *American Journal of Mental Deficiency, 68*, 320–335.

Baumeister, A. A. (1967). Problems in comparative studies of mental retardates and normals. *American Journal of Mental Deficiency, 71*, 864–875.

Borgman, R. D. (1969). Intelligence and maternal inadequacy. *Child Welfare, 48*, 301–304.

Brandon, M. W. G. (1957). The intellectual and social status of mental defectives. *Journal of Mental Science, 103*, 710–738.

Budd, K. S., & Greenspan, S. (in press). Parameters of successful and unsuccessful interventions with mentally retarded parents. *Mental Retardation.*

Budd, K. S., & Greenspan, S. (1984). Mentally retarded mothers. In E. A. Blechman (Ed.), *Behavior modification with women,* New York: Guilford Press.

Budd, K. S., & O'Brien, T. P. (1982). Father involvement in behavioral parent training: An area in need of research. *The Behavior Therapist, 5*, 85–89.

Edgerton, R. B. (1967). *The cloak of competence: Stigma in the lives of the mentally retarded.* Berkeley: University of California Press.

Fotheringham, J. B. (1980). Mentally retarded persons as parents. Unpublished manuscript. (Available from North York General Hospital, 4001 Leslie Street, Willowdale, Ontario M2K 1E1).

Greenspan, S. (1978). Maternal affect-allowance and limit-setting appropriateness as predictors of child adjustment. *Genetic Psychology Monographs, 98*, 83–111.

Greenspan, S. (1979). Social intelligence in the retarded. In N. R. Ellis (Ed.), *Handbook of mental deficiency: Psychological theory and research* (2nd ed.) (pp. 483–531). Hillsdale, NJ: Lawrence Erlbaum.

Greenspan, S. (1981). Defining childhood social competence: A proposed working model. In B. K. Keogh (Ed.), *Advances in special education* (Vol. 3). Greenwich, CT: JAI Press.

Griest, D. L., & Forehand, R. (1982). How can I get any parent training done with all these other problems? The role of family variables in child behavior therapy. *Child and Family Behavior Therapy, 4*, 73–80.

Grossman, H. (1973). *Manual on terminology and classification in mental retardation.* Washington, DC: American Association on Mental Deficiency.

Heber, R. A. (1961). *Manual on terminology and classification in mental retardation.* Washington, DC: American Association on Mental Deficiency.

Heber, R., & Garber, H. (1975). The Milwaukee project: A study in the use of family intervention to prevent cultural-familial mental retardation. In B. Z. Friedlander, G. M. Sterritt & G. E. Kirk (Eds.), *Exceptional infant: Vol. 3. Assessment and intervention* (pp. 399–433). New York: Brunner/Mazel.

Hertz, R. A. (1979). Retarded parents in neglect proceedings: Erroneous assumptions of parental inadequacy. *Stanford Law Review, 31*, 785–805.

Kinney, J. M., Madsen, B., Fleming, T., & Haapala, D. A. (1977). Homebuilders: Keeping families together. *Journal of Consulting and Clinical Psychology, 45*, 667–673.

Mercer, J. R. (1973). *Labelling the mentally retarded: Clinical and social system perspectives on mental retardation.* Berkeley: University of California Press.

Mickelson, P. (1947). The feebleminded parent: A study of 90 family cases. *American Journal of Mental Deficiency, 51*, 644–653.

Mira, M., & Roddy, J. (1980). Parenting competencies of retarded persons: A critical review. Unpublished manuscript. (Available from Children's Rehabilitation Unit, University of Kansas Medical Center, Kansas City, KS 66103).

Peterson, S. L., Robinson, E. A., & Littman, I. (1983). Parent-child interaction training for parents with a history of mental retardation. *Applied Research in Mental Retardation, 4*, 329–342.

Plomin, R., DeFries, J. C., & McClearn, G. E. (1980). *Behavioral genetics: A primer.* San Francisco: W. H. Freeman.

Pomerantz, D. (1982, June). Programming effectively for mentally retarded parents and their families. Paper presented at American Association on Mental Deficiency, Boston. (Available from Special Education Dept., State University College at Buffalo, Buffalo, New York 14222).

Ramey, C. T., Holmberg, M. C., Sparling, J. J., & Collier, A. M. (1977). An introduction to the Carolina Abecedarian Project. In B. M. Caldwell & D. J. Stedman (Eds.), *Infant education for handicapped children* (pp. 101–121). New York: Walker.

Robb, W., & Weiss, F. C. (1981). Training retarded parents as behavior change agents. Unpublished manuscript. (Available from Eunice Kennedy Shriver Center, 200 Trapelo Road, Waltham, Mass. 02154).

Schilling, R. F., Schinke, S. P., Blythe, B. J., & Barth, R. P. (1982). Child maltreatment and mentally retarded parents: Is there a relationship? *Mental Retardation, 20*, 201–209.

Shaw, C. H., & Wright, C. H. (1960). The married mental defective: A follow-up study. *Lancet, 30,* 273–274.

Sheridan, M. D. (1956). The intelligence of 100 neglectful mothers. *British Medical Journal, 1,* 91–93.

Skeels, H. M., & Dye, H. B. (1939). A study of the effects of differential stimulation on mentally retarded children. *The Journal of Psycho-Asthenics, 44,* 114–136.

Thorndike, E. L. (1920). Intelligence and its uses. *Harper's Magazine, 140,* 227–235.

Wahler, R. G. (1980). The insular mother: Her problems in parent-child treatment. *Journal of Applied Behavior Analysis, 13,* 207–219.

Wald, M. (1975). State intervention on behalf of "neglected" children: A search for realistic standards. *Stanford Law Review, 27,* 985–1040.

Wolfensberger, W. (1975). *The origin and nature of our institutional models.* Syracuse, NY: Human Policy Press.

Zetlin, A. G., Weisner, T. S., & Gallimore, R. (in press). Diversity, shared functioning, and the role of benefactors: A study of parenting by mentally retarded persons. In S. K. Thurman (Ed.), *Children of handicapped parents,* New York: Academic Press.

Chapter

8

Families Who Adopt Mentally Retarded Children

Who, Why, and What Happens

Laraine Masters Glidden

ALTHOUGH BOTH psychologists and sociologists have studied families with retarded children for several decades now, it has become commonplace for recent reviews to suggest that we still know little about the functioning of such families (Crnic, Friedrich & Greenberg, 1983). Sometimes this knowledge gap is blamed on the dearth of studies in this particular area and sometimes on the field in general, which has failed to focus its efforts on combining the study of the individual within the family ecological system (Belsky, 1981; Lerner & Spanier, 1978). Both developmental psychologists and family sociologists have been faulted for not engaging in the sort of cross-fertilization that would produce a vigorous interdisciplinary approach to the study of families with mentally retarded children.

Recent work in the field has attempted to address these criticisms by focusing on the re-

tarded child as a member of a dynamic family unit that is itself a member of a still larger dynamic societal/economic/political network (e.g., Chapter 1, Chapter 9). This work will undoubtedly begin to prove fruitful as models are developed that incorporate the complex interaction of individuals with family members, and family units with other societal institutions and networks.

The work described in this chapter, however, is a reformulation in a different sense. It does not take a broad ecological approach to the study of families, but it does depart from the traditional stress models that prevail when studying families with retarded children. Because the families of interest—those who have adopted rather than biologically borne retarded children—undergo a rather different life experience involving the entrance of a retarded child into their family, it is reasonable to pre-

Preparation of this chapter was supported in part by faculty development grants from St. Mary's College of Maryland. Data were collected while the author was on sabbatical leave and affiliated with The Family Research Unit, London Hospital Medical College, London E.1, England. Appreciation goes to my colleagues there for their support and advice and to the many fine agency workers and adoptive families whose cooperation was essential to the conduct of this research.

dict that their subsequent life experiences are also different from families with biological retarded children. Before turning to the adoptive families who are the focus of the research described in this chapter, the literature on family reactions to biological handicapped children is briefly reviewed. This review, as well as a summary of prior work in the adoption of handicapped children, provides a context for interpretation of the results of the current study.

FAMILY REACTIONS TO BIOLOGICAL HANDICAPPED CHILDREN

Investigators have traditionally viewed the presence of a retarded child in the family as crisis-producing, often inducing lifelong stress and distress. The literature is replete with terms such as "chronic sorrow," Olshansky's (1962) label for the presumably pervasive and enduring reaction suffered by parents of a mentally retarded child. Other writers have focused only on the initial reactions of shock, disbelief, anger, denial, despair, and mourning for the fantasized, but lost, perfect child (see Parks, 1977, for a summary of this work) and have suggested that the end of the process comes when parents start to accept the child, become attached to it, and begin to meet its needs, as well as those of the rest of the family. If and when this final adjustment is made, it precipitates a crisis of a different sort, one involved in the reality of caring for a difficult-to-care-for child. Writers have separated these two types of crises by referring to the former as a tragic crisis or a personal values crisis and the latter as a role organization crisis or a reality crisis. Existential crisis may be the best label for the initial reaction because there seems to be general agreement that its components include feelings of despair, meaninglessness, questioning of identity, and so forth. Reality crisis seems appropriately descriptive of the latter reaction.

There seems to be little general consensus in the literature about how profound and long lasting the existential crisis is and what parental, child, or circumstantial factors operate to ame-

liorate or prolong it. For example, Olshansky's proposal that parents of retarded children feel chronic sorrow has little substantive data to support it. His original paper was an essay based on personal, clinical experience, and others have written from a similar perspective (Ballard, 1978; Wright, 1976). Indeed, later work indicates that the greatest distress is at the initial diagnosis of mental retardation and that, although stress and sadness do also occur later, they tend to be experienced periodically, rather than continuously (Wikler, Wasow, & Hatfield, 1981).

In addition to the lack of consensus, there has been a general tendency to treat tentative and unreplicated findings as conclusive and to overstate the negative impact of the retarded child. For example, the now classic work of Farber and his colleagues usually has been cited as indicating a more negative reaction to a severely mentally retarded child than the data warrant. Farber (1959) compared the marital integration of families who had institutionalized their retarded children with that of those who kept them at home. The only near-significant result he found was that, for parents with low marital integration before the child was born (marital prediction score), institutionalizing a boy was associated with higher marital integration than keeping the boy at home. This finding did not pertain for girls nor for families with high marital integration before the birth of the retarded child. Similarly, in Farber (1960) there were no overall significant differences in mean marital integration of parents with a retarded child in an institution and parents with a retarded child at home.

Another of Farber's (1959) findings that has been often quoted and somewhat overemphasized for its negative impact is the effect of a retarded child on the normal siblings. He found that the maternal ratings of personality traits of normal sisters of the retarded child are significantly higher if the retarded child is institutionalized. What rarely is reported, however, is that this effect holds only if the retarded child is under 10 and that the reverse effect occurs for normal brothers (i.e., their personality ratings are higher if the retarded sibling stays at home). Because none of Farber's work uses non-retarded controls, it is impossible to draw any conclusions about stress and negative adjustment in comparison to what the normative family experiences. Indeed, a number of investigators have questioned, given the clinical nature of many of the studies in this field, the biases of those conducting them, and the scarcity of work utilizing comparison groups, whether there is any chronic negative impact on the family of having a retarded child (Booth, 1978; Friedrich & Friedrich, 1981; Voysey, 1975).

One of the better and more recently conducted studies in this area attempted to compare parents of handicapped children with those of matched, nonhandicapped children on a number of psychosocial measures. Friedrich and Friedrich (1981) studied 34 families of children who were either mentally and/or physically handicapped and a control group of 34 families matched for family income, maternal age, and family size who had nonhandicapped children of a similar age (mean CA≅9 years). Mothers completed five different self-rating scales, including the Holroyd Questionnaire on Resources and Stress (QRS), which measures 15 different dimensions relevant to families caring for a dependent member (Holroyd, 1974). Friedrich and Friedrich concluded that the mothers with handicapped children reported a less satisfactory marriage, less religiosity, and less psychological well-being than the mothers with nonhandicapped children. They reported significantly more child problems, such as difficult personality characteristics, social obtrusiveness, and occupational limitations; significantly more parent problems, such as poor health/mood, excess time demands, and negative attitudes; and significantly more difficulties in family functioning, such as lack of family integration and limits on family opportunity. Indeed, of 19 different dependent variables measured, only 3 failed to demonstrate significant group differences: Mothers of handicapped children did not report more pessimism, more financial problems, nor more lack of social support on

the Holroyd than did mothers of nonhandicapped children.

In contrast, Gath (1977), studying only Down syndrome children, found very few differences between their families and families with normal children matched for child age, social class, and family structure. Physical health, psychiatric illness, and family activity were comparable for the two groups. There was a significantly higher rate of marital breakdown or serious marital disharmony among the families of the Down syndrome children, but positive measures of the marital relationship were also higher. Gath points out that almost half of the parents of Down syndrome children indicated that their marriage had become stronger, rather than weaker, following the birth of the handicapped child. This finding would be consistent with a model that suggested that preexisting family and individual characteristics strongly influence the impact a retarded child will have on the adaptation of the family unit. Friedrich (1979) examined some of these preexisting characteristics in his attempt to predict the coping behavior of mothers of handicapped children. Using the Holroyd QRS as the criterion variable, and 19 predictor variables (e.g., severity of child's disability, child's sex, religiosity, marital adjustment), he found only three variables that significantly predicted coping behavior and that accounted for 46% of the total variance. The most significant of these three was the mother's degree of marital satisfaction and feelings of security in the marital relationship. In addition, less stress was reported by mothers whose handicapped child was at home, rather than in an institution, and more stress was reported by mothers of a female, rather than a male, handicapped child. Not only were more severe disabilities not associated with more stress, but, in fact, there was a significant negative correlation between these two variables. The finding relating to marital satisfaction is not surprising and is comparable to the findings of Farber's early work. The findings on institutionalization and sex of child are not congruent with previous work, and although they might be explained on a post hoc basis (e.g., stressed families are more likely to institutionalize a handicapped child) they clearly need replication before they can be taken seriously.

Holroyd's own work with her questionnaire has consistently demonstrated that the scale discriminates among different types of caregivers and dependent mothers. For example, in Holroyd (1974), mothers, more than fathers, reported poorer health or mood and limitations in freedom and personal development. Mothers of retarded children were more concerned about overprotection or dependency problems than mothers of emotionally disturbed children. Holroyd and McArthur (1976) compared mothers of autistic, Down syndrome, and outpatient clinic children. The mothers of autistic children reported more personal and family problems than mothers of children in the other two groups, but mothers of Down syndrome children did not report more problems than mothers of outpatient clinic children. This last finding is of particular interest, because it suggests, along with Gath's (1977) data, that the reality of caring for a Down syndrome child may not be as stressful as many writers have assumed it to be.

These reality concerns or crises, also, may be neither unending nor immutable. For example, Birenbaum (1971), in an interview study of 103 mothers of retarded children, found, as others have done, that the women described many difficulties in both adjusting to the birth of a handicapped child and to the strain of raising a handicapped child. They also, however, described benefits. One respondent said, "Well, at times I felt like the sacrificial lamb. And at other times I felt very happy. It brought my husband and I very close" (p. 60). Another mother described the satisfaction she received in watching her retarded daughter develop and learn. In response to a question about changes in the situation since the child's retardation was first diagnosed, 75% of the respondents said things were better or much better than before, usually because the child was increasingly able to fit into family routines. Burden (1980) conducted a longitudinal study of 25 mothers who received home-based therapy for their severely handicapped infants. Whereas almost half (46%) of the mothers had been depressed immediately after the birth of their handicapped child, only 21% were still depressed 2 years later. Furthermore, although the author is properly cautious given the nature of the data and the comparison group, there is the suggestion that the mothers who received extra support services showed greater improvement than did the control mothers.

Darling (1979) also discusses these themes in her book about 22 families with children having birth defects, most of whom were retarded. She reports that, although the initial reactions of guilt and self-pity that follow the diagnosis are usually intense, they are also usually short-lived. For example, one mother said, "As time goes on, you fall in love. You think, 'This kid's mine, and nobody's gonna take her away from me!' I think by the time she was 2 weeks old I wasn't appalled by her anymore" (p. 136). Although some mothers reported having a breakdown when the child was young, they all reported an improvement in mood and health that seemed related to their involvement in either formal or informal support groups. Some parents said that initially they had wanted their handicapped child to die, but all described the gradual growth of love. Darling concludes that, although marital and family disintegration may be one consequence of the birth of a handicapped child, the opposite effect is just as probable. She analyzes this effect as in part a result of the creation of the family with a handicapped child as an in-group, in contrast to the out-group of the rest of society. The negative reactions of the out-group may serve to create in-group cohesiveness.

In summary, then, many studies have described the immediate negative impact on the parents of discovering their child is handicapped, an impact that frequently precipitates an existential crisis. Other studies have looked at the way families adjust and cope in the long run to the reality crises of rearing what may be a more-difficult-to-rear-than-normal child. This latter work has frequently found both positive and negative effects of having a handicapped child in the family. Often-reported positive effects include strengthening marital and family relations; increasing compassion, love, meaning, purpose, and understanding; and enhancing life for the sibling. Negative effects are frequently extensions of the reactions during the existential crises (e.g., unresolved guilt, anger, lowered self-esteem), but also include reality demands of time involvement, expense, and extensive and unrelenting physical caregiving. None of the published work has attempted to untangle the adjustment to the existential crises from the adjustment to the reality crises. This untangling, of course, would be most difficult to accomplish in the biological family where the reality crises begin almost immediately after the diagnosis of handicap while the family is embroiled in the acute stages of its existential crisis. It is not only a temporal simultaneity, however, that creates the inextricability. Clearly, parents who are guilty, embittered, grieving, and angry are not going to perceive and react to reality crises in the same way as parents who are not so suffering. Thus, the realities of caring for a mentally retarded child, for example, may seem far more burdensome to the parent who is still mourning her or his perfect baby and finds it difficult to form an attachment to the marred substitute that took its place.

Nonetheless, there are methods that should help differentiate the results of the existential and reality crises. One technique is to study the existential crisis as an independent variable and examine its relationship to the reality crisis. For example, if one could rate the intensity and duration of distress of the biological family following the diagnosis of handicap and then also measure the amount of stress and strain in actually caring for the handicapped child, the relationship between the two might be clarified. To the author's knowledge, no investigator has used this method.

A second approach is, in a sense, a subset of the first. If one could locate families who are rearing mentally retarded children and thus would be involved with the reality concerns, but who had not experienced any existential crises following the diagnosis of their child,

then the two reactions would be readily separable. Such parents would be highly unusual and perhaps nonexistent among the biological families of retarded children, but should be very common, indeed virtually universal, among those families who had adopted retarded children. Such families would have made a conscious and voluntary decision to rear a handicapped child; they would have known about the handicap and would have some information about how to cope with it before their reality concerns began. Thus, whatever reality crises adoptive parents experience should be a "pure" consequence of the reality of caring for a difficult child and not a result of unresolved existential conflicts. Despite the potential power of this approach, there are very few published reports studying families who have adopted handicapped children.

FAMILIES WHO ADOPT MENTALLY RETARDED CHILDREN: PREVIOUS WORK

The need for adoptive parents of handicapped children has been recognized for several decades. Fradkin, writing in 1958, described both the negative characteristics (e.g., being rejected for a normal child), as well as the positive ones, (e.g., extreme flexibility), that might motivate parents to consider adopting a handicapped child. Yet, as late as 1977, Krisheff wrote that essentially no information was available on the attitudes, policies, or practices of agencies regarding the adoption of mentally retarded children. Nonetheless, retarded children are being adopted in increasingly greater numbers than in previous years. Although there are no accurate national data available in the U.S., some representative data from Great Britain are of interest. Between 1979 and 1981 the British Agencies for Adoption and Fostering, a national clearinghouse for hard-to-place children, reported more than a doubling of the number of retarded children placed through them. More particularly, the number of Down syndrome children placed quadrupled in that 2-year period (British Agencies for Adoption and Fostering, 1983).

Given then that there are families adopting mentally retarded children, do we know from previous work what characteristics, if any, typify those families and whether they experience the difficulties of rearing a retarded child reported by the biological parents of retarded children? The answer is a dramatic and resounding "no." Based on her experiences in social work, Gallagher (1968) described what *should* be the characteristics of parents who adopt retarded children. She listed such qualities as patience, flexibility, reasonable expectations, and knowledge of mental retardation. Although her list has face validity, there is very little published research that describes what, if any, characteristics are shared by parents who do adopt retarded children. Indeed, an extensive bibliographic search uncovered only two studies, published or unpublished, that provided any empirical data.

Gath (1983) described 11 families who knowingly adopted or were long-term foster parents for mentally retarded children. Seven of the children had Down syndrome. The parents were older; the mothers' mean age would have been 44 at the time their adopted/fostered child was born. Three of the 11 parents were widowed women; the remainder were married couples rated as having a good quality marriage. Five of the 11 families had fostered children before, and 2 had a biological handicapped child. Eight of the families had biological children, and in five of these cases, the children were already adult and independent. None of the 11 mothers was rated as having significant psychiatric problems. In contrast, 20% of the mothers in a comparison sample of families with biological mentally retarded children had significant psychiatric problems. Indeed, Gath described the foster/adoptive parents as ones who have "unusually strong personalities, stable relationships and an outward-looking attitude combined with a high degree of determination" (p. 39).

De Leon and Westerberg (1980) examined the records of one agency to compare 21 families who had adopted retarded children with 58 families who had adopted nonretarded children over a 3.5-year period. They examined nine variables, all of which were adoptive parent characteristics: physical handicap, unusual appearance, religious behavior, experience with children, marital status, educational status, occupational status, working/nonworking at time of application, and age. They found that persons adopting retarded children tended to be more unusual in appearance (e.g., over- or underweight, having severe dental problems, to be less well educated, and not to be two-parent working families). The authors concluded that the people who usually may not be favored by adoption agencies may be the ones most likely to adopt retarded children. They do not speculate whether this finding may be the result of agency policy (i.e., giving "less qualified" parents "less desirable" children), or parental self-selection.

Two other studies have examined the adoption of children with medical problems. In Franklin and Massarik's work (1969 a, b, c), mentally retarded children were specifically excluded. However, some of their findings may be relevant, particularly those pertaining to the children with severe medical conditions, where extensive rehabilitation and home treatment may be needed. For example, children with severe medical problems were more likely to be adopted by families where the mother was over 40, where there were biological children already in the family, and where the families were in a lower social class. It is important to note, however, with regard to the social class finding, that 31% of the families who adopted severely impaired children were in the professional/managerial classes. Indeed, the authors concluded that there are two rather different prototypical adoptive families. One is less well educated and less achievement-oriented, seeing their child as just a child. The other is highly educated, affluent, and very achievement-oriented. Parents in this latter family type saw themselves as being motivated by the desire to help a child who needed help.

Wolkind and Kozaruk (1983) also studied the adoption of children with medical problems, but they did not exclude retarded children from their sample. Indeed, of the 84 families that they interviewed, 12 children or 14%, were considered to be either retarded or significantly developmentally delayed at the time of placement. A number of family characteristics of this subset of 12 deserve mention. First, in comparison to the "usual" adopter, these families were less likely to be in the professional classes. No family was in the highest social class in Great Britain, Registrar General (RG) 1, and three families were in RG 4, semiskilled work. Second, most of the families had prior familiarity with handicap, either through work or personal experience. This characteristic was particularly true for the families who adopted children whose retardation was definite and likely to be moderate or severe, (e.g., Down syndrome). In fact, all these families specifically wanted to adopt a handicapped child, in contrast to many of the other families who wanted to adopt a child, but were willing to consider a handicapped child.

Some of the above work also looked at the outcome of the adoption. Gath (1983) reports that the foster/adoptive parents of the Down syndrome children in her sample found great rewards in what they were doing and that the children had fewer behavior problems than those who had been institutionalized. Franklin and Massarik (1969b) reported that 71% of the adoptive parents of children with severe medical problems felt that the family had not been adversely restricted nor influenced by the child's condition. However, parents of children with more severe medical problems, in contrast to less severe ones, were more likely to indicate the defect as a cause of stress in the family. Hockey (1980) reports a similar finding. In his study of 137 mentally retarded adopted children, almost 25% of the families were experiencing serious problems. He also states that this finding is particularly true for the more severely retarded children. His sample size for these categories is very small, however, so that his conclusions should be regarded with caution.

In Wolkind and Kozaruk's study (1983), the responding parents were asked some specific questions that pertained to the success of the adoption. Raters were able to categorize the adoption outcome as being at one of three success levels: 1) highly successful, would definitely do it again; 2) uncertain success, some regrets about doing it; and 3) definite regrets, would not do it again. Of the 12 families described above, 11 were scored as category 1, and 1 was scored as category 2. Thus, these families viewed the adoption of their children in a very positive way.

In summary, then, although there is very little substantive work by other researchers on the adoption of retarded children, there are suggestions that people who adopt such children are: 1) usually familiar with handicap; 2) not as highly educated as other adopters; 3) experienced child rearers; and 4) frequently motivated to adopt a handicapped child specifically. Other characteristics have not been systematically studied. In addition, all three studies that have looked at outcome found that the large majority of parents view the adoption as successful and the relationship between parent and child as positive.

FAMILIES WHO ADOPT MENTALLY RETARDED CHILDREN: THE PRESENT STUDY

The present study is an outgrowth of this previous work. Its major objectives were to: 1) describe demographic characteristics (e.g., age, educational level, social class, religious affiliation, and so forth of families who adopt mentally retarded children); 2) explore the preadoption motivation of the parents (i.e., how and why did they come to be adoptive parents of retarded children); and 3) assess the postadoptive adjustment of the families.

Subjects

The subjects were 43 British families who had among them adopted 57 retarded children. One family refused to participate, leaving 42 families and 56 children in the final sample. Thirty-six of the families were married couples at the time of interview; six were headed by single women.

All but five families were identified through the adoption agencies that had been instrumental in placing the children. The remaining five families were referred by one of the other families in the sample. Although the participation rate was 98%, the sample cannot be considered either random or unbiased. Agencies with a reputation for placing handicapped children were contacted more than were others. Because more severely handicapped children are usually more difficult to place, the sample consists almost entirely of children who are retarded because of a definite organic etiology. Thirty-three of the children were Down syndrome, and 19 others had some other chromosomal, genetic, or organic problem directly relating to the mental retardation. In only four of the children was there no diagnosed exogenous retardation, and even in these children, there were family and medical histories that were not inconsistent with organic involvement (e.g., epilepsy).

The children went to live with their adoptive families when they were, on average, 54 months old. This mean, however, masked a wide range of 0–198 months. Similarly, although the children were, on average, 79 months at the time of this study, their ages ranged from 8 to 210 months. There were an almost equal number of girls (27) and boys (29).

Method

All interviews, except one, were done in the homes of the adoptive families. All 42 mothers were interviewed either alone or with the fathers. The present report, however, focuses only on data obtained from the mothers.

The interview was semistructured, focusing on three primary areas of interest. The first section was concerned with preadoption motivation and how the mother or family had made the decision to adopt and how that decision led to the adoption of the target child or children. The second section dealt with the background of the family, particularly the parents and their extended family. The third section contained many detailed questions about the impact of the adopted retarded child on family functioning. The completion of the interview schedule itself took from about 1.5 hours to 5 hours, depending on the number of target children in the family, how elaborative the respondent(s) was, and how many interruptions were necessary. Although some coding of the interview schedule was done at the time of interview, with the permission of the respondents all interviews were tape recorded and coding was also done from tapes.

Following completion of the interview schedule, the respondents were asked to complete two questionnaires. One, an adaptation of that designed by Farber (1959), consisted of 10 multiple-choice questions, assessing functioning of the respondent after the placement of the child in the family. This short questionnaire was completed by respondents immediately following the interview. The second questionnaire was the Questionnaire on Resources and Stress designed by Holroyd (1974) to assess functioning in families caring for a handicapped, dependent member. It consists of 285 true-false statements and was analyzed along the 15 different dimensions suggested by Holroyd. These questionnaires were left with the respondents, along with a stamped, addressed envelope for return. They were completed and returned by the mothers for 88% of the 56 children.

Results and Discussion

Demographic and Background Characteristics Social status was measured by the Registrar General's index of occupations. Father's occupation was used, except in the six instances where the adopter was an unmarried woman, in which case her occupation was used. The Registrar General system has six divisions, RG 1 and 2 being professional; RG 3 being skilled work either nonmanual (3 NM) or manual (3 M); RG 4 being semiskilled work; and RG 5 being unskilled work. As in other adoption studies (Raynor, 1980; Wolkind & Kozaruk, 1983), the majority of the families were in RG 1 or 2 (55%); 33% of the families were in RG 3, and the remaining 12% were in RG 4. Although this sample is more professional than the British population in general, it is also less skewed toward RG 1 than the general adoptive population. Only 5 of the 42 families (12%) were in RG 1 at the time of the placement, whereas other adoption studies report higher percentages (e.g., Jaffee & Fanshel, 1970 = 38%; Raynor, 1980 = 22%). As would be expected, given the occupational status of the adopters, educational level was also high. In England, a three-tier classification system is most appropriate to categorize education: 1) school leaving without passing any examinations; 2) certification by some examination system (there are several); and 3) college or university education. Using this tripartite system, 67% of the mothers had passed some school examinations, and 64% had some college or university training. The fathers were similarly well educated, with 76% of them having passed school examinations and 61% having some college or university training.

Most of the families lived within 125 miles of London, but with 90% living in either suburban or rural areas and only 10% in urban areas. Sixty-nine percent of the adopters owned the home in which they were living.

The majority of the respondents—57% of the women and 58% of the fathers—described their religious affiliation as Church of England. The next largest group—14% of the mothers and 11% of the fathers—were affiliated with Roman Catholicism. Four couples and one wife preferred the designation Christian to any denominational affiliation, four couples were members of other Christian churches, and three couples said that they had no religious affiliation.

Most families had either work or personal experience and familiarity with handicap. Four of the 42 families had had at least one biological handicapped child, and one family had previously adopted a "normal child" who turned out to have a handicapping condition. In 28 of the families, either one or both parents had work experience with handicapped persons, (e.g., nursing, special education). In only six cases, or 14% of the sample, was there neither a personal nor an occupational familiarity with handicap.

Twenty-two of the 42 families, or 52%, had at least one living biological child. However, in four families those children were the moth-

er's by a previous marriage. These adoptive couples had no biological children with each other. Including these four couples and five unmarried women, 24 adoptive parents had no biological children.

Preadoption Motivation   There were various motivations to adopt. Twenty-six of the 42 adopters, or 60%, had specifically wanted a handicapped child. Of these 26 adopters, 9 had no biological children, although one couple had already adopted two other children who were nonhandicapped at the time of their adoption. Of the 16 adopters who did not initially seek a handicapped child, 11, or 69%, were childless, in contrast to the 42% of the childless adopters who wanted a handicapped child from the beginning. Table 1 presents the frequencies for families with and without biological children (excluding three families with previously adopted nonhandicapped children) and whether they initially sought to adopt a handicapped child. A chi-square analysis of these data confirms the impression that the ratios of initially wanting or not wanting a handicapped child were different for families already with biological children in comparison to families without biological children.

The 26 adopters who initially wanted to adopt a handicapped child had many different idiosyncratic reasons for their preference. One mother had worked in a residence for physically handicapped children 15 years before her child's placement and had vowed that if ever in a position to do so she would adopt such a child. The child placed with her was both physically and mentally handicapped. In another family, both husband and wife worked as nurses' aides in an institution for the retarded and decided that they specifically wanted to

Table 1. Preadoption motivation: Biological children and initial desire to adopt a handicapped child

Initially wanted handicapped child	Families with biological children	Families without biological children
Yes	17	8
No	3	11

adopt a Down syndrome child, because they so enjoyed the residents with Down syndrome with whom they worked. One couple, with two biological children, had talked for several years about their desire to provide a loving family life to a child who desperately needed one. Then the mother saw a newspaper advertisement for a particular handicapped child, and called the adoption agency to make an inquiry; although that advertised child was already unavailable, they eventually adopted a different retarded child.

The 11 childless adopters who did not seek a handicapped child initially had a primary motivation of wanting a family, but in contrast to many persons who want a family, they were willing to consider a retarded child as a family member. Sometimes this willingness clearly came from a familiarity with handicap, sometimes from a religious or world view of the importance of nurturance for all humans, and sometimes from a seemingly naive or matter-of-fact perception of the child as "not all that different from normal."

Religion was a motivating factor for a substantial minority of adopters. Twenty-four percent of the adoptive mothers mentioned it as an important influence. These same mothers also attended church at least once a week and saw themselves as more religious than the average Briton.

Postplacement Adjustment Although the semistructured interview contained several dozen questions relating to postplacement family functioning, only the results of the two global assessments of the placement are considered here:

1. All things considered, has _____'s adoption worked out: Better than you expected, about as well as you expected, or less well?
2. Thinking back over your entire experience with _____, and all the good times and the bad times—if you had it to do over again, do you think you'd adopt _____, would you not adopt him/her, or are you unsure?

Each of these questions was coded on a 3-point scale, with 3 being the best outcome category and 1 being the worst. Of the 56 children placed, 33, or 59%, received a total score of 6, indicating that their mother thought that the adoption had worked out better than expected and she would do it again. An additional 15 children (27%) received combined scores of 5; of these, 13 were rated a 2 on question 1 (adoption had worked out as well as expected) and a 3 on question 2. Thus, it can be concluded that the adoptions of 46, or 82%, of the children were definitely successful. In two of the remaining ten cases, the combined scores were only 2, meaning that the adoption was worse than expected and the family would not do it again. Indeed, in one of these families the placement was disrupted, and the child had left the home just prior to the interview. Interestingly, in both of these "worst" cases, the children were over 10 at the time of placement. The remaining eight cases are less extreme. In six families, the target child was one of two or more mentally retarded children who had been adopted. In five of these six families the adjustment to the first child had been fine, with the adjustment to the second, more recently placed child, being somewhat problematic. In regard to the overall success of the placement, only two mothers, the ones who received scores of 2, said that they would not adopt the target child again. For 86% of the children, the mother indicated she would definitely adopt the child if she had it to do over again.

Responses to the Farber questionnaire also show remarkably little difficulty in coping with the problems of a handicapped child. This questionnaire consisted of 10 items, 8 of which could be scored on a positive-neutral-negative 3-point scale. The questions consisted of the general format, "Since _____ was placed, I'm (more, less, about as *patient*) as I was before." The author assigned a -1 for change in negative direction, 0 for no change, and a $+1$ for change in a positive direction.

Table 2 presents the mean ratings for each of the eight items that were scored in this way. Mothers perceived themselves as generally becoming more patient, having more friends, being happier, having generally changed for the better, and getting along better with their husband. For worry, nervousness, and anger,

Table 2. Adoptive mother responses to Farber Questionnaire for 55 target children

Item	Mean[a]	Percentage of responses with no change
Patient	.40	36
Friends	.31	69
Worry	.05	65
Nervous	−.05	73
Angry	.00	67
Happy	.55	38
Global change	.30	37
Marital	.40	51

[a]Based on a 3-point, −1, 0, +1 scale. Thus, a mother who responded that she was less patient received a −1; no change received a 0; and more patient received a +1.

most mothers saw no change, and for those that did, the number who perceived the change as negative was balanced by those who saw it as positive. In fact, for 15% of the children, mothers indicated that no change had occurred on any of the variables queried. For the other families there were many more changes in the positive than in the negative direction. Indeed, 55% of the forms had no negative changes indicated.

The present results based on the Holroyd QRS are a bit more difficult to interpret without a comparison group. However, Holroyd has made means available for a number of different groups, and although these groups can certainly not be considered controls because the children differ on a number of characteristics from the children in the present sample, including age, culture and possibly social class, it is informative to examine the pattern of differences. Table 3 presents the means and standard deviations (SD) for all 15 scales of the Holroyd questionnaire for the 49 retarded children in the present sample for whom questionnaires were returned, along with the means and SDs for the two comparison groups from Holroyd's research—normal controls and developmentally disabled (DD) 10-year-olds. Higher scores on the Holroyd questionnaire indicate problem areas as the scale labels (e.g., poor health/mood, excess time demands), suggest.

As can be seen in Table 3, the present sample has significantly lower scores, indicating more successful functioning, than the Holroyd DD sample on 10 of the 15 subscales. In fact, the sample does not differ significantly from the normal controls on many of the subscales that involve psychological and attitudinal variables, such as poor health/mood, negative attitudes, and lack of family integration. This closer resemblance to the normal controls in parent and family functioning is especially noteworthy given that the children themselves are markedly different from the normal controls, with all five scales relating to child problems being significantly higher. Indeed, the adopted children are even more physically incapacitated than the Holroyd DD sample, probably because they are younger in age.

Although great caution should be exercised in overinterpreting these data because the present sample was drawn from a population different from that of Holroyd, one may speculate that adoptive parents, as do biological parents, experience some difficulties in rearing mentally retarded children but that: 1) these difficulties are not experienced in as psychologically damaging a way for them and/or 2) their psychological mood and attitudes are different as a result of the very different circumstances surrounding the entrance of the retarded child into the family. As one mother said when talking about the differences in the reaction of biological and adoptive families, "When you're talking about fostering or adopting a mentally handicapped child, it is a completely different relationship. You chose the child; you took it because you felt you could do something for it, whereas the poor mother is presented with this child . . . completely different altogether."

SUMMARY, CONCLUSIONS, AND IMPLICATIONS

In summary, the present work suggests a number of tentative conclusions, as well as a number of interesting areas for further exploration. The type of family who is likely to adopt a mentally retarded child: 1) is familiar with handicap; 2) is more likely to be middle-class than the average person, but less likely

Table 3. Comparison of groups on Holroyd Questionnaire on Resources and Stress (QRS)

Category/QRS subscale $\overline{X}$	(1) Glidden Adopted MR		(2) Holroyd Normal controls		(3) Holroyd DD		t-test values for (3)−(1)	t-test values for (1)−(2)
N	49 6.5 $\overline{X}$	SD	21 10.4 $\overline{X}$	SD	143 9.8 $\overline{X}$	SD		
Parent problems								
Poor health / mood	1.46	2.24	2.05	1.94	4.95	3.05	6.71**	−1.10
Excess time demands	4.35	2.58	3.67	2.63	5.53	2.86	2.64**	0.97
Negative attitudes	5.55	3.68	4.24	2.32	10.98	4.59	8.28**	1.77
Overprotection / dependency	3.90	2.43	3.14	2.03	6.17	2.68	5.51**	1.32
Lack of social support	4.12	1.27	2.52	1.33	4.45	1.51	0.58	4.62**
Overcommitment/ martyrdom	2.88	0.97	2.24	1.26	3.50	1.32	3.58**	2.03*
Pessimism	3.63	2.15	2.71	1.38	3.53	2.72	−0.26	2.06*
Family functioning								
Lack of family integration	2.84	2.71	2.86	1.82	5.23	3.84	4.78**	−0.04
Limits on family opportunity	0.57	1.17	0.43	0.75	1.80	2.06	5.02**	0.57
Financial problems	3.16	2.03	2.57	1.96	5.49	3.36	5.66**	1.12
Child problems								
Physical incapacitation	4.24	2.54	1.00	1.14	2.81	2.03	−2.80**	7.25**
Lack of activities	1.16	1.09	0.52	0.81	2.47	1.89	5.85**	2.86**
Occupational limitations	3.30	1.47	1.05	1.20	3.43	1.26	0.53	6.50**
Social obtrusiveness	1.90	1.18	0.48	0.68	2.41	1.37	2.55**	6.34**
Difficult personality	13.98	4.70	3.38	2.80	15.33	5.56	1.64	11.50**

*$p < .05$.
**$p < .01$.

to be the highest social class than the average adoptive family; and 3) has a variety of reasons for wanting to adopt, including biological infertility, religious conviction, and personal/professional experience with handicap. The present numbers, however, are too small and the sample too nonrandomly selected to state these conclusions firmly.

Many adoptive families do experience reality crises, or, at least, difficulties, although most of them seem to cope with these problems quite well. Of course, because no direct comparison has been made between adoptive and biological families who are matched on family and child characteristics, this conclusion is very tentative. An additional reason for being tentative about the conclusions is that the children in the present sample were only in their adoptive homes, on average, 15 months, and 26 children or 46% were still under 5 years old at the time of interview. Thus, it is a young and recently adopted sample. Others (e.g., Wikler, 1981) have suggested that, when the retarded child enters puberty and young adulthood, the family is likely to experience stress as there are new reality crises with which to cope. Clearly, the present study, time-bound as it was, could not assess the probability of such difficulties.

The present work thus describes families who have chosen to rear retarded children and has characterized them in terms of demographic and motivational characteristics. It also suggests that they may cope better than the biological families of retarded children. However, even if the latter conclusion remained true after additional research, its cause is not patently obvious. Do adoptive families have an easier time because they do not suffer existential crises, or are they, to begin with, very special families, high on such characteristics as family integration, commitment, and responsibility?

Clearly, further investigation is necessary. We need to study more families who adopt mentally retarded children, as well as to compare them with matched families who have biological retarded children. These comparisons, to yield maximally fruitful data, should examine age of adoptive child and length of placement as predictor variables. In addition, as Gallagher, Beckman, and Cross (1983) have recommended, longitudinal as well as cross-sectional data are needed. It is only such carefully controlled comparison that will be able to untangle the effects of the existential crises from the reality crises and begin to assess a cause-effect relationship between the two.

REFERENCES

Ballard, R. (1978). Help for coping with the unthinkable. *Developmental Medicine and Child Neurology, 20,* 517–521.

Belsky, J. (1981). Early human experience: A family perspective. *Developmental Psychology, 17,* 3–23.

Birenbaum, A. (1971). The mentally retarded child in the home and family cycle. *Journal of Health and Social Behavior, 12,* 55–65.

Booth, T. A. (1978). From normal baby to handicapped child: Unravelling the idea of subnormality in families of mentally handicapped children. *Sociology, 12,* 203–221.

British Agencies for Adoption & Fostering. (1983). *Annual review: 1982–83.* London: Author.

Burden, R. L. (1980). Measuring the effects of stress on the mothers of handicapped infants: Must depression always follow? *Child: Care, Health & Development, 6,* 111–125.

Crnic, K. A., Friedrich, W. N., & Greenberg, M. T. (1983). Adaptation of families with mentally retarded children: A model of stress, coping and family ecology. *American Journal of Mental Deficiency, 89,* 125–138.

Darling, R. B. (1979). *Families against society: A study of reactions to children with birth defects.* Beverly Hills: Sage Publications.

De Leon, J., & Westerberg, J. (1980). *Who adopts retarded children?* Unpublished manuscript.

Farber, B. (1959). Effects of a severely mentally retarded child on family integration. *Monographs of the Society for Research in Child Development, 24,* (Whole No. 71).

Farber, B. (1960). Family organization and crisis: Maintenance of integration in families with a severely mentally retarded child. *Monographs of the Society for Research in Child Development, 25,* (1, Whole No. 75).

Fradkin, H. (1958). Adoptive parents for children with special needs. *Child Welfare, 37,* 1–6.

Franklin, D. S., & Massarik, F. (1969a). The adoption of children with medical conditions: Part I—Process and outcome. *Child Welfare, 48,* 459–467.

Franklin, D. S., & Massarik, F. (1969b). The adoption of children with medical conditions: Part II—The families today. *Child Welfare, 48,* 533–539.

Franklin, D. S., & Massarik, F. (1969c). The adoption of children with medical conditions: Part III—Discussions and conclusions. *Child Welfare, 46,* 595–601.

Friedrich, W. N. (1979). Predictors of the coping behavior of mothers of handicapped children. *Journal of Consulting & Clinical Psychology, 47,* 1140–1141.

Friedrich, W. N., & Friedrich, W. L. (1981). Psychosocial assets of parents of handicapped and nonhandicapped children. *American Journal of Mental Deficiency, 85,* 551–553.

Gallagher, J. J., Beckman, P., & Cross, A. H. (1983). Families of handicapped children: Sources of stress and its amelioration. *Exceptional Children, 50,* 10–19.

Gallagher, U. M. (1968). The adoption of mentally retarded children. *Children, 15,* 17–21.

Gath, A. (1977). The impact of an abnormal child upon the parents. *British Journal of Psychiatry, 130,* 405–410.

Gath, A. (1983). Mentally retarded children in substitute and natural families. *Adoption & Fostering, 7(1),* 35–40.

Hockey, A. (1980). Evaluation of adoption of the intellectually handicapped: A retrospective analysis of 137 cases. *Journal of Mental Deficiency Research, 24,* 187–202.

Holroyd, J. (1974). The Questionnaire on Resources and Stress: An instrument to measure family response to a handicapped family member. *Journal of Community Psychology, 2,* 92–94.

Holroyd, J., & McArthur, D. (1976). Mental retardation and stress on the parents: A contrast between Down's syndrome and childhood autism. *American Journal of Mental Deficiency, 80,* 431–436.

Jaffee, B., & Fanshel, D. (1970). *How they fared in adoption: A follow-up study.* New York: Columbia University Press.

Krisheff, C. H. (1977). Adoption agency services for the retarded. *Mental Retardation, 15(1),* 38–39.

Lerner, R. M., & Spanier, G. B. (1978). A dynamic interactional view of child and family development. In R. M. Lerner & G. B. Spanier (Eds.), *Child influences on marital and family interaction.* New York: Academic Press.

Olshansky, S. (1962). Chronic sorrow: A response to having a mentally defective child. *Social Casework, 43,* 191–194.

Parks, R. M. (1977). Parental reactions to the birth of a handicapped child. *Health & Social Work, 2,* 51–66.

Raynor, L. (1980). *The adopted child comes of age.* London: George Allen & Unwin.

Voysey, M. (1975). *A constant burden: The reconstitution of family life.* Boston, MA: Routledge & Kegan Paul.

Wikler, L. (1981). Chronic stresses of families of mentally retarded children. *Family Relations, 30,* 281–288.

Wikler, L., Wasow, M., & Hatfield, E. (1981). Chronic sorrow revisited: Parent vs. professional depiction of the adjustment of parents of mentally retarded children. *American Journal of Orthopsychiatry, 51,* 63–70.

Wolkind, S., & Kozaruk, A. (1983). *Children with special needs: A review of children with medical problems placed by the Adoption Resource Exchange from 1974–77.* (Report to the Department of Health and Social Services). London: London Hospital Medical College Family Research Unit.

Wright, L. S. (1976). Chronic grief: The anguish of being an exceptional parent. *Exceptional Child, 23,* 160–169.

Chapter

9

Immediate and Continuing Adaptations in Parents of Handicapped Children

A Model and an Illustration

Dale C. Farran, Joyce Metzger, and Joyce Sparling

THE BIRTH OF AN IMPAIRED child is an unexpected event that occurs at a time of already heightened physical and emotional awareness on the part of the parents. At this vulnerable time, parents are faced with the unalterable loss of the anticipated normal child, in addition to the overwhelming demands of coping with the new situation. Such an event can be thought of as a crisis for the family, a precipitous stress forcing parents to adapt and cope. Researchers, service deliverers, and policy-makers have been intensely interested in the process that parents go through in adapting to the stress of having a handicapped child. Too often, service deliverers and policy-makers have been forced to adopt a reactive position toward these families. Services are demanded and policies are created to take care of problems that occur in families of handicapped children. Thus, siblings of handicapped children are provided counseling because of the shift in the roles they play in these families. There is concern about depression in mothers and fa-

thers and about the possibility of higher divorce rates in families with handicapped children.

This chapter argues that, as worthy and as needed as these services and concerns are, they generally occur after the fact. They are dealing with problems that have emerged in families over time. Some of these problems could have been prevented if the *process* of adaptation, both short- and long-term, had been understood. Research can and should make a contribution to our knowledge of this process.

Research into stress and its effects can make a strong contribution to our understanding of the process of adaptation. Several important models of adaptation to stress have already been developed; one of them has been adapted specifically for parents with handicapped children. These models are important, not because of their theoretical contribution, but because they provide precision in selecting services and policies. A working model of adaptation to the stress of having and raising a handicapped child should delineate where in the process services could be offered most effectively. It should enable service providers to work *proactively* with parents, anticipating and thereby reducing the impact of stress points.

Several models of stress representing various points of view are presented here. One model is then discussed in more depth. Finally, a parent of a child who was severely damaged by a DPT shot describes the process of her family's adaptation to this continual strain.

HEALTH MODELS OF STRESS

The investigation of stress, its causes, and its consequences has a long and continuing history. Yet, despite many efforts to determine the exact nature of stress, our understanding remains fragmentary. As Cox (1978) argued:

> The concept of stress is elusive because it is poorly defined. There is no single agreed upon definition in existence. It is a concept familiar to both layman and professional alike, it is understood by all when used in a general context but by very few when a more precise account is required, and this seems to be a central problem. (p. 1)

Over the years, models have been developed to trace the ways in which external events produce stressful reactions in individuals. Some models have focused on the *response* of the organism; Selye (1980), one of the better-known theorists, developed the notion of a General Adaptation Syndrome, "a non-specific response of the body to any demand" (p. 12) made upon it." Thus, according to Selye, change of any kind produces a response in the organism that renders it more vulnerable to illness. Selye's (1956) pioneering work in this area led to studies of stress-related diseases and to the sophisticated epidemiologic work of John Cassel (1978).

Other models have focused more on the nature and number of the external events themselves, the *stimulus for the stress*. (See Cox, 1978, for a summary.) All events are somewhat stressful, but some events are more stressful than others. Individuals have a harder time adapting to more stressful events. The more events there are, the more stress is ex-erted and the more likely are negative reactions. In the response-based models, one studies stress as a reaction ("I feel distressed"); in the stimulus-based models, stress is the pressure exerted on an individual by an event ("I am *under* stress"). Both views are commonly expressed.

Another health model of stress has attempted to go beyond both of these one-dimensional views of stress. Cox (1978) has proposed a transactional model of stress in which the organism and the environment are undergoing continual readjustments to each other. Cox is interested in the individual's perception both of the demands of the event and his or her ability to meet those demands. Thus, individual variability plays a major role in this model. Some people, for example, tend to exaggerate the demands that situations place on them; others downplay the demands. The estimate of what adjustments are required is an important determinant of how much stress one feels. Moreover, people differ in their estimates of their own ability to deal with different demands; some have conservative estimates, whereas others have quite inflated ones. According to Cox, stress results from a perceived imbalance between the demands of an event and an appraisal of one's skills to meet or contend with the event. This perception leads to behaviors to reduce the imbalance; the results of those attempts feed back to influence one's perceptions of personal skills and to alter the demand characteristics of the event.

Although a great deal of research has been stimulated by these various models, including attempts to develop Life Event Scales so that there would be a common metric for evaluating levels of stress (Coddington, 1972; Holmes & Rahe, 1967), there is no agreement yet about the interaction of psychological demands and physiological reactions, such as illness or disease. This lack of consensus may be due to insufficiencies in all the models so far proposed—that is, none of them captures enough of the truth to supplant the others—or it may be due to there actually being more than *one* path by which adaptation to stress occurs.

These paths may be altered somewhat depending on the nature of the event, the nature of the respondent, and the number of times that the path has been recently taken. The following model was originally developed to chart the course of adaptation to sudden job loss by the primary wage earner in a family. It has recently been adapted specifically for families of handicapped children.

STRESS-ADAPTATION MODEL FOR PARENTS OF HANDICAPPED CHILDREN

The Stress-Adaptation model is presented in Figure 1. It is a linear model with three major components (represented by boxes), each of which must be understood before the impact of any event on the individuals involved can be determined. This model is both a stimulus- and a response-based depiction. The demands (the first two boxes) on the parents when there is a major event are examined in great detail. The middle or central box in the model examines the individual's capacity to adapt to the event, including all the components relating to that capacity. Farran and Margolis (1984) assert that much of both research and service delivery has focused on the end-state or the impact of demanding events on individuals. Such an approach will always lead to a less-than-adequate understanding and inadequate services because it does not take into account the various ways individuals can have reached the same end-state. Without knowledge of individual differences, anticipatory services cannot be developed.

Although the Stress-Adaptation model is linear and appears to terminate in that it reaches an "impact" state, it is applicable to chronic conditions. Individuals existing in a state of chronic strain cycle periodically through the pathway depicted by this model. A new cycle is trig-

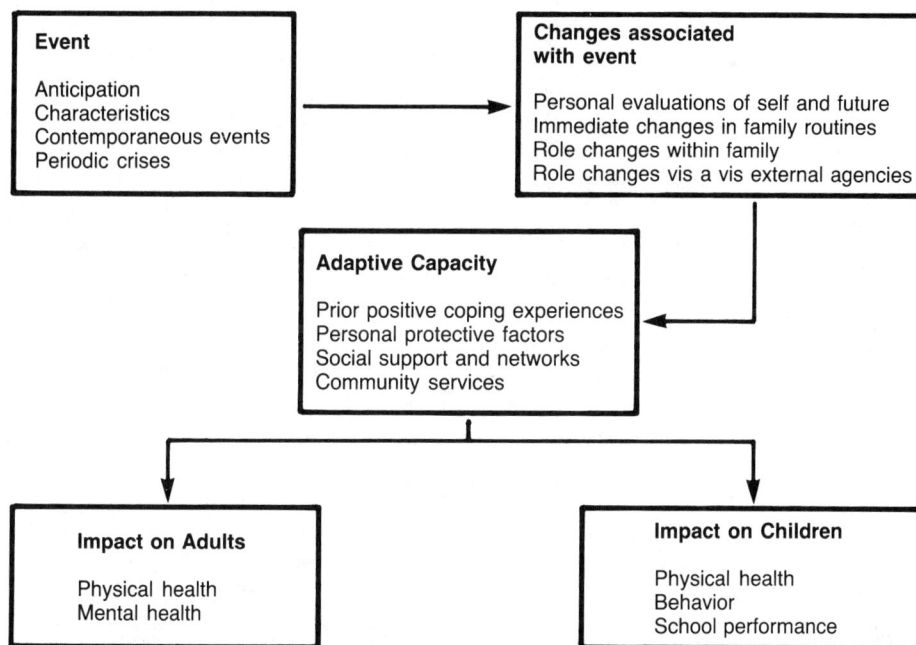

Figure 1.   Stress-Adaptation model. (Adapted from Farran, D. C., & Margolis, L. (1984). Integrative model for analyzing the effects of a precipitous stress such as unemployment of families. In L. Margolis & D. Farran (Eds.), *The North Carolina work and family life project: An investigation of the health and behavioral consequences for families of paternal job loss*, 12–24: Final report submitted to the WT Grant Foundation.

gered each time new events occur that demand changes on the part of the family. (Sometimes, in fact, the adaptations parents made initially in an attempt to cope with demands can themselves bring about new demands on the family.) The middle component, the individual's capacity to adapt, does not remain static, but must be assessed with each new cycle through the process. Unfortunately, resources can be strained by coping with chronic conditions, leaving the family in a weakened condition for handling new demands. The next several sections of this chapter describe each component of the Stress-Adaptation model in turn.

The Event

Initial Occurrence   The first component of the Stress-Adaptation model relates to the event itself and its immediate demand characteristics, such as the loss of a job or the birth of a handicapped child. An analysis of the nature of the event is an important part of the Cox interaction model as well; but Farran and Margolis (1984) also include within this component an assessment of what *other* demands are being placed on the family at the same time. Thus, if the birth of a handicapped child occurred at the same time the family had just changed houses or experienced the death of a grandparent or had a teenager with serious difficulties in school, those factors would increase the demands being placed on the family at the time of the event of interest. In order to understand what the family or the individual is experiencing, it is critical to have information not only about a particular event but also about other occurrences in the family's life. Moreover, the event itself must be thoroughly described. Divorce, job loss, or the birth of a handicapped child are all significant events in a family, but the definition of the event and the way it actually occurred can be quite different from family to family. For a parent with a handicapped child, the child's disorder can range from being sudden and completely unexpected to having been preceded by an ultrasound diagnosis; at first glance the child could be normal in appearance, or his or her appearance could be startling to the parent. These

variations are significant and must be noted in order to understand individual reactions.

Predictable Periodic Crises   Several authors have pointed out that parents do not reach a terminus in their adaptation to the stress of having a handicapped child (Blacher, 1984; Wikler, 1981). New major events continue to occur throughout the child's lifetime that trigger a new cycle of upset, changing demands, and new adaptations. This recycling through the stress process does not occur in response to some internal and therefore unobservable state of the parents. Primarily, it is brought on by situations and events that involve the child. In a very important article on mentally retarded children, Wikler (1981) divided these events into two main types, and although her focus was on retarded children, these two types of events are experienced by all parents of handicapped children. The two types are: 1) those that represent a discrepancy between parental expectations for their child's development and what the child was actually achieving and 2) those experiences that are unique to families of retarded children. This first type of crisis relates to the psychological adjustment in expectations. Without necessarily being conscious of it, parents have expectations for their children's development based on their own development and on the developmental patterns of other children they have come into contact with who are not handicapped. Handicapped children's development will not proceed according to normal expectations; they may not walk at the right time or walk correctly; they may not talk correctly or at the right time, and in general they violate parental expectations for the achievement of developmental milestones. As each milestone approaches, is passed, and is not reached by the child, it can be expected that parents will cycle through a new grief and adaptation process.

Wikler (1981) also argues that there are unique events experienced by families of handicapped children. Parents have no models to help them learn how to cope with such events as receiving the diagnosis of chronic, long-lasting impairment; undergoing a serious discussion of placing one's child in an institution; and worrying about who will take care of the child once they no longer can. Parents of nonhandicapped children do not experience these events. Each of these events may well be the start of a new cycle of upset and distress for parents of handicapped children.

In addition to the events that Wikler describes, Minde, Hackett, Killou, and Silver (1972) note the event of the child's becoming aware of the irrevocable nature of his or her disability. Minde et al. found that children themselves went through a severe crisis at adolescence in the development of their self-concept. Many of the children they interviewed expected miraculously to be free of their impairment once they were adolescents and certainly by the time they were adults. When this transformation did not occur, severe bouts of depression were experienced by many of the adolescents. Coping with the adolescent's own depression about the situation adds a tremendous burden to the families and places demands on them for skills in counseling their children through this period.

Demands of the Event

Immediate Changes   The second component of the Stress-Adaptation model assesses what the event actually requires of the one who is experiencing it; that is, how much change does the individual or the family have to undergo as a result of this event? Changes can be both psychological and physical or external.

Certainly, parents of handicapped children must alter their perceptions of the child they expected to have. Drotar, Baskiewicz, Irvin, Kennell, and Klaus (1975) proposed a sequential process of adaptation that parents go through in adjusting to the news that they have a handicapped child. The psychological adjustment does not occur immediately; rather, it appears to take place in stages. (This proposed sequential process has been criticized by Blacher, 1984, among others, for its lack of understanding of the cyclic nature of adjustment.)

In addition to the need for a psychological adjustment, other external demands are placed on the parents. These demands are different from the ones they expected and planned for. Parents of a handicapped child must coordinate their care of the child with professionals. Frequently, the child is sick or weak and must be cared for in the hospital for a lengthy period; parents' lives are constantly disrupted until the child is home. Once there, the child may need special provisions that the parents must arrange; the child may need therapy on an intense and regular basis, which parents must also arrange. The number of such demands affects parents' ability to adapt to them. Although this may seem self-evident, the *number* of demands are infrequently assessed when determining reactions to the stressful event of having a handicapped child.

Changing Demands Through The Years   As Blacher (1984) pointed out, parents' adaptation to having a handicapped child is cyclical. Parents do not reach the Drotar et al. (1975) stage of reorganization and then proceed smoothly for the rest of their child's life. The demands of having a handicapped child are not constant. Different skills are required of parents when the child is an infant than when he or she is older. The "small" events that surround the large event of having a handicapped child are not the same throughout the child's lifespan. During infancy it appears that the largest demand on the parents relates to taking care of the child within the home. Beckman (1983) interviewed 31 parents and observed their handicapped infants. The factor most related to the degree of stress experienced by parents was the level of caregiving difficulty presented by the child.

Because of the extra caregiving demands, many early intervention projects for handicapped infants see as one of their goals helping parents develop skills to care for the infant physically and to stimulate him or her appropriately. Kasari and Farran (1984) observed 18 mothers of handicapped infants, half of whom experienced early, systematic, and home-based intervention with this focus. The other half received periodic evaluations of their infants and suggestions for therapeutic procedures from professionals in their offices. When the infants were about 12 months of age, parents who had experienced intense intervention that focused on parent-child interactions received higher ratings on the appropriateness and the qualitative aspects of their interactive behaviors from observers who were unaware of the type of intervention the parents had received.

In 1982, Suelzle and Keenan reported data from interviews conducted with nearly 300 families of handicapped children of varying ages. The concerns of the parents interviewed changed with the age of their children. The parents of preschool-age children were rather optimistic about neighborhood acceptance of their children, and fewer than half of them were concerned about special schools, alternative living arrangements, or service needs for their children at an older age. With parents of older children, there was a steady decrease in the amount of acceptance the parents expected from their neighbors and in the number of possible playmates for their child. There was also a steady increase in their concern about special education and alternative schools being provided for the child. As might be expected, parents of older adolescents had great concern about community living facilities and sheltered workshops for their children. It is possible to imagine parents who cope well with the demands of a handicapped child in infancy but who find the demands of dealing with a recalcitrant school system and an indifferent community overwhelming as the child gets older. What this suggests, obviously, is that the services offered to families of handicapped children must be in tune with the demands they are facing at any one point in time.

Role Changes   The demands of having a handicapped child frequently alter the roles played by all the members of the family (Agathonas & Valaes, 1982; Gallagher, Beckman, & Cross, 1983). In 1983 Kasari and Farran developed the Child Care Role Scale. It has been used to interview parents of handicapped children about the type and degree of help they receive in day-to-day care for their children and to compare those patterns to families where the child was free from handicap (Kasari, Farran, & Harber, 1984). In families with young handicapped children, mothers clearly carried most of the burden of care. Many activities in which mothers engaged with their handicapped children were the mothers' exclusive province; there was never a substitute for them. This was especially true of parents with severely handicapped children; the help the mothers did receive was frequently in the form of assistance with the task, rather than substitution.

Breslau, Salkever, and Staruch (1982) investigated the labor force participation rate of parents with handicapped children and found that mothers' work status interacted with the disability level of the child and the income level for the family. In low-income families of a handicapped child, mothers were 10% less likely to be working than in low-income families of nondisabled children. In high-income families, mothers were about 7% more likely to be working than in families of the same income level whose children were not disabled. This finding suggests that the changes in the role status of women in the family vis-a-vis working or staying home is a function of degree of economic support received by the families. Families with greater income are more likely to be able to afford the mother some relief in the day-to-day care of her child by allowing her to set up care for the child so that she can work. Therefore, the demands of caring for a handicapped child may be differentially experienced by families with different income levels, and further, the level of help they need from professionals will be different as well.

Adaptive Capacity

The final component of the Stress-Adaptation model relates to the adaptive capacity on the part of the individuals involved. This is a complex area that itself can be divided into many subparts. In effect, the first two components of this model dissect the event itself and the initial adjustments required of the parent. The process of adaptation—the third component—is composed of a number of different dimensions. One of them involves the individual's prior experience at coping with demanding events. Prior positive coping experiences give parents an initially positive attitude toward their ability to cope with new events. This is very similar to Cox's (1978) idea of an individual's perception of his or her ability to handle the event. The Stress-Adaptation model also takes into account individual personality characteristics. There is no doubt that some people enlarge and exaggerate an event, whereas others diminish it. A final aspect of this third component of the model relates to social support. Social support can be both emotional and instrumental; it can derive from intimate sources, from family, and/or from a larger community. All these factors together—prior experience, personality, and social support—interact and affect the way parents cope with the event and its subsequent demands on them.

Personality Characteristics Personality has always been a difficult construct both to define and to measure accurately. It is especially difficult to handle in models depicting reactions to stress-producing events. Frequently, there is no way of knowing to whom these events will occur. Crnic, Friedrich, and Greenberg (1983) argued that there were no prospective studies "designed" to look at the characteristics of parents before the birth or diagnosis of their handicapped child. This is certainly true, but it is not, however, an indictment of the research community for lack of forethought. Rather, one cannot know who will produce the handicapped child, and thus there is a true inability to do a prospective study. (The authors of this chapter are working on a study to examine the effects of an ultrasound diagnosis of impairment on the parents involved. In some ways, this can be viewed as a prospective study. However, parents who seek an ultrasound diagnosis at 6–7 months prenatally do so only because they are thought to be at risk for producing an impaired infant. According to a survey by Sparling in 1984, 20% of them do receive a diagnosis of impairment. Their psychological states at the time of the ultrasound experience may well be affected by their concerns about the likely outcome of that procedure).

Although not dealing with the parents of handicapped children, Heinicke, Diskin, Ramsey-Klee, and Given (1983) did conduct a prospective study examining maternal characteristics prenatally, and infant characteristics and maternal behavior 4 months postnatally. It is a complex study that is not easy to summarize. Adaptation, as might be expected, consisted of both maternal characteristics and infant characteristics. The maternal characteristics that seemed to be important in predicting subsequent adaptation to the birth of a child were such factors as confidence and "ego strength" as measured by the Minnesota Multiphasic Personality Index (MMPI). In a recent large-scale study of handicapped infants in North Carolina, Comfort-Smith and Bailey (1984) found that mothers with a high degree of internal control were rated higher in their behavioral interactions with their children by home visitors. The rating scale used, the Parent Child Interaction Scale developed by Farran, Kasari, and Jay (1983), is one measure of the parents' adaptation to the handicapped child.

The Carolina Institute for Research on Early Education of the Handicapped in North Carolina has been conducting three longitudinal studies to investigate how parents cope with their handicapped children (Gallagher, 1983). Early discussions among members of that institute suggest that such parental skills as a sense of humor and resilience are critical. Unfortunately, there is no accepted measuring device for determining individual differences in these particular parental characteristics.

Prior Experience If parental personality is a relatively unresearched phenomenon, the idea of prior experience in coping with stress-producing events is virtually untouched by research. Prior positive coping experiences may, of course, be a factor in increasing parental confidence as measured by Heinicke et al. (1983). Unfortunately one of the few studies related to this issue is not concerned with handicapped children. Boyce, Jensen, James, and Peacock (1983) investigated the number of family routines in which families engage, and the relationship between how routinized the family is and its ability to ward off illnesses. Unexpectedly, the most heavily routinized families had the least resistance to illness; they apparently had not developed the flexibility to deal with external influences and forces. Although it seems somewhat tangential to the subject at hand, the Boyce et al. study suggests an avenue worth exploring with families of handicapped children. Once again, however, researchers are faced with the inability to conduct a prospective study on this issue. Family routines are necessarily disrupted by the birth of a handicapped child and may take some time to settle down to regular patterns. It would be important to investigate family routines before the child was born and diagnosed as impaired.

Social Support   The role of social support in mediating the effects of life events (Williams, Ware, & Donald, 1981) or in indirectly affecting emotional well-being (Lin, Simeone, Ensel, & Kuo, 1979) is well established. The *process* by which socal support exerts such influence is not clear, however. It may be a buffer between the family and upsetting events so that the family has fewer adjustments to make (McCubbin, Joy, Cauble, Comeau, Patterson, & Needle, 1980), or it may serve to help the family adjust more quickly to the changes brought about by the event (Pearlin, Lieberman, Menaghan, & Mullan, 1981). Turner (1981) argues that social support becomes most critical in stressful circumstances; that is, until one needs to test the level of support, its existence is not as important.

Margolis and Farran (1984) conceive of support as existing in a set of nested environments beginning with intimate support. Several other investigators have also commented on the importance of intimate support for adaptation to child rearing in general and to handicapped children specifically. Belsky (1984) found that the level of support the husband gave the wife was the most important source of support. It is important, therefore, in single-parent families that those mothers already identified as being both low income and nonworking parents of handicapped children are also likely to have the least amount of social support.

Although there are many difficulties in studying the concept and utility of social support—detailed at some length by Thoits (1982)—one important issue is whether social support should be viewed as a state or a trait.[1] If social support is a *state,* then one can determine individuals' levels of social support by counting the number of people with whom they interact and on whom they feel they can rely in an emergency. Simplistically, then one would increase the availability of such people to families who were low on those measures. However, that strategy will likely not work because individuals seem to vary in the degree to which they need support. For some people, one close friend is sufficient, whereas for others one close friend would suggest severe isolation. Social support must in some ways be seen as a *trait* that will vary with individuals. It is important to look at the degree of satisfaction that individuals feel with the level of support they are receiving and not only at the absolute number of people in their support network.

Community Services   Unfortunately, for families of handicapped children there are no universally available services for children at a single age and no comprehensive set of community services covering the family's and the child's needs as they grow older. The authors are familiar with cases where families have relocated (fathers changed jobs, in one case left the military, mothers gave up careers) in order to move into an area where better services were available for the particular handicap their child had. In North Carolina, for example, the services offered vary county by county, despite the existence of a statewide early intervention program. In some counties that program has been stable and well run and is coordinated with services for older preschoolers. Families in those counties feel much more confident about the future; ambiguity about future decisions has been removed. In other counties parents feel a constant, looming dread because the intervention team is not well run and future services are fragmented and depressing to consider.

Community services are a crucial factor in how well the family adapts to having a handi-

---

[1]The authors are grateful to Emily Arcia for this distinction.

capped child. Sometimes the service itself becomes a part of the family support network. There are problems when families are too dependent on community services, however. One family with whom the authors are familiar relocated to be near a particular service; as a result, they lost close contact with extended family and friends. The family became so attached to the service and detached from their family and friends that when their second child was born, they had no one who could stay in the home with the older handicapped child. A worker from the agency providing the service stayed with the handicapped child until the mother was discharged from the hospital with the new baby. It would be more beneficial in the long run for service providers to help parents and families establish ongoing and permanent support systems of their own, rather than allowing the family to become dependent on the service providers alone.

Finally, community services could become an important factor in mediating the parents' reactions to the periodic, predictable crises they will face rearing a handicapped child. Wikler (1981) termed this sort of intervention as "proactive" (p. 281). Interventionists who are familiar with Wikler's definition of the various crises that parents undergo can anticipate times when parents will need help. For example, a new crisis may be triggered in a family as their handicapped adolescent gets ready to leave his or her placement at age 17 or 18. Many counselors who are dealing with handicapped youngsters placed in regular high schools have no information about available community services, are unaware of sheltered workshops, and do not see it as their role to advise parents of these services. Who is to perform that function?

Many interventionists are trained to provide such guidance to parents only in the preschool years or the early elementary school period. Yet clearly, late adolescence is a very distressing time for parents and also a time at which they feel very uncertain. Programs that parents may desire for their children in the future have long waiting lists and must be signed up for

years in advance. Parents need someone to advise them of these steps at the proper time, some years ahead of when they will actually use these services. Such efforts will prevent or at least reduce some of the changing demands through the years and thus reduce the amount of distress parents experience. However, with services as fragmented as they are, handled by so many agencies with no coordinating body, it is unlikely parents will receive this kind of proactive help.

Summary of the Stress-Adaptation Model

The value of analyzing in detail the various models for parental adaptation to a handicapped child is to enable the development of better services and policies for families. The authors argue that these models are in fact critical to the development of services and policy. What is apparent from these models is that it is less effective to deal after the fact with parental and family reactions to the event. For example, parents who are similarly depressed may have reached that state by quite different routes. Helping alleviate the depression for one family might be quite a different endeavor from helping reduce the same degree of depression for another family. Moreover, helping alleviate the depression after it has developed is almost too late. If service providers and policy-makers understand the way an event exerts its influence, they can intervene earlier in the process of adaptation. In the Stress-Adaptation model there are two clear places for intervention: 1) One can attempt to alter the demands of the events, reducing the number of changes families must undergo both immediately and through the years; and 2) one can intervene at the level of individual adaptability through such efforts as parent support groups and individual counseling.

One thing is certain—the adaptation process for families of handicapped children is an ongoing one (Shapiro, 1983). Too often the services provided are fragmented and age-related. The service system works against preparing parents for what lies ahead and does not give them the skills and the relevant information they need to cope with those subsequent demands. Coordination across service delivery systems is extremely important. Frequently, the parent must become his or her own advocate, carrying with him or her all the relevant information, *going from professional to professional, and in many ways contributing more than he or she is receiving.* Stress models are valuable in that they enable *professionals* to work together and to plan in a prospective way how to provide the best help to families of handicapped children.

AN ILLUSTRATIVE EXAMPLE

The following brief case history traces one family's adaptation to two handicapped children. The first child was a spina bifida child who lived 15 months. Two children who developed normally were then born. The fourth child in the family was a normally developing boy who developed severe seizures 10 days after being given a DPT inoculation at 8 months of age. This boy is now 10 years old; his impairment is extensive. This retrospective report by Joyce Metzger is written in the first person and details her point of view of the family's adjustment to the chronic strain of raising a severely handicapped child. It is difficult to move from the theoretical to the concrete, and the reader may be highly aware at first of the change in style and immediacy. The authors believe, though, that *both* the abstract summarization across families and the vivid intensity of a single case are essential to understanding the process families undergo.

Although there has been no attempt to delineate point by point where Joyce Metzger's family's experiences fit the model proposed in the earlier part of the chapter, the situations she relates here are directly relevant to it. The authors did not force this condensation of 10 years into shorter episodes that might have demonstrated the efficacy of the Stress-Adaptation model more clearly. Instead, the story is told in summary form as it is remembered, and events have been clustered under headings that derive from the model.

Background

Don and I, married 5 years, moved to Hawaii from New Jersey 1 year before Karen's birth. Because our residency was to be for only 1 year, we took advantage of every opportunity to enjoy Hawaii's beautiful outdoors and night life. We became outdoor-oriented. The newness of our home, jobs, and environment was still present when our first child arrived.

Karen Ann was born with spina bifida, with myelomeningocele, shunt hydrocephalus, and multiple other complications. Throughout her brief life, Don was my most important support. He was my strength. Our closest relatives were thousands of miles away. Mutual friendships were established through work, with a few friends especially close.

Although we had prior knowledge of the "possibility" that our child might have some complications, Karen's degree of physical and mental disability was still devastating. In my 8th month of pregnancy, the doctor informed us that our child "might not be able to walk." With very little information given to us, we found ourselves at the medical library researching spina bifida. We *thought* we were prepared, but with each new development came its own new pain.

The doctor's first comment after Karen's birth—"Well, we're lucky. Her head hasn't started to grow yet"—started the series of crises we weren't prepared for. No matter how much reading we had done, having prior information did not buffer the shock. For 3 days I could not bring myself to meet my brand new daughter. Her being given just 1 week to live cautioned me about not getting attached to her. I was also very fearful of what I would see. Finally, I was moved to walk down the hallway toward her room. I don't know how long I stood outside her door, terrified to go in. I went in. With great surprise, joy, and relief, I found my beautiful, blond little girl sleeping! I was overwhelmed with love for her. She was beautiful, just as Don had been telling me all along! Visitations were exhausting for me as I recovered from childbirth itself. But being away from Karen was emotionally draining. Many times Don and I would visit her in the middle of the night to calm our anxiety about her dying alone. We wanted so much for her to know that her parents loved her dearly.

Having the nursing staff, doctors, and equipment within Karen's reach was our support system. Their professional skills, gentleness, and encouragement were our only comfort. After 1 month of new crises each day (it seemed), we were told we could take Karen home. The thought of taking our Karen home was truly exciting, but it was overshadowed by our fear of our inexperience and lack of knowledge and skills.

The time came when Karen needed equipment at her side to keep her alive. After the third hospital trip in 1 day, the inevitable alternative came to our tired minds and bodies: institutionalization. We didn't want to give up. Karen never had. She had always come through every crisis. The day that she was released into our care with a high fever, seizures, and kidney infection because "we could watch her more closely" proved to be our breaking point. The responsibility was too great. For months doctors had urged us to consider placing her in a home, but we refused. I guess they knew we would come to understand why such a decision would be wise. They just waited. Once she was there, feelings of emptiness, guilt, and love propelled my daily visits to the home. Having her in someone else's care did not alleviate the stress and worry.

Karen died 1 month after being admitted to the institution. The moment I saw her take her last breath, a "heaviness" in my chest, one which I was never really aware of before, lifted. I physically felt lighter. We cried and kissed her good-bye.

I know God has a Master Plan for all of us. We all are here to love, grow, and be Agents of God. Throughout Karen's short life, I questioned her purpose. Here's a tiny human being—blind, retarded, paralyzed, deformed—why was she here? As the pain and grief diminished with time, positive feelings about her being came into our awareness. Re-

flecting back on that year, it seemed that we made quite a team! We did have good days. We did have that warm feeling as a family. We did laugh. All three of us were God's Agents. Karen came to us purely for love, which we wholeheartedly gave her. From Karen, Don and I received strength, confidence, and pride. Yes, we were proud of Karen, and of ourselves, too.

God works in so many ways. One week before Karen died we were blessed with the news of our second child. Where there's a void, God will fill it.

The Event: Another Handicapped Child

Contemporaneous Events After Karen's death, three absolutely normal births occurred in the Metzger family. Glen, our third, was an infant, the other two were preschoolers, and we loved each other greatly.

If one wished to contact the Metzger family, an appointment was necessary. The minute Don finished his day's work at 3:30 P. M., the family sped off to the beach, parks, friend's homes. Plans were seldom made. Excursions, picnics, and so on just happened at any given moment. What a happy, happy family. A part-time job opened up for me (4:00 P.M. to 9:00 P.M.). With the dinner prepared by 3:30, I would dash off to work as Don took over his role of "superdad," taking the kids all over. At 9:30 P.M. when I returned, all still remained awake eager to tell me their latest experiences with their Dad.

The Occurrence On that Sunday morning, a strange feeling came across me as I read the Sunday paper, enjoying a cup of coffee in peace. Glen was usually awake babbling in his crib. I heard nothing. Upon checking him I found him lying limp and white on his saturated sheet. Instantly, thoughts of our first daughter flashed through my mind. Seizure! Glen had had a seizure! His coloring and limpness told me so. The family raced Glen to the hospital where he remained for 1 week recovering from never ending pre- and postseizure states. Despite numerous tests, no cause was found. No reason. The doctors were baffled. From that day on, our youngest son has suffered from an uncontrollable seizure disorder.

Our normal, healthy, thriving son is now struck by powerful lightning bolts electrifying his brain with tremendous surges of wild energy, leaving him exhausted and unprepared for the next attack. Each bolt shatters his world and ours. Thunderstorms hit again, and again, and again . . . propelling our search for answers from the doctor, eventually many doctors. "Why can't you stop these? Why don't you know what causes these? Why does your knowledge stop with us?" Or did they know? Were they protecting us from the truth . . . tumors, terminal illness? How could we build our defenses if we didn't know our enemy and its power? Without medical solutions, we began to look at ourselves. Was it genetic? Was it hereditary? Having previously had one physically and mentally deficient child provided strong evidence that genetic factors could very well be the cause. However, the doctors eliminated these as possible causes.

I asked God, "Did I not learn enough through Karen? Was there a particular lesson I missed? Were my errors so great? Did I stop the process of commitment by giving her away? Is Glen an extension of that process? Is Glen Karen?" I remember sitting in church one evening, tired, confused, and angry. I was angry with God. I demanded answers, immediate answers. Why was I obsessed with that one-word question "why"? A bowl filled with tiny slips of paper with brief messages from God was passed around for each to draw from. My message was one word typed in all capitalized letters with an exclamation mark: ACCEPT! My response to God's message was: WHY should I accept? (How cynical I was becoming.)

Preoccupation with unanswered questions subsided as the years passed. Understanding the reasons why or how would not obliterate the problem. Perhaps God's message ACCEPT came through. We stopped trying to control what was beyond our control. Our violent colleague demanded our respect and acknowledgement. Gradually, through routines specifically designed to work around and with the

Thunderstorm, love, joys, and pleasures silently crept back into our world.

Then, suddenly, like the Thunderstorm, a gigantic boulder came crashing into our living room. Engraved on it in large letters;

> DPT . . . Seizure disorders with an onset immediately after DPT immunization are generally topic-clonic, resistant to routine anticonvulsant therapy, and have poor intellectual prognosis . . . . Make sure your doctor gives your child a careful examination before each shot . . . . Any child with a history of previous seizures should not be given more pertusis!

We calmly lived with the Boulder for 6 months (by this time new developments were everyday routines), walking around it and occasionally questioning its existence, its purpose. Curiosity, investigation, and suspicion grew into new fears, angers and chaos. Did God send this Boulder with this message? What were we supposed to do with it? Could we handle any more psychological stress? Years ago we used all the resources—doctors, ourselves, God—to find answers, finally accepting "Because that's life." The possibility that a vaccine that saves millions of young lives could be the producer of our son's suffering had generated emotional confusion. Our present situation: Hovering over our home is the powerful, unpredictable Thunderstorm. Inside the home is a life-style compatible with the storm. In the living room lies the mysterious Boulder. What do we do with the Boulder?

Changes Associated with the Event

Reorienting the Family's Focus Prior experience helped Don and me through Glen's seemingly endless seizure activity. We knew that the attacks eventually cease and the postseizure states take over. But even with this understanding, our new situation was much more difficult than with our first daughter. Karen was bedridden so we never had to worry about injuries sustained during seizures. With Glen being active and mobile, he would crash to the floor hitting any object on the way down. His safety became our greatest concern. Soon, the family's focus was constantly on Glen's activities, Glen's whereabouts, Glen's surroundings, Glen's behavior, Glen's eating, Glen's safety at all times.

Anticipation of seizures occurring anytime and anywhere (which they did) drastically altered this outdoor-oriented family's life-style. Added to concern over Glen's seizures themselves was public reaction. People became frightened, understandably so; thus we found ourselves having to calm them down. This public attention on the family was extremely uncomfortable. Quick trips to drug stores frequently turned into major events. Picnics were cancelled minutes before departure time. Family outings became more stressful than enjoyable.

To avoid robbing Jill (age 5) and Jay (age 3) of normal childhood experiences, a new system developed. The family unit split. Don or I would stay home with Glen. Thus, our "duty system," a system that has been in effect for almost 9 years, became our pattern of life. This system is used for Jill and Jay's school programs, sports activities, birthday parties, and even vacations. One parent relates events to the other through photos, scrapbooks, souvenirs, and words.

Periodic Crises: An Example   At age 3 Glen's seizure activity remained uncontrolled. Medications (13 different drugs) proved ineffective. Behavior management became a problem. To counteract Glen's hyperactivity and to reduce seizures, a ketogenic diet was introduced to the family. I say "family" because the diet affected every one of us as much as it did Glen.

To prepare Glen's little body for this diet, hospitalization was required. One week for fasting and another for gradual introduction to the special foods. This desperate effort to help Glen cost $4,000 in laboratory work alone, not to mention hospitalization costs. Each pea, lettuce leaf, spoon of applesauce had to be weighed in grams. All sugar and starches were eliminated. One bite of any restricted food would erase all initial efforts, and back to zero we would go. The refrigerator and cupboards were tied shut. Snacks were eaten privately.

Meals were often served before or after Glen's. Neighbors and Glen's school personnel monitored the diet when Glen was away from home. Two years on this stringent routine brought little improvement in Glen's behavior or seizure activity.

Surprisingly, each family member's active involvement in this ridiculous inconvenience brought positive feelings. Personal contribution, personal effort, personal sacrifice raised the family's spirits . . . we cooperated willingly and understandingly with our silent partners, the pills and syrups. Participation in this common project bonded the family unit, making up for the "separated feeling" created by the duty system.

Changing Roles and Demands   Our duty system provides respite for one parent and time with Jill and Jay for the other parent. Perhaps this system is not unique. Families with normal children follow similar patterns, but when the youngsters grow up the system ends. With time Jill and Jay joined the system, each being responsible for Glen's care for a specific time. Again, this sibling responsibility is common in families with normal children. However, our situation differs in complexity and extended use. Glen's condition and demands remain the same. Glen is still 2 years old no matter what his chronological age. With this extended "familyhood" come roles not normally played until later years, if ever.

By the time Glen was 3 years old, each family member played roles with bits and pieces belonging to that of doctor, olympian, educator, and psychologist.

1. *Medical Doctor*   Seizures and the required caregiving became normal routine even for the children, who handled episodes with confidence. However, bouts with asthma attacks, pneumonia, bronchitis (common childhood illnesses) increased in severity with his disorder. When sick and not eating, Glen's daily medication became so heavily concentrated in his blood, he easily came close to comas. Judgments were and are left up to

us: How many seizures constitute an emergency?

2. *Olympian* Glen's hyperactivity permitted only the healthy and strong to supervise his activities. His constant motion was physically exhausting at times.

3. *Educator* The task of educating Glen to achieve his developmental milestones was performed by trial and error. Oh, how we needed that developmental psychology degree! Breaking down learning processes for simple tasks, step by step, was difficult for us. Unaware of the developmental setbacks produced by each seizure, we took Glen's slow progress personally and as a reflection of our teaching skills. Conflicting professional opinions and family experiences created much psychological and emotional stress. After sharing our concerns over Glen's behavior and slow progress, the following professional reports were received:

> *The pediatrician:* Glen is developing normally.
>
> *The neurologist:* Treat Glen no differently than the other children. He is a normal child with seizures. You must not let him feel different.
>
> *The child psychologist:* Glen is a normal 2½-year old child. Mom has to get her act together.

Efforts intensified to MAKE GLEN NORMAL. We were doing something wrong. But what?

4. *Psychologist* Without formal training, experience, or models to follow, the family searched for successful behavior management techniques—reward systems, time-outs, exaggerated praise—and appropriate responses to Glen's actions.

How should one respond when finding seven bologna slices stuck neatly in a row on the outside of the refrigerator door, especially when the focus for that month was placing objects in a line? What is the maximum number of time-outs in one day? What behaviors brought on seizures? (While shopping, Glen's determination to get out of the cart ended in grand mal seizures . . . on 2 consecutive days. Did he have that much control over his seizures? Did our behavior have that much control?) Oh, where was the psychologist! How were we supposed to act? Respond? Live normally?

5. *Individual roles* In time each family member found his or her comfortable role with Glen. Interestingly, after examining these roles, each person selected a role opposite his or her natural interests. Jay, a child who must work hard in academics and needs lots of coaxing to do homework, chose the "teacher" role. When he is in charge, he schedules structured activities (i.e., puzzles, paints, matching games). Because of Glen's short attention span, Jay lines up projects allotting specific time periods for each.

Our 15-year-old daughter, Jill, who still insists on having her mom tuck her in bed every night and who repeatedly states, "I don't want to grow up," takes on the "mother" role when alone with Glen. Time passes quickly as she bathes him, washes his hair, and bakes cookies with him.

A comfortable role for Don is that of a "coffee mate." He and Glen spend many afternoons in restaurants drinking coffee and reading the paper. An athlete, outdoor person, and physical education teacher, Don finds his comfort zone in a restrictive environment with little physical activity.

As for myself, my role changes, too. My favorite pastime is reading and writing. Where do I find myself with Glen? On the basketball court shooting baskets and playing Horse. I elected to be Glen's "coach."

Relating to External Agencies Meeting the expectations of the above professional roles was attempted by the family before receiving educational and community intervention. We were very optimistic and excited for the time when Glen would receive the state's special education services. Our responsibilities would finally be shared with professionals—teachers, therapists, and psychologists—people with answers!

Preparation for Glen's schooling started with social workers, psychometrists, and psychologists. Oh, what welcomed intervention! At last, we would have help the medical profession could not provide. So confident was I that the first day Glen went off to school I started my working career outside the home. Adjustments within the family unit were difficult enough. Little did we know of the new demands waiting for us outside the home.

Assisting educators, nurses, and bus drivers in feeling comfortable with Glen's seizures was our first task. So many were frightened. Some, concerned over the slightest behavior change in Glen, anticipated seizures and would call me at work. Their adjustment process mirrored ours. Time and experience brought confidence.

Stressful events began accumulating, causing much frustration and anger. A lesson learned very early was that, when special education services increase, so do our responsibilities. We were informed by a child psychologist working closely with school systems that parents of handicapped children must become assertive, even obnoxious advocates for their children. Well, we qualify. For Glen to reach his maximum potential in growth and development, close monitoring, open communication, and persistence are required of us. First-hand experience has taught us that. A brief recap of Glen's 5-year educational experience explains why.

We requested Glen's first transfer out of a program due to the teacher's abuse of Glen (and the other children) and the sterile teaching environment. Other teachers encouraged us to go as far as to demand the teacher's release. We went as far as the superintendent. What he wanted to do with his staff was up to him (he retained her).

However, our major intent was to have Glen placed in an appropriate classroom. Glen's second transfer came about because the classroom size would be increasing from 5 to 14 students. Glen would be lost. Trusting the Department of Education specialist's expertise, we agreed to another recommended program. Glen was then placed with the profoundly retarded population with a rotation to 10 teachers a year, plus class rotation each day. Glen needs consistency. He needs routines. He needs models. Our great disapproval led to a third transfer. Presently, Glen is in a classroom of 14, all much higher-functioning students (reading and solving math problems). Glen, a 10-year-old boy functioning at a 2-year level, is again grossly misplaced. Glen's placement was based on our negative reactions to educational decisions, not on Glen's needs. This present teacher is known for his ability to handle "problem parents."

Demands outside the home have proven to be just as trying, if not more emotionally upsetting, than those inside the home. Faith in our "expected" educational support system has been shattered, but we continue to rebuild. We have to. We see future demands that will require just as much energy . . . . What does Glen do after 21? What facilities will be available for him in 10 years? Will I have to quit a career to stay home with him? What happens to him when we can no longer care for him? The demands will not change, but will grow in number and magnitude.

Some Aspects of Adaptive Capacity

Self-Esteem It is difficult to think about our personal skills as being unitary; our evaluations of ourselves and hence our self-esteem appear to be on a roller coaster, varying with the situations with which we are dealing and with how much control we have.

Parenting itself has brought so many rewards and satisfactions to Don and me as we see our children grow and succeed in school, sports, and social acceptance. Pride in ourselves and in our parenting skills comes mostly from Jill and Jay. Books, doctors, other parents, other children, relatives all provide us with guidelines in parenting and teaching. Applying our knowledge (what we instinctively know and what we learn from others) to our parenting skills permits us to play an active role in their achievements; thus, their successes are our successes.

Glen's successes evolve through an entirely different process. No one knows how Glen learns; hence, no guidelines are available. Glen determines what, when, and how to learn. At times quiet seizures unknown to us erase our efforts. The degree of satisfaction we receive with Glen's successes is as great as that of Jill and Jay. Perhaps, however, our disappointments stem from the level of the end product. Glen's number and level of end products are not even comparable to Jill's and Jay's. Thus, we feel more disappointed and less successful.

Glen's Individualized Education Program (IEP) conferences produce stress for us. Anxiety builds as we prepare for the meeting, updating our knowledge of appropriate goals and objectives, laws pertaining to transportation, special services, and so forth. This preparation for my teacher role often seems worthless as the conference itself is transformed into a hearing, an evaluation of our teaching skills. My mother role dominates to protect my teacher role, which lacks confidence to begin with. Here is where my overly protective, overly defensive instincts seep out. Silent conversations with myself help me get through the evaluation conducted by seven or more professionals.

Teacher:	Glen rarely completes tasks other than puzzles.
Mother:	He loves puzzles.
Teacher:	Glen has an aversion to table work.
Mother:	You should see him out on the basketball court. He made 100 baskets in 1 hour!
Teacher:	Glen drools. Children have an aversion toward socializing with him due to his touchiness.
Mother:	The drooling comes with his handicap. Everyone in Glen's world is okay, great. We're working on the hand shaking. Why are you teaching?
Teacher:	Glen is an affectionate little boy eager to start his day in school.
Mother:	Thank you. We like you, too.

Teacher:	Glen can sit for only 10 minutes.
Mother:	Wow, that's 5 minutes longer than last year! Great!
Teacher:	Children bring their life-style to school. Much of Glen's energies are spent in "avoidance behaviors."
Mother:	Now just wait a minute young man! Do you have 20 hours to hear what the family, especially Glen, has gone through for the past 10 years!

We are truly grateful and appreciative for the special education Glen receives. Beautiful, skillful people have rescued us. Positive thoughts do outweigh the negative ones; however, once a year we experience extreme apprehension toward our roles as teacher.

Constant Support Systems   We are truly fortunate. Even before Glen's disorder manifested itself, love, health, emotional stability, financial security, and education were all present. My heart cries out for families lacking any one of these at the onset of hardships such as ours. In this "special parenthood" every faculty is put to ultimate testing; each needs support. Our continuum of support systems evolved in different manners. Some systems had to be sought out, others automatically came. Within our support network I found three kinds of help: constant (family, friends, doctors); intermittent (community); and individualized.

Nuclear Family   Mental, emotional, and physical help has come from the family itself through common experiences. The intense highs and lows that the family share create strong understandings that each is not alone. When Glen stops, we stop. After returning from middle-of-the-night emergency runs, the family often slept together in one bedroom just to stay close. When Glen is hospitalized, the children choose to wait at the hospital, rather than stay with friends (in one instance they waited patiently for 6 hours). We all reach our natural highs when Glen recovers from another bad spell; adds a new word to his vocabulary; learns a new behavior or drops an annoying one; and then Glen keeps us child-like as he reminds us of the flowers, garbage trucks, buses, bubbles, and birds.

Effects of the continuous influx of conflicts seep out even in minor attitude changes, and the family again works with these changes. For example, I've made buying presents for me somewhat challenging for the other family members (an attitude I'm working on to reverse). Perhaps to spare myself from even the slightest pain or disappointment, I've set up strange criteria for them to follow when selecting gifts: nothing that breaks, nothing that wears out, nothing that dies. What's left? Intangible gifts—dinners out, time with friends, time for classes, vacations, and solitude. Memories last. My most memorable Mother's Day gift was an evening under the stars at the Waikiki Shell with Andy Williams, while the family dashed home to scrub floors, clean bathrooms, and do laundry before picking me up after the show. Intangible gifts are respite for me. Marvelous biking and camping trips through Alaska with their adventurous father have given Jill and Jay their special respite. Time set aside for cycling, running, and coaching provides Don with respite. We give free time to each other. Our understanding through common experiences and teamwork in providing respite gives us the emotional and mental support we need.

Friends As with any team, the spectators' spirit and encouragement energize team effort. Loyal friendships, which are many, have furnished us with this support throughout the years. Even though they themselves cannot fully comprehend or feel the impact of our situation, their availability comforts us. Sharing their struggles and pleasures with us has relieved our periodic feelings of isolation, reminding us that every family, not just the Metzgers, has its own mountains to climb. Special friends have entered into our lives recently. These few people are not spectators but teammates because they too have children like our Glen. They too live with seizures and mental retardation. Our meeting was perhaps spiritual for me as we just sat in silence looking at each other. At last, no words were needed. The understanding and compassion were already present. Now, no lengthy descriptions are nec-

essary in replying to "How are things going?" Just "good" or "bad" is enough to receive encouragement or hurrahs. Sharing experiences has allowed each of us in our own way to help the other with the present problems and to anticipate future demands on the family as time passes.

Doctors During the first 3 years, the medical profession was the family's primary support. We needed them desperately at any given time, and they were there. We still do need them. Their expertise provides assistance with medical needs—seizures, medications, illnesses; thus, they have become Glen's primary support. Secondary to that are the family's needs for emotional, mental, and physical guidance that are met through other people.

Intermittent Support *Church Support* Before Karen's arrival, we were "periodic" church goers, each still in the process of formulating our own beliefs. Being new church members when Karen was born provided immediate ministerial and prayer support. Don and I were able to attend church regularly because much of Karen's brief life was spent in the hospital. Having this spiritual support did help us through our crises with Karen. However, shortly after her death, the minister stated, "Karen is in Heaven, but in the same physical and mental states as she was on earth." Confusion and sadness that was generated from this particular theological belief started our search for other theories, other churches. We did find another church. However, Glen's seizures and hyperactivity proved too much for the nursery staff and ourselves. Trying to sit attentively and calmly in a service, still being very anxious about the activities in the nursery, was extremely difficult. Soon, our duty system touched this routine. We began attending church separately.

One of my favorite childhood Bible passages, I Corinthians 13:4, began flashing over and over in my mind as time passed:

Love is very patient and kind, never jealous or envious, never boastful or proud, never haughty or selfish or rude. Love does not demand its own way. It is not irritable or touchy. It does not hold grudges and will hardly even notice when others do it wrong.

Strong ambivalence between the church's description of Love and what I was actually feeling created inner turmoil. Because I found myself unable to meet many of these expectations, I felt unlovable and thus sought church counseling. Ambivalence with my anger (over Glen's suffering and its effect on our lives) and love was intense. I did not have kind feelings. Patience, put in laymen's terms as "the admirable endurance of a trying situation or person, usually through a passiveness which comes out of understanding," was not present. Trying to comprehend our situation—even the doctors and clergy didn't understand—brought everything but passivity, patience. I was irritable. I was touchy. I was jealous and envious of "normal" families. I did hold grudges. I did have resentment. Resentment, "the ill will and suppressed anger generated by a sense of grievance," allowed me little space to forgive. The counselor told me that I would forgive when I released my resentment after my grieving stopped. We were grieving the slow death of our child's promising future . . . our grieving process is still in progress. When will our grieving stop so resentment can leave to allow forgiving feelings to occur?

I was told that the feelings we were experiencing were the same as everyone else's—which placed us in the "normality" bracket again. I was not told that, along with intense situations, intense feelings arise—that my profound struggles were understandable and okay. The counselor's last words, "Glen has the problem. Glen has the seizures, not you," offered little comfort. Yes, Glen has seizures. But so did the family members. Seizures controlled our lives! I suspect the physical and mental demands in caring for Glen became higher priorities over my spiritual understanding as I grew tired of "thinking spiritually." Perhaps the church did help all it could, and I was not open enough. Whatever the reason, spiritual support via personal reading, personal conversations with God, and personal thinking took over the role that once belonged to the church. Church became merely an hour of respite.

Community Support   As Glen approached eligibility for schooling, tangible and concrete help began to clear our confusion. Home visits by social workers personalized their services. Help was finally coming to us, rather than our seeking it. Glen's psychological testing and our parent interviews established a basis from which we could start monitoring any progress, Glen's and ours. The Easter Seal Society provided Glen with his first schooling experience. Its first goal, which took a year to achieve, was to have Glen remain in the room—not just on a chair or activity—but in the room. Mother rap sessions guided by the society's psychologist alleviated the isolation and frustrations felt and elevated our spirits. Throughout Glen's schooling, despite our periodic disappointments and struggles with the system, many kind, understanding, and skillful teachers brought much encouragement and hope to the family. We will always need their support.

The support system having the most impact on our lives has been the Easter Seal Society's respite program. Respite provides us with temporary relief; it provides after-school care for Glen daily and all day on holidays. Respite staff's expertise in supervision, discipline, and structured activities not only helps us but contributes much to Glen's social development. Its existence enables both Don and me to maintain full-time employment, and Jill and Jay to participate in after-school activities. Glen's need for "independence" is fulfilled at Respite through his interaction with other children, outside the demanding classroom and his family supervision. He loves Respite! We love Respite! We need Respite!

Individual Support Systems   Not only is life a continuous process of adjustments, it is a process of changing roles—hats I call them. After 15 years of wearing a Don hat, Jill hat, Jay hat, Glen hat, and Family hat, the time came when I wanted my own hat. The absurdity of adding another hat to my crowded wardrobe was overpowered by my tremendous urge to do something for myself, Joyce. The first day Glen went off to school, I put on my own

Career hat. Of course, this action added another dimension to our already unpredictable life-style, but the rewards have been many. No other "therapy" has had such an impact on my psychological well-being as my own career. Time devoted to developing my own skills and creativity has raised my self-esteem to new and important highs. It has made me a happier wife, mother, and individual. My colleagues and work stimulate my mind! Casual conversations range from the latest recipes to such questions as "Does thought come before language, or does language come before thought?" However, Glen seldom leaves my mind. As I do at home, I work minute to minute, not really knowing when the next emergency will strike. My own career has brought about a new perspective on my life. Life is not one big seizure! Life is not only to give of oneself, but it is also okay to take for oneself. This balance voids my feelings of self-denial and self-pity.

Along with my involvement with the "normal" population at work, another support system is my involvement with agencies working with the "special" population. Hope for Glen's future has risen through my exposure to such service-providing agencies as I learn about their joint efforts to improve life for handicapped persons and their families. Knowledge acquired about services available through these agencies would not have come easily through social workers and teachers alone. Experience has shown me that most of these people are familiar only with their own specialty.

A support system I wish had entered our lives much earlier than it did is individual and family counseling. Inevitable repercussions from our unnatural duty system have appeared. Psychological intervention could have corrected misperceptions and approved sad feelings. Jill and Jay love Glen and are extremely protective of him, but they too experience ambivalent feelings. "My friends tease me and say I'm mental like Glen." "I don't want Glen near my friends because he scares them." "Where will you take Glen when my friends come over?" "Don't let them see him with his helmet on." "Honestly, won't he ever grow up!" Don—the provider, the father, and husband—responsible for everyone's well-being, silently struggles with his own emotions. As close as we are, we all possess our own private anxieties, fears, and pain. Counseling with all of us, telling us that our negative feelings are normal, should have started when we were a young family. Oh, how I wish we all could have gone through these years emotionally, as we did physically, together.

Summary of Case History

We experience the same emotions with Glen as we did with Karen—love, joy, sadness, fear. Reflecting back on Karen's brief 15 months, sadness seemed to have been the paramount emotion felt. A quiet sadness. Crises seemed to have appeared and disappeared quietly, perhaps the reason being there were just the three of us. However, with Glen, time intensified these same feelings.

> Time added new feelings—anger, disillusionment, self-doubt, isolation.
> Time brought the normal growth demands to each member: each one struggling through life stages, each one working hard to achieve dreams, each one striving to become the best he or she can be.
> Time brought other significant events in life:
> "Joyce, your father passed away."
> "Don, your mother has cancer."
> "Don, your father passed away."
> "Don, your mother passed away."

Ten years of "normal" living filled with the continuous recycling of crises attached to Glen's handicap—illness, failure, disappointment, fear—have tested our strength and endurance as individuals and as a family unit.

We anticipate Jill's and Jay's future with enthusiasm. Success has already come to them in academic achievement and social acceptance. We look forward to their promising careers, their marriages, and our grandchildren. In contrast, apprehension smothers our view of Glen's future. As hard as he tries, he is still destined for scholastic failure, social rejection and an inability to live independently, marry, or have children. Preparing Jill's and Jay's future comes with time. Planning Glen's future starts today. As one of his teachers said, if we want Glen to be a sweeper at "McDonalds" 10 years from now, the broom has to be placed in his hands now. Glen's total dependence on Don and me will remain, and recurrent crises will continue. We wonder who will outlast whom? How many more seizures can his little body take? What will the family do when Glen becomes 21 and ineligible for school programs? When we die or are unable to care for him, who will assist him with his self-help skills? Whose heart will overlook his inappropriate behavior, his failure to learn, his seizures? Who will love our 2-year-old son?

SUMMARY: A FINAL WORD

The Stress-Adaptation model presented in this paper has been under development since 1980. The Metzgers have been living with Glen for 10 years. Model and case study have come together in this paper to illustrate *general* principles with *specific* instances. No model can capture a single family's experiences with absolute fidelity; each family will uniquely experience the stresses with which they cope. Yet, models have a great usefulness in enabling us to analyze families with somewhat different

experiences so that more appropriate services and policies can be generated. In the Metzger's case, for example, many of the *demands* associated with having Glen were actually created by the various service agencies with whom the family interacted. The family had to become its own case manager, mediating the demands and figuring out how to respond.

This case history was summarized over a 10-year period. It would not be possible to trace how many times the family cycled through the process described by the Stress-Adaptation model. It is clear that both individually and as a unit the family's adaptive capacity became strained through this repeated recycling. It is also clear, however, that this family was able to muster new resources as older ones became dysfunctional. Not all families may be that strong.

Both parts of this chapter should serve to alert professionals concerned with families of handicapped children to the areas where they can do the most appropriate research, provide the most effective services, and generate the most potentially useful policies. Somehow, in addition, there needs to be the resolve and the wherewithal to accomplish these tasks.

REFERENCES

Agathonas, H., & Valaes, T. C. (1982). Families of children with Down's Syndrome in Greece. *Journal of Comparative Family Studies, 13,* 221–229.

Beckman, P. J. (1983). Influence of selected child characteristics on stress in families of handicapped children. *American Journal of Mental Deficiency, 89,* 150–156.

Belsky, J. (1984). The determinants of parenting: A process model. *Child Development, 55,* 83–96.

Blacher, J. (1984). Sequential stages of parental adjustment to the birth of a child with handicaps: Fact or artifact. *Mental Retardation, 22,* 55–68.

Boyce, W. T., Jensen, W. W., James, S. A., & Peacock, J. L. (1983). The family routines inventory: Theoretical origins. *Social Science and Medicine, 17,* 193–200.

Breslau, N., Salkever, D., & Staruch, K. S. (1982). Women's labor force activity and responsibilities for disabled dependents: A study of families with disabled children. *Journal of Health and Social Behavior, 23,* 169–183.

Cassel, J. (1978). The contribution of the social environment to host resistance. *American Journal of Epidemiology, 104,* 107–123.

Coddington, R. D. (1972). The significance of life events as ideologic factors in the disease of children. *Journal of Psychosomatic Research, 16,* 7–18.

Comfort-Smith, M. & Bailey, D. (1984, April). *Maternal*

characteristics that influence mother-child interaction. In D. C. Farran (Chair). *Rating maternal interactions with handicapped and at-risk infants: A new clinical and research instrument.* Symposium presented at the Eighth Biennial Meeting of the Southeastern Conference on Human Development, Athens, GA.

Cox, T. (1978). *Stress.* London: Macmillan.

Crnic, K. A., Friedrich, W. N., & Greenberg, M. T. (1983). Adaptation of families with mentally retarded children: A model of stress, coping, and family ecology. *American Journal of Mental Deficiency, 88,* 125–138.

Drotar, D., Baskiewicz, B. A., Irvin, N., Kennell, J., & Klaus, M. (1975). The adaptation of parents to the birth of an infant with a congenital malformation: A hypothetical model. *Pediatrics, 56,* 710–717.

Farran, D. C., Kasari, C. & Jay, S. (1983). *Parent-Child Interaction Scale Training Manual.* Chapel Hill, NC: Frank Porter Graham Child Development Center.

Farran, D. C., & Margolis, L. (1984). Integrative model for analyzing the effects of a precipitous stress such as unemployment of families. In L. Margolis & D. Farran (Eds.), *The North Carolina work and family life project: An investigation of the health and behavioral consequences for families of paternal job loss.* Final report submitted to the WT Grant Foundation.

Gallagher, J. J. (1983). The Carolina Institute for Research. Early Education of the Handicapped. *Journal of the Division for Early Childhood, 1,* 18–24.

Gallagher, J. J., Beckman, P., & Cross, A. H. (1983). Families of handicapped children: Sources of stress and its amelioration. *Exceptional Children, 50,* 10–19.

Heinicke, C., Diskin, S., Ramsey-Klee, D., & Given, K. (1983). Pre-birth parent characteristics and family development in the first year of life. *Child Development, 54,* 194–208.

Holmes, T. H., & Rahe, R. (1967). The Social Readjustment Rating Scale. *Journal of Psychosomatic Research, 11,* 213–218.

Kasari, C. & Farran, D. (1983). *Child Care Role Scale.* Unpublished instrument. (Available from the Carolina Institute for Research in Early Education of the Handicapped, University of North Carolina, Chapel Hill, NC 27514).

Kasari, C. & Farran, D. (1984, December). Relationship between early intervention and mother-infant interaction. Poster presented at the National Conference on Comprehensive Approaches to Handicapped and At-Risk Infants, Toddlers and Their Families, Washington, DC.

Kasari, C., Farran, D., & Harber, L. (1984, March). *Variability of infant social-communicative behavior in caregiver-infant interactions.* Paper presented at the 1984 Gatlinburg Conferences on Mental Retardation/Developmental Disabilities, Gatlinburg, TN.

Lin, N., Simeone, R., Ensel, W., & Kuo, W. (1979). Social support, stressful life events, and illness: A model and an empirical test. *Journal of Health and Social Behavior, 20,* 108–119.

Margolis, L. & Farran, D. (1984). *The North Carolina work and family life project: An investigation of the health and behavioral consequences for families of paternal job loss.* Final report submitted to the WT Grant Foundation.

McCubbin, H., Joy, C., Cauble, A., Comeau, J., Patterson, J., & Needle, R. (1980). Family stress and coping: A decade review. *Journal of Marriage and the Family, 42,* 855–871.

Minde, K. K., Hackett, J. D., Killou, D., & Silver, S. (1972). How they grow up: 41 physically handicapped children and their families. *American Journal of Psychiatry, 128,* 104–110.

Pearlin, L. I., Lieberman, M. A., Menaghan, E. G., & Mullan, J. T. (1981). The stress process. *Journal of Health and Social Behavior, 22,* 337–366.

Selye, H. (1956). *The stress of life.* New York: McGraw-Hill.

Selye, H. (1980). The stress concept and some of its implications. In V. Hamilton & D. Warburton (Eds.), *Human stress and cognition.* Chichester, England: Wiley.

Shapiro, J. (1983). Family reactions and coping strategies in response to the physically ill or handicapped child: A review. *Social Science and Medicine, 17,* 913–931.

Sparling, J. (1984). *Parental adaptation to prenatal diagnosis of impairment.* Unpublished manuscript. (Available from Joyce Sparling, Dept. of Special Education, University of North Carolina, Chapel Hill, NC. 27514.)

Suelzle, M., & Keenan, V. (1981). Changes in family support networks over the life cycle of mentally retarded persons. *American Journal of Mental Deficiency, 86,* 267–274.

Thoits, P. A. (1982). Conceptual, methodological, and theoretical problems in studying social support as a buffer against life stress. *Journal of Health and Social Sciences, 23,* 145–159.

Turner, R. (1981). Social support as a contingency in psychological well-being. *Journal of Health and Social Behavior, 22,* 357–367.

Wikler, L. (1981). Chronic stresses of families of mentally retarded children. *Family Relations, 30,* 281–288.

Williams, A., Ware, J., & Donald, C. (1981). A model of mental health, life events and social supports applicable to general populations. *Journal of Health and Social Behavior, 22,* 324–336.

Section
III

SOCIAL ECOLOGY OF FAMILIES WITH HANDICAPPED CHILDREN

Chapter

10

Family Stress Theory and Research on Families of Children with Mental Retardation

Lynn McDonald Wikler

INTEREST IN STRESS in families of children with mental retardation has increased dramatically in recent years. In both 1983 and 1984, federal agencies dealing with mental retardation designated ''family support'' as a priority for funding of research programs. Seventeen state legislatures, concerned with averting the need for institutionalization, have initiated tax-supported family support programs to bolster family functioning; two years ago, there were only four such programs (Bates, 1984). The number of research reports on family functioning presented at American Association on Mental Deficiency meetings is two to three times that of previous years, and journals in the field recently carried major review articles or published special issues (Crnic, Friedrich, & Greenberg, in *American Journal of Mental Deficiency*, 1983; Gallagher, Beckman, & Cross, in *Exceptional Child*, 1983; Earhart & Sporakowski, in *Family Relations: Special Issue on Families of Children with Handicaps*, Janu-

ary, 1984; Blacher, in *Mental Retardation*, 1984; and Hansen & Coppersmith, in *Family Therapy Collections: Special Issue on Families of Handicapped Children*, 1984).

The rather sudden attention devoted to the mentally retarded person's family is a consequence of the normalization movement. Normalization begins with withdrawal from, or avoidance of, institutionalization. The best alternative to institutions, for children, is the family; yet the family environment will not serve as a reliable milieu for mentally retarded children if their presence is perceived as overly burdensome and, in particular, if their inclusion proves so stressful that adequate family functioning becomes impossible. It is a telling, although often forgotten, fact that one of the institution's original functions was to relieve the family of the perceived burden of caring for a child with mental retardation. The institutions may disappear, but the families' needs do not. Yet, as the movement away from institutions became a stampede, little was known of the families' capacities, resources, and limits in providing care.

As a result, clinicians, special educators, and researchers, who until only recently studied the individual child with mental retardation in a social vacuum, are now scrambling to expand their knowledge about the child's immediate psychosocial context, the family. Unfortunately, some of the current writing reflects a further academic violation as no notice is taken of the extensive literature on family stress existing in journals of such disciplines as sociology, social work, social support, and family therapy. Too often, studies of stress in mental retardation families do not make their theoretical framework explicit, and some seem to lack one altogether. On the other hand, with the notable exception of Bernard Farber and a few others, the major writers on family stresses have paid little attention to mental retardation. An interdisciplinary approach is called for to address this deficit, so researchers, planners, and clinicians may better respond to the current public concern.

Sociologists of family development theory deal with family change by dividing family life over time into a series of eight stages (Duvall, 1957). Role reciprocities and role conflicts at different periods in the family's development depend on structural features of the family. The assumptions are that there is high member interdependence and that families are forced to change the rules for interaction as roles shift. These theorists do not, however, address the process of developmental change by which families differentiate and transform their interactional structure. It is the family stress theorists that offer perspectives on the ways in which these transitions would proceed. Family stress theorists have elaborated on how both normative and nonnormative stressors provoke disequilibrium in stable familial responses (Adams, 1968, 1975; Farber, 1968; Hill, 1949).

Family stress theories that have been proposed have not received sufficient elaboration and testing. Nevertheless, one theory in particular is both plausible in its own right and

rich in its implications for understanding the functioning of families with mentally retarded children. Its potential for summarizing the literature on family stress in this area and for assessing that literature's strengths and shortcomings makes it ideal for use in the present review. The particular theoretical framework used in this discussion is based on work by the sociologist, Reuben Hill (1949, 1958, 1970, 1983) and on its elaboration (particularly in the important dimension of stress in families over time) in recent work by McCubbin and Patterson, (1983): Hill's "ABCX" Model. It must be emphasized that the theory is not "proven" and may not be capable of substantiation; the author refers to it for its heuristic value, and the remarks that follow do not presuppose its acceptance.

The goal of this chapter is to demonstrate the usefulness of existing theories of family stress in organizing our knowledge of stress in families of children with mental retardation. There are five sections in this chapter directed toward this goal. First, a family stress theory is summarized and discussed in relation to mental retardation. Second, two separate literature reviews are presented using that theory. Third, two recent research projects applying the theoretical framework are described. Fourth, the familial perceptions about mental retardation are emphasized as a research challenge. Fifth, future directions of research in family stress and mental retardation are suggested.

HILL'S ABCX MODEL ON FAMILY STRESS

Attention to families' reactions and adjustment to stress has been a long tradition in family research. Much of this work assesses the impact on the family of "stressor" events in relation to a host of variables, ranging from the individual's psychological condition to interpersonal relations both within the family and between the family and the outside world. These interactions have been studied both synchronically and diachronically and in relation to both single stressor events and series. Hill's conceptualization of the process of a familial reaction to stressor events in his ABCX model of family crisis, in particular, has provided the foundation for much of the family crisis research in the past two decades.

Hill's schema begins with the identification of four components of the family's experience of stress:

A (The stressor event)—interacting with
B (The family's crisis-meeting resources)—interacting with
C (The definition the family makes of the event)—procedure
X (The family crisis)

Each of these elements exists in the kinds of familial response to mental retardation on which research is currently focused. However, these elements are not always satisfactorily identified and distinguished. Even the most important distinction, that between the stressor event(s) and the family's crisis, is sometimes blurred. Some elaboration on these elements is thus needed before proceeding with the present view.

The stressor event (A) can be defined as a problem situation that presents itself to the family for resolution.

> Stressor is the life event or transition impacting upon the family unit which produces, or has the potential of producing, change in the family social system. This change may be in various areas of family life such as its boundaries, goals, patterns of interaction, roles or values. (McCubbin & Patterson, 1983)

The definition of stressor events as problem situations that present themselves to the family for resolution directs attention to the process of stress. This enables the researcher to make observations of both adaptive and nonadaptive responses to stressors in families. "Stressor" would be an event or a state that arises from a "demand-capability" imbalance in the family's functioning, which is characterized by a nonspecific demand for coping behaviors, with distress or crisis (X) being the unpleasant dysfunctional or maladaptive responses to that demand (McCubbin & Patterson, 1983). Hill drew attention to the importance of distinguishing normative stressors (e.g., developmental milestones, transitions, death) from nonnormative stressors (e.g., war, floods, earthquakes) and stressors having their source within the family system from those arising outside the family system (1949, 1958; Mederer & Hill, 1983).

Although these distinctions about stressors have yet to be incorporated into the research on families of children with mental retardation, there is evidence that the categories of stressors have differential impacts on family functioning. For example, an essential feature of the normative/nonnormative distinction is the extent to which the stressor can be anticipated. If the stressor is anticipated and preparations can therefore be made, the impact of the stressor on the family is likely to be significantly reduced (Golan, 1981).

The significance of the normative/nonnormative distinction in mental retardation seems to be mediated by social class. For middle-class families, mental impairment in the child is ordinarily a nonnormative (i.e., unanticipated) stressor, regardless of the level of retardation. For the lower-class family, the child's mental retardation is always a nonnormative stressor if it is moderate or severe (see Farber's (1975) eloquent discussion of this point); however, for a lower-class family, the level of functioning of the person with mild mental retardation may be seen as normative. Multiple threats to normal development continuously exert themselves on a poor family and thus increase several-fold the likelihood of having a mildly mentally impaired child (see Begab, Haywood, and Garber, 1983; Ramey and Finkelstein, 1981). Even if it were perceived as nonnormative by the poor family, the mild mental retardation may be perceived by the caregiving members of the family as having less impact than other stressors that present a threat to survival (e.g., eviction, hunger, unemployment or severe illness). The relative weight of the stressor is thus contextually determined. Farber (1968) distinguishes the "role reorganization crisis" of the lower-class family with a mentally retarded child from the "tragic crisis" of the middle-class family.

The distinction between intra- and extra-familial source of the stressor (arising in connection with mental retardation) is equally rich in its implications for analysis of the family's situation. Generally, the stressor event of mental retardation in a child is classified as internal to the family. The child who is afflicted with the disability is a member of the family, and the origin of the stressor is perceived to be the child's internal make-up, whether resulting from genetic disease or unspecified. Occasionally, however, mental retardation presents itself as having an extrafamilial source, as in the case of a child who becomes brain damaged as a result of a collision with a car driven by a drunk driver, or that of a child who becomes mentally retarded because of poor medical treatment. In both of these cases the cause of the mental retardation is external. Future research may find it useful to distinguish between internal and external sources of the handicapping condition of the child.

Nonnormative stressors, although unexpected, do not long remain unexplained by family members, and their personal understandings of the origin of the stressor affect their responses to it. Fate, or God, or else the family genetic tree on the one side or another may be blamed, or the blame may be placed on the person with the disability. An example that illustrates this dimension of blame in families is autism. Autism fulfills the criteria of being a nonnormative familial stressor. When Kanner (1957) first identified the disorder, he characterized the mother as typically being cold and disengaged from the child. The causality of autism was quickly labeled as INTERNAL by professionals, and for years families suffered stresses beyond those of raising an unresponsive, difficult, developmentally delayed child, that is, stresses of being blamed by the helping professionals (see Wasow & Wikler, 1983).

Although Hill's stressor categories apply directly and helpfully to the study of family functioning in relation to mental retardation, they constitute only the first items on a long list of factors that have been shown to have a differential effect. The degree of severity of the child's mental disability has already been mentioned as a factor; so too are the number of handicapping conditions, the age and sex of the child, and the behavioral and social characteristics of the mentally retarded child. A recent study, for example, investigated the relationship between such interactional and social dimensions as the child's temperament, responsiveness, repetitive behavioral patterns, and caregiving demands with level of stress reported by mothers (Beckman, 1983). The results help illustrate the variability inherent in the stressor of mental retardation, going beyond the IQ scores themselves.

Hill's model dismisses the notion of a direct relationship between the stressor event (A) and the resulting family crisis (X). He proposes instead that there are two major buffering variables, which could protect the family from becoming dysfunctional following exposure to the stressor event. The B factor comprises various types of family resources available to that particular family; the C factor is the subjective meaning assigned to the stressor event by the family. Hill assigns equal weights to the two factors and suggests that they either increase a family's vulnerability toward the stressor or resilience against the stressor.

Hill summarizes the B factor as the "adequacy-inadequacy of family organization" (1958). Burr (1973), in his synthesis of family stress research, describes the B factor as the family's ability to prevent a change in the family social system from creating a crisis or disruption in the system; that is, the capability for resisting crisis. The B factor has received a great deal of attention by stress researchers in recent years. The following list identifies some essential features of a family's resources:

1. **INDIVIDUAL** variables, such as current and historical coping skills, health, mental health, educational level, and intensity of religious beliefs of each family member
2. **MARITAL** variables, such as marital status, marital satisfaction levels, role consensus; and the couple's negotiation skills,

communication styles, their patterns of sharing of roles and workloads and providing emotional support

3. **FAMILY** interactional variables, such as the family's level of adaptability and cohesion, their history of managing with transitional or nonnormative stressors; the structure of their interaction, their sharing of affect, the autonomy of family members, the congruence of their mythology, the efficiency of task negotiation (Beavers, 1982), and the extent to which they give support to one another, promoting self-esteem

4. **EXTENDED FAMILY** variables, such as frequency of contact, type of contact, function of contact, and satisfaction with contact, all of which help define the impact of the extended family in buffering the nuclear family from the impact of both chronic and acute stressors

5. **INTIMATE FRIENDS,** their frequency of contact, the intensity of the relationship, and the functions of these exchanges

6. **FRIENDS AND NEIGHBORS,** the number of such relationships, the functions served in these relationships, and the degree of reciprocity and maintenance of the relationships over time

7. **COMMUNITY GROUPS, CLUBS, WORKPLACE ACQUAINTANCES,** number of involvements, functional exchanges, reciprocity, maintenance over time

8. **PROFESSIONALS AND HUMAN SERVICES ORGANIZATIONS,** the number and type, the type of service performed, length of involvement, and satisfaction with services delivered

Family resources can be classified into three levels: personal supports, the informal support network and the formal support network (McCubbin, Joy, Cauble, Comeau, Patterson, & Needle 1980). Support networks are currently being studied with avid interest because interaction with a good support network when faced with acute stressors is so repeat-

edly and significantly correlated with better functioning (Bruhn and Philips, 1984). The most recent research studies are attempting to define further the most beneficial types of support networks. These studies suggest that it is better to have one intimate with whom you have daily contact, rather than several acquaintances; it is better when not everyone in your support network knows everyone else (because of the risk of losing all if any judge you badly); it is better if your support network satisfies multiple needs, including financial and other forms of assistance, as well as companionship and emotional support; and it is better to reciprocate with your own functional contributions to the support network, in the interest of maintaining that support network over time. Families with more personal resources and strong interpersonal informal support networks cope better with high stress than do those without these family resources (Ell, 1984).

The formal support network consists of professionals and community agencies used by the family. Although these are professional helpers, they are not necessarily the main source of help; in one study inquiring into the sequence with which families under stress report how they choose family resources, the professional was turned to last (Vincent, 1983). When a person requests help from the professional, it may well be because all the previous attempts to engage support from informal support have failed.

The C factor of perception, in contrast to the B factor, family resources, has received too little attention from family stress researchers (Boss, 1986) as a variable that could buffer the impact of the stressor on the family. Hill (1949) defined the C factor as the degree to which the situation is seen by the family as a threat to family status, family goals, or family objectives. The subjective meaning that members of a particular family assign to the stressor event will, Hill suggests, weigh as a mediating variable in predicting the course of events for that family. This perceptual factor affects the degree to which family members make an effort to coordinate their interaction as a group response to the stressor (Mederer and Hill, 1983). Family members may view the stressor as easy or difficult to manage, as "fate" or as an aggression against the family unit, as an opportunity to grow from a challenge or as an overwhelming load necessitating escape. As a result, they may perceive themselves as helpless victims or achieve the role of active agents in their effort to survive and to overcome the stressor's effects. According to Burr (1973), "the best label for this phenomenon is probably the subjective definition of the severity of the change."

Stressor events are events that demand accommodation from the family; in McCubbin's terms, tension that needs to be managed.

Family stress (AS DISTINCT FROM STRESSOR) is defined as a state that arises from an actual OR perceived demand capability imbalance in the family's functioning and which is characterized by a multidimensional demand for adjustment or adaptive behavior. Stress, then, is not stereotypic, but rather varies depending upon the nature of the situation, the characteristics of the family unit, and the psychological and physical well-being of its members. Stress becomes distress when it is subjectively defined as unpleasant or undesirable by the family unit. (McCubbin & Patterson, 1983)

Crisis (the X factor) comprises any sharp or decisive change for which old family patterns are inadequate (Hill, 1949), the amount of disruption in the family system, and the extensiveness of the impact of the stressor on the family's functioning. "It denotes variation in the amount of disruptiveness, incapacitatedness, or disorganization of the family social system, and it varies continuously from no crisis to a high amount of crisis" (Burr, 1973). "As distinct from stress, which is a demand-capability imbalance, crisis is characterized by the family's inability to restore stability and by the continuous pressure to make changes in the family structure and patterns of interaction. In other words, stress may never reach crisis proportions if the family is able to use existing resources and define the situation so as to resist systemic change and maintain family stability." McCubbin and Patterson (1983), as did Hill (1949, 1958), proposed that a "period

of disorganization" would characterize the family as it accomodated to the stressor event.

Hill's ABCX model is based on an assumption that the stressor event is a discrete event with a beginning and an end. As such, his theory pertains to acute rather than chronic stressors: Hill's portrait of a family's adjustment has been called the roller coaster model (as can be seen in Figure 1 on page 186). A period of disorganization occurs following the stressor event. Thereafter, the family restructures and reestablishes its equilibrium. The new level might be better or worse than the previous level of family functioning (Mederer & Hill, 1983). The angle of the dip (to continue the roller coaster metaphor)—that is, the abyss of family dysfunction during the crisis—would be determined by the B and C factors. Thus, by assessing the resources the family has available for handling a stressor event, as well as the meaning that it makes of that stressor event, one should be able to predict the extensiveness of the family crisis that would result from the stressor event. Alternatively, interventions that altered the number and quality of family resources and/or the cognitive attributions shared by the family about the stressor event could alleviate the severity of the impact of the stressor event.

McCubbin and Patterson (1983) have recently added a new dimension to the ABCX model: Their "Double ABCX Model" focuses on the family efforts over time to recover from a crisis situation. Using Hill's original ABCX model as its foundation, it adds postcrisis variables in an effort to describe: 1) the additional life stressors and life strains that shape the course of family adaptation; 2) the critical psychological, intrafamilial, and social resources that families acquire and employ over time in managing crisis situations; 3) the changes in definition and meaning assigned by families to the process of adjustment as families develop a description of their efforts to overcome their predicament; 4) the coping strategies families employ; and 5) the range of outcomes of these family efforts (McCubbin and Patterson, 1983). This elaboration of the ABCX model is an effort to describe additional concurrent stressors affecting recovery from the original crisis, both the new and previously existing resources used by the families in the recovery process, their perceptions and evaluation of their postcrisis situation, and the family outcome or degree of adaptation (Mederer & Hill, 1983).

The ABCX models may take on a greater potential utility in examining the processes of stress in families of a child with mental retardation because mental retardation is such an extremely stigmatizing feature of a person in this society. Not all societies perceive mental retardation as so totally negative. (See Edgerton, 1970, for a commentary on various societal perspectives toward people with mental retardation in his review of anthropological studies.) The family of the retarded person feels the brunt of these prejudices, but it also may share them. It is critical, therefore, when examining how the stressor event of mental retardation, which is so harshly stereotyped, would affect a family, to include an examination of how the family perceives and values the person with mental retardation and its associated hardships.

The subjective meaning (C) accorded to this stressor by almost everyone who interacts with the child and the parents is uniformly discrediting. And the problem starts early. The stigma associated with mental retardation affects the infant and its family from diagnosis onwards, and for an infant with Down syndrome, the process of alienation probably begins at birth. Nurses whisper, doctors avoid coming into the room, parents decline to send out announcements, and friends and family fail to visit and welcome the new baby or congratulate the mother. The perception of the stigmatizing condition inhibits people who ordinarily might rejoice in a new baby's arrival from their usual behavior. Whether out of fear, sadness, or lack of information on how to handle the novel situation, the most common behavioral response may be to withdraw, rather than approach.

The long-term effect of social stigma is, in many instances, to diminish severely the family's informal support network, thereby causing them to lose a vital family resource (see Darling, 1981). Thus perceptions about men-

tal retardation may not only affect family outcome (X) but also interact with the family resources (B) from the outset, as well as over time. For example, an often-found characteristic of families of children with mental retardation is that they are socially isolated when compared to families of normal children matched for social class (Davis & Mackay, 1973; McAllister, Butler, & Lei, 1973). Because poor informal support systems combined with high stress is a combination that jeopardizes families (Ell, 1984; Egeland, Breitenbucher, & Rosenberg, 1980; Lin & Ensel, 1984), the interaction of the B and C factors for families of children with mental retardation should be more intensively studied. Hill's model may contribute to the formulation of potentially fruitful research questions for determining risk for crisis in families of mentally retarded children.

Although the Hill theory, because of its emphasis on the buffering power of both the family's resources and the subjective meaning of the stressor, is uniquely suited to studying the stress in these families, few studies have included the subjective component (C) in their interviews with families, and many have not even examined the support networks and family resources (B). Most studies have instead simply correlated the stressor (A) of mental retardation with some definition of family impact/crisis (X). These studies have not generally made distinctions about types of stressors, nor have they acknowledged the process of adaptation over time in family systems. In the next part of this chapter. the family stress and mental retardation literature are reviewed using the ABCX model as an organizing framework.

TWO LITERATURE REVIEWS ON FAMILIES OF CHILDREN WITH MENTAL RETARDATION

This section presents two separate reviews of the research literature on stress in families of children with mental retardation. Each builds on the ABCX model, but each serves different ends. The first review considers ways in which family resources and family perception (factors

B and C) were or were not incorporated into the methodology and/or the discussion sections of 12 studies on families of children with mental retardation. None of these studies was explicitly guided by the Hill/McCubbin model, yet several either collected data on some aspect of the family's resources as a mediating factor or referred in their discussions to the impact of such factors. Table 1 describes each study's research questions, samples, instruments, and reported results.

In contrast, the second review identifies reported findings concerning the B and/or C factors from many studies published over the years on families with mentally retarded children.

Attention to Family Resources (B) and Perception (C) Factors in Studies on Families with Mentally Retarded Children (See Table 1)

An advantage of using a theoretical framework in reviewing literature is that it enables one to specify the domains that need attention. A theoretical framework also facilitates a critique of the treatment or neglect of those domains by the researchers being reviewed.

The author has selected a dozen studies for review, each published in refereed journals during the recent past. They were chosen for their relative methodological sophistication and for their prominence in the field. Each examined some aspect of the relationship of a child's developmental disability to family functioning. Although none of the studies mentioned Hill or McCubbin, because they were addressing the issue of stressful impact on the family of raising a mentally retarded child, one can assume that they were struggling at some level with the issues conceptualized by the ABCX model. For this reason, it seems acceptable to consider what they studied from this perspective: Family resources and family perceptions may have a powerful interactive effect with the probability as well as the intensity of a family crisis. Although ultimately the topic was the same for all the studies presented here, the specific focus of each was unique; that is,

the part of the construct being examined was different for each one.

There was, for example, considerable variation in the operational definitions of the stressor event (A), as well as of the family crisis (X). In the studies by Miller and Keirn, by Cummings, and by Davis and MacKay, the (X) was as follows: Cummings (1976) and Miller and Keirn (1978) each contrasted parents (one, mothers and the other, fathers) of disabled children with parents of nondisabled children (A) on psychological indicators of individual functioning (X). The purpose of each study was to explore the impact on the parent's mental health of having a mentally retarded child; thus, the parent's mental health was considered by them to be the (X) factor. The impact on the family (X) was defined by Davis and MacKay, using a survey questionnaire, by the number of mental health and/or health-related hospitalizations, by reported alcohol abuse, by the number of divorces, and so forth. In their study, the parents of normals and subnormals were compared (Davis and MacKay, 1973).

Reflecting on Hill/McCubbin's model, one could raise some issues about these three studies. First, because the parents were not matched with one another on the B and C factors, the full meaning of the reported differences (X) remains unclear. Had those variables been controlled for, the findings might have been stronger, with the range of reported problems potentially being smaller. In most studies the failure to consider the variable of social class in comparing two samples is seen as an important omission. Using the Double ABCX model of family stress would lead one to insist on either controlling for B and C, or including data on these variables in the analysis. Second, one could argue that, rather than defining the X factor, the results of these studies really helped elaborate on the constellation of the B factor (i.e., family resources). Or one could suggest that, in order to define the parameters of the B or C factors, one would first have to identify the extent to which raising a handicapped child affects the availability of

Table 1. Attention to family resources (B) and perception (C) factors in studies on families with mentally retarded children

Author(s)	Focus of study	Sample	Dependent variable	Components of ABCX model examined	Results
Beckman, 1983	To examine the relationship between child characteristics and stress reported by mothers, e.g., Rate of development Social responsiveness Temperament Repetitive sterotypic behaviors Additional or unusual caregiving demands	Handicapped infants and their mothers ($n = 31$) Age range 6.6–36.6 months	Mothers determined by Questionnaire on Resources and Stress (Holroyd, 1974) Holmes and Rahe Schedule of recent experience	A,B,X	Four of the child characteristics (temperament, responsiveness, repetitive behavioral patterns, and care giving demands) were significantly related to the amount of stress reported by mothers on QRS, but not significantly related to the amount of stress reported on the Schedule of Recent Experience. Also the number of parents in the home was associated with the amount of stress reported on QRS and the Schedule of Recent Experiences. (Single parents had more stress.) No significant difference between amount of stress was reported by mothers of boys or girls. No significant difference between child's age and stress was reported.
Cook, 1963	Compare child-rearing attitudes of mothers of handicapped children with various types of disabilities	Mothers of blind ($n = 4$) deaf ($n = 20$) cerebral palsied ($n = 53$) mongoloid ($n = 25$) organic ($n = 66$)	Mother's child-rearing attitude (PARI) by questionnaire	A,X	No significant difference was found in warmth scores among handicapped groups or between moderate-severe group. Significant differences were found in authoritarian

(continued)

Table 1. (continued)

Author(s)	Focus of study	Sample	Dependent variable	Components of ABCX model examined	Results
					scores among the handicapped groups and between moderate-severe group.
Cummings, 1976	Compare psychological adjustment of fathers of mentally retarded with chronically ill and healthy children	Fathers of mentally retarded (n = 60) chronically, physically ill (n = 60) healthy (n = 60) Common demographics in following areas: Intact family status Natural father More than 1 child Child is 4–13 years old Socioeconomic status	Fathers' prevailing mood Self-esteem Standard measures including Sentence completion test Self-Acceptance Scale of the Berger Inventory Shoben Parental Attitudes Inventory Edwards Personal Preference Schedule	A,X	Fathers of the mentally retarded had: 1. More depressive feeling and more preoccupation with child. 2. Inferiority as fathers and general lack of relationship gratification + low enjoyment of the child 3. Higher for order and lower dominance, plus more heterosexuality. 4. Greater negative impact from fathering than those of chronically ill children.
Davis and MacKay, 1973	Compare indicators of family problems in families of normal child with families of subnormal children	Families with subnormal child (n = 70) Families with normal child (n = 28) These families were matched on basis of SES; religion; family size; sex, age, and ordinal position of the index child.	Marital status, separation or divorce Physical health of parents Mental health of parents Alcoholism in parents Employment of either mother or father Social outings Number of family vacations	A,X	Following factors failed to differentiate the matched groups: Incidence of separation or divorce Physical health of parents Mental health of parents Alcoholism Employment of mother or father Factors that significantly distinguished matched groups: Social outings significantly fewer in families of sub-

Author/Year	Purpose	Variables/Measures	Sample	Code	Findings
Friedrich and Friedrich, 1981	Compare parents of handicapped children with parents of normal children with regard to stress and the variables that can mediate that stress	Stress (QRS) in parents Holroyd's Questionnaire on Resources and Stress Marital Satisfaction Lock-Wallace Marital Adjustment Inventory Psychological well-being Psychological Well-Being Index Social Support Index Nukolls, Cassell, and Kaplan, 1978 Religiosity Index Zuk, Miller, Barham, & Kling, 1961	Families with a handicapped child (n = 34) Families with a nonhandicapped child (n = 34) Child age range 2–16 years Handicapped children 15 mentally retarded 8 motor difficulties 11 combination of motor difficulties and mental retardation	A,B,X	normal children Significantly fewer families with handicapped child were able to go on vacation. More stress if child is handicapped Significant differences found on all subscales of QRS except social support, (pessimism and financial problems) Significant group differences on scores on remaining instruments.
Holroyd and McArthur 1976	Compare mothers of autistic with Down syndrome children in terms of their attitude toward the child and the effects of the child on themselves and their families	Mother's attitude toward child Effect of child on mother Effect of child on family (Measured with QRS)	Autistic children (n = 22) Down syndrome (n = 22) Clinic (n = 32)	A,X*	Autism group scored higher than the Down syndrome group and the clinic group on all scales except financial problems. Mothers of clinic children had higher mean scores on 3 scales than mothers of Down syndrome children.
McAllister, Butler, and Lei, 1973	Compare patterns of social interaction in families with behaviorally retarded child and families of a normal child	Frequency of intrafamily patterns Frequency of extrafamily patterns	Parents of children who are behaviorally retarded (using Vineland Scale scores) (n = 281) Normal children and parents (n = 784)	A,X	Less interaction within families with behaviorally retarded child No effect on formal community organizations affiliations Visit people outside immediate family less frequently with behaviorally retarded child

(continued)

Table 1. (continued)

Author(s)	Focus of study	Sample	Dependent variable	Components of ABCX model examined	Results
Miller and Keim, 1978	Compare MMPI profiles of parents of emotionally disturbed with mentally retarded and nonclinic children.	Mothers and fathers of mentally retarded ($n = 50$) emotionally disturbed ($n = 50$) Normal ($n = 50$) Age of child = 6	Parental adjustment (MMPI)	A,X	Mothers of mentally retarded and emotionally disturbed had elevated scores. Mothers of emotionally disturbed had most difference from normal group. Fathers had no significant difference in any group.
Nihira, Meyers, and Mink, 1980	Examine the reciprocal relationship between home environment and social competency of moderately-severely retarded children	Mentally retarded children and their families ($n = 120$) Age of child 8–14	Home environment assessed using battery of questionnaires and with observation inventories to the primary caregiver. Instruments: 1. Home observation of measure of environment. 2. Family Environment Scale. 3. Environmental status variable. Child development measures 1. Adaptive behavior scale 2. Primary Self-Concept Inventory 3. Other child-related variables	Double ABCX	Home environment has significant correlation with social and psychological adjustment over time. Psychosocial climate of the home correlated with emotional adjustment of mentally retarded adolescent. Adjustment of mentally retarded adolescent correlated with social and emotional aspects of parenting behavior.
Suelzle and Keenan, 1981	Contrast the support networks utilized by parents of partially retarded children at four different stages over the life cycle	Sampling population: parents of developmentally disabled children age 0–21 classified in mild or educable range	Personal and professional supports were explored in a questionnaire including: 1. Manner in which parent found out child developmen-	A,B,C,X	Type of health care professional seen by family varies with life-cycle stage of child. Locating appropriate services differs by life-cycle

178

Study	Purpose	Sample	Variables	Codes	Findings
			tally disabled 2. Availability of extended family and community supports 3. Severity of disability 4. Manner of securing community service 5. Professional services utilized 6. Attitude toward direct service 7. Involvement in child's program and 8. Parent's organization 9. Opinions and public policy 10. Long-term plans and objectives for child Life-cycle stage of child: preschool, elementary, teenage, young adult.		stage: Preschool parents rely on doctors and personal support; parents of older child rely on school personnel. Utilization of personal support declines over life cycle. Parents of older children are less supportive of normalization concept.
Waisbren, 1980	Compare parental attitudes toward self and child after birth of a developmentally disabled child versus after birth of a nonhandicapped child, in United States and Denmark.	United States developmentally disabled ($n = 30$) nonhandicapped ($n = 30$) Denmark developmentally disabled ($n = 30$) nonhandicapped ($n = 30$) Child = 1.5 years	Parental attitudes Impact on family relations Impact on relationships outside family Interview as shown through: 1. Events surrounding birth 2. Initial concerns and attitudes 3. Explanation of the handicap 4. Parent-child relationship 5. Parents' ideas and plans for the future 6. Parents' thoughts	A,B,C,X	Parents of handicapped and nonhandicapped children were similar in coping with new baby. Parents of developmentally disabled expressed more feelings of hopelessness, anger, rejection. Parents of developmentally disabled felt changed in more negative ways. No significant national difference was found between Danish and U.S. parents. Fathers of developmentally disabled child who felt

(continued)

Table 1. (continued)

Author(s)	Focus of study	Sample	Dependent variable	Components of ABCX model examined	Results
			about interview Standard 1. Daily Activities Checklist. 2. Social Network Form (Adapted from Bott, 1957) 3. Family Relationships Marriage Form (Locke and Wallace, 1959) 4. Family Relationships Parents and Inlaws Forms (Adapted from Barsch, 1963) 5. Health Questionnaire. 6. Change Scale (Adapted from Farber, 1959)		their parents were supportive had better attitude about marriage and more stress. Mothers of developmentally disabled who felt they had high support network had more positive feelings about child but more stress.
Weller, Chanan, Cohen, and Rahman, 1974	Examine the effects of social variables of social class and country of origin on parental attitudes and feelings about having a child with mental retardation	Israeli population Asian-African origin (n = 38) European origin (n = 38) Children mildly retarded (n = 38) Children severely retarded (n = 38) Mean age = 9 years	Parental guilt feelings Accuracy of perception of retardation Acceptance-rejection of child.	A,B,C	Middle-class parents held more realistic perceptions of the retardation. Parents of severely mentally retarded were more realistic in evaluating child capabilities than those of children with mild mental retardation. No difference in parental guilt or acceptance-rejection was found by social class or level of mental retardation.

180

each of these family resources. For example, the effect over time on the exhausted parent might be to reduce some of the personal-level family resources available for managing the chronic stresses. This would be particularly relevant to the Double ABCX model.

Rather than using a control group, some investigators have chosen to compare disability types in children or to compare their levels of impairment as a way of further defining the stressor event itself (A). Their research question posed was whether there are certain specific attributes or specific disabilities that provoke a uniquely stressful response in the caregiver. Cook (1963) explores attitudes toward parenting as his dependent variable (X) by contrasting parents of children with various types of developmental disabilities (A). He examines each disability in terms of how it interacts with both the warmth and authoritarian dimensions of parenting (using the PARI, by Schaefer & Bell, 1958). Holroyd (1976) analyzes the responses on a stress questionnaire, Holroyd's Questionnaire on Resources and Stress in Families of a Handicapped Person, (QRS) of parents of autistic children contrasted with parents of mentally retarded children and parents of clinic children. (Her questionnaire, which is the most widely used instrument in this field today, assesses amount of family stress (X), with a sum score and 15 subscale scores.) Beckman (1983) also examines the individual child's characteristics (e.g., responsiveness of the child, irritability of the child) and their differential impact on the reported stress levels of the caregiving mother.

In the Cook, Holroyd, and Beckman studies, the effect of the stressor event (A) was determined by contrasting parents of children with different types of handicapping conditions, rather than by comparing parents of children with disabilities with parents of children who were nondisabled. This study design helps to delineate not whether there are more stresses when one raises a child with mental retardation in the family, but rather how the stresses manifest themselves in relation to specific aspects of the child's disability. These studies help explore the variability inherent in the stressor (A).

The studies of Holroyd and McArthur (1976), Beckman (1983), and Friedrich and Friedrich (1981) operationalized the family crisis (X) by a score from the QRS; however, each used a different methodology. Except for Beckman's analysis on single parents (considered here to be an acknowledgment of the B factor) none considered any buffering factors. Holroyd contrasted parents of children with three types of disabilities. Her cluster analysis looked for patterns fitting each disability type on her 15 face-valid scales. Beckman contrasted mentally retarded children in terms of their caregiving characteristics and used sum scores on the QRS for her dependent variable. She also included in her analysis the life events checklist to control for other non-mental retardation-related stressors. Friedrich and Friedrich (1981) contrasted disabled children's mothers with those of nondisabled children, also using the QRS sums scores as the dependent variable indicating family stress (X). However, they made clear that they conceptualized the "family resource" (B) variables as interacting with (A) to affect the impact on the family (X). They operationalized several levels of family resources; they used standardized questionnaires to assess psychological well-being, religiosity, marital satisfaction, and availability of social support; and they included these variables in a regression to explain the variation of QRS scores. Rather than simply relating A versus Non-A to X, they essentially entered factor B into the equation. There was, however, no mention of the C factor in this study.

Two studies included in their definition of (X) the number of family social contacts with the community (Davis and MacKay, 1973; McAllister et al., 1973). The social isolation that was indicated by their data was seen as showing the deleterious impact on the family. However, given the Hill/McCubbin model, it seems equally salient to consider these findings as reflective of diminished family resources (B), whose variability for each family would have implications for their individual capacity for family coping. These interactive concepts are not mentioned by these authors.

In contrast, two other studies did not define (X) at all and instead examined variables that they designated as buffering in their function. Suelzle and Keenan (1981) contrasted four separate stages across the life cycle of a child with mental retardation, and although they did not specifically identify the B and C factors as such, they collected data and then analyzed them. Comparing the different age groups of children, they surveyed the extended family and community supports, as well as the utilization patterns of professional services (B factor), and they also gathered data on the parents' attitudes toward the child, attitudes toward the services, and attitudes toward normalization policies (C factor). Although the discussion section showed sensitivity to these dimensions of family stress, the interactive nature of these buffering factors with the stressor event of mental retardation over time (Double ABCX) eluded the authors. Similarly, Weller, Chanan, Cohen, and Rahman (1974), studied social class and ethnicity (both could be labeled as family resources—B) in terms of their impact on the parental accuracy of perception of mental retardation, on their acceptance or rejection of the mental retardation, and on their guilt (factor C). They too omitted any characterization of (X), but did attempt to determine the interactive nature of these variables of social class and background on perception. However, the implications for the long-term management of the chronic stress of A were not noted.

In two other studies the researchers collected all the data that would be needed for an analysis according to Hill/McCubbins' model, but did not analyze it or organize it around that model. The first study, by Waisbren (1980), assessed the disabled versus nondisabled child's mother and father (A versus Non-A) on health, marital satisfaction, family relationships, and social network (Factor B); measured the perception of changes by the parents, including a contrast between Danish parents and American parents (factor C); and collected reports on stress (X). However, in Waisbren's analysis, all these findings are treated as simply (X) impact on the family. Only in the discussion does the author begin to mention the interrelationships of these various domains, and in the conclusion the author refers to correlations among stress levels, social support, and perception.

Nihira, Meyers, and Mink (1980), in the only longitudinal study included here, analyzed the relationship over time of the disabled child's social competence to its home environment and family dynamics. Their measures of these variables incorporate both perception questions and family resources questions. Their discussion is unique because it suggests a reciprocal influence between A and X; they open the concept of bidirectionality over time. This formulation moves us away from linear causality into an interactional framework similar to that suggested by McCubbin and Patterson (1983). As with Waisbren, Nihira et al. collect all the data accorded relevance by Hill/McCubbin; however, because they do not use that theoretical model, they do not analyze their data accordingly. One could speculate that such an analysis of their data might be a most intriguing test of the theoretical model.

In summary, twelve studies have been briefly presented and discussed in respect to the ABCX model of stress in families. None of them indicated familiarity with this theoretical perspective. Some included measurements of the B and C factors; however, none of them assigned equal weight to these factors. In those studies in which all of the "relevant" data were already collected, one might speculate that these theoretical underpinnings would strengthen the results of their research enterprise.

Data on Buffering Variables B and C from Studies on Families with Mentally Retarded Children

Despite the lack of direct attention paid to the B and C factors in these dozen studies of the impact of a child's mental retardation on families, a wealth of available data can be organized around the B and C concepts. Some can be gleaned from the studies just discussed; other information that has held up well over time is available in older studies of the familial impact of mental retardation. Further data are available in studies of related issues, such as the correlates of institutionalization among families with children who are mentally retarded.

Few of the studies in this second literature review involved direct or clinical observation or interviews with family members. There is, accordingly, a dearth of what seem intuitively to be important behavioral interactional patterns, family dynamics, or data on the parents' ability to work together in solving emotional and practical problems caused by their child's condition. The data collected and reviewed here concern for the most part relatively stable, nonsubjective sociological variables, such as social class, gender, level of the child's impairment, and frequency of contact with family and other associates.

Still, the studies are a mixed lot. They vary considerably in methodological rigor, scope, and specificity to the problem of stress, and they investigate a number of quite different issues and hypotheses. Although not all these disparities are duly noted in the data presented below, the author has exercised a number of cautions; for example, no variable is presented unless found important by two or more investigators working independently. In keeping with the reliance on Hill's framework, these findings are presented in two sections, the first being the family's resources/social support system (B factors) and the second relating to familial perception of the stressor event (C factors).

Family Resources (B Factors) The review of the research on families of mentally retarded children pinpointed several variables that were frequently reported and that could be classified as family resources. With these resources a family would be expected to cope more effectively with the stressor (A); without them the family would be more likely to be at risk for family crisis (X).

The first variable is the complex variable of social class. The higher one's social class, the greater are one's financial resources and the more skills one has in negotiating the service delivery system. Middle-class families with a child who is mentally retarded are more likely to utilize the available services than are lower-class and minority families (Justice, O'Connor, & Warren, 1971; Stone, 1967). Middle-class parents more frequently organize formal support networks, such as parent associations, for themselves (NARC, 1975; Waskowitz, 1959). These involvements would decrease stress. The financial stress of raising a mentally retarded child can result in downward mobility in the father's career status *if* the child is born early in his career; that is, before he has established himself (Culver, 1967; Downey, 1963; Gumz & Gubrium, 1972).

On the other hand, families without financial resources, career ladders, or access to formal service systems in order to survive must rely heavily on informal support networks. The kin systems of poor families are often extraordinarily strong and supportive. In this respect lower-class families have advantages over middle-class families, given that regular supportive involvement with extended family members is also reportedly associated with decreased stress. In families of mentally retarded children, frequent contacts with grandmothers are especially significant in increasing coping ability (Farber, 1960; Holt, 1958; Waisbren, 1980).

Frequency of church contacts, as well as the intensity of one's personal belief (i.e., religiosity), has also been associated with decreased stress in families of mentally retarded children (Farber, 1960; Levinson, 1975; Saenger, 1960; Zuk, Miller, Barham, Kling, 1961). (It might be interesting to analyze the extent to which church and religious beliefs provide informal support through a community as opposed to personal support through a positive empowered perspective on life. These would both be features of the B factor. Religious beliefs might also function as C factor variables in which God's wishes, rather than bad luck, are attributed causality—the one being empowering, the other being helpless.)

Social isolation in families of mentally retarded children is an often-reported finding (Carver & Carver, 1972; Davis & MacKay, 1973; Dunlop & Hollingsworth, 1977; Farber, 1959, 1960, 1964; Holt, 1958; Jacobs, 1974; Legaay & Keough, 1966; Levinson, 1975; McAllister et al., 1973; Meyerwitz & Farber, 1966; Schonnell & Watts, 1956). The family seems to have a diminished circle of acquaintances and contacts, belongs to fewer organizations, and shares fewer leisure-time activities. The lack of integration into their community, the impoverished social life, and lack of vacation time deprive these families of intra- and interfamilial resources.

Studies of families in which the parents are not stressed also show siblings to be adapting well; nevertheless, the adolescent normal female sibling is reportedly at increased risk for stress. She experiences a greater risk for problems at school, for sexual acting out, and for mental health clinic visits (Gath, 1973; Grossman, 1972; Ruseman, 1981). This risk may be related to the burden of care on the family of raising a mentally retarded child. The teenager may contribute in major ways to child care of the retarded sibling because of the difficulty in obtaining babysitting help from apprehensive neighbors, friends, or relatives. The child care demands can interfere with the pursuit of a ''normal'' teenage social life at a critical developmental period.

The quality of the marriage is a family resource. The stability and satisfaction of the marital relationship are related to the experience of stress in the family (Waisbren, 1980). Contrary to popular belief, the divorce rate for families of mentally retarded children is *not* increased when the families studied have been matched for social class (Korn, Chess, & Fernandez, 1978; Longo & Bond, 1984; Davis & MacKay, 1963). However, those couples who report a *low* level of marital satisfaction *prior* to the diagnosis of mental retardation experience a *higher* rate of marital stress than do those who reported a high level of satisfaction prior to the diagnosis (Farber, 1960; Levinson,

1975). Wives who report that their marriages are supportive are better able to cope with the stress (Friedrich, 1979). Individual functioning—mental and physical health—is not affected by raising a child with mental retardation, despite increases in stress.

Familial Perceptions (C Factors)   The familial *perception* (C) of the stressor event of mental retardation as reported by researchers varies in many ways. First, parents have generally been found to have accurate perceptions about the child's level of functioning, although there are some dramatic exceptions (Pollner & Wikler, 1977; Wikler, 1976). Mothers perceive the mentally retarded child as more of a hardship in direct proportion to the child's incapacitation and helplessness (Barsch, 1968; Beckman, 1983; Burnett, Tymchuck, and Smith, 1974; Cummings, Bayley, and Rie, 1966; Dingman, Eyman, and Windle, 1963; Erickson, 1968; Farber, 1975; Holt, 1958; Levinson, 1975; Routh, 1970; Stevenson, 1954). In addition, the mother's ability and enthusiasm for functioning in the maternal caretaker role are adversely affected by the developmentally disabled child who is *not* affectionate or *not* demonstrative (Beckman, 1983; Holroyd, 1976; Marshall, Hegrenes, & Goldstein, 1973; Ricci, 1970; Rutter, 1975; Seitz, Hoekenga, & Goldstein, 1977). Mothers appear *less* affected by the IQ level per se or by the sex of the child than do fathers.

Fathers generally have increased difficulty in coping with mental retardation when the afflicted child is male (Chigier, 1972; Farber, 1962; Farber, Jenne, & Toigo, 1960; Gorelick & Sandhy, 1967; Grossman, 1972; Gumz & Gubrium, 1972; Tallman, 1965). Their perception of the mental handicap seems to be related to concerns about the eventual performance of their boys in roles outside the home.

Several characteristics of the mentally retarded child are reported to contribute to negative perceptions for *both* parental figures:

1. The increased visibility of the child's deviance (i.e., unusual physical appearance) is related to increased strain (e.g., higher rates of institutionalization) (Anderson,

Schlottman, & Weiner, 1975; Graliker & Koch, 1965; Hammond, Sternlicht, & Deutsch, 1969; Saenger, 1960; Zuk, 1959).

2. Lower IQ levels of the child are related to increased strain, including more frequent placement (Anderson et al., 1975; Graliker & Koch, 1965; Hammond et al., 1969; Levinson, 1975; Mercer, 1966).

3. The increased age of a moderately, severely, or profoundly mentally retarded child (particularly a male child over 9 years old) is related to increased marital problems (Birenbaum, 1971; Farber et al., 1960; Stone, 1967).

4. The birth order of the mentally retarded child, specifically being the first born, increases the parental report of the severity of the stressor event (Farber, 1960; Graliker & Koch, 1965; Sternlicht, Staaky, & Sullivan, 1975).

The parents' social values and social standing, in addition to socioeconomic class position, affect the ways in which they perceive mental retardation. The most significant of these characteristics is level of education. The *more* educated parents tend to have *more* difficulty adjusting to what is perceived as the "tragedy" of mental retardation in their offspring (Dunlap & Hollingsworth, 1976; Farber, 1959, 1960; Garfield & Helper, 1962; Holt, 1958; Levinson, 1975; Weller et al., 1974).

The impact of the child's retardation may be triggered less by the child's capacity as measured on an absolute scale than by the discrepancy between the *actual* performance and the *expected* performance. This discrepancy asserts itself, moreover, periodically over the lifespan of the mentally retarded person (Farber, 1968; Olshansky, 1962; Wikler, 1981). There may be particular periods when these perceived discrepancies are most acute: 1) those generally acknowledged points where one would normally expect significant *developmental* gains in a child and 2) those *transitional* points in service delivery systems when the need for extra resources reminds the parent

of the differences that exist between their lives and those of parents of normal children. (Peterson & Lippa, 1978; Suelzle & Keenan, 1981; Wikler, 1981; Wikler, Wasow, & Hatfield, 1981).

The normal siblings in the family perceive and adjust to mental retardation in the family in ways similar to those of their parents (Begab, 1968; Grossman, 1972; Schreiber & Fealey, 1965). Their parents offer a model to them of how to respond to the stressor. The exception to this is the normal sibling who shares the same sex as the handicapped child; he or she may be at increased risk in terms of social functioning (Farber & Jenne, 1963; Grossman, 1972; see Vadasy, Fewell, Meyer, & Schell, 1984 for a review of research on siblings).

This partial review of the literature, which categorizes the B or C factors variables salient to family adaptation to mental retardation, includes the first steps toward a theoretically adequate approach to a complex and dynamic area of research on stress in families with a mentally retarded child.

USING THE ABCX FRAMEWORK IN FAMILY RESEARCH

Two recent studies using the ABCX framework deserve more detailed exposition, both for their intrinsic interest and as examples of what can be done in this field when research is informed by a theoretical perspective.

Peterson (1981)

Peterson applied Hill's theoretical model in his dissertation research (1981). He operationalized the ABCX factors as follows:

(A) Factors: Peterson composed a 46-item questionnaire to reveal the specific nature of the handicap (e.g., "Have you had to modify your car?" "Does your handicapped child have difficulty in his or her sexual maturation and expression?"). These responses produced a stressor score.

(B) Factors: A one-page questionnaire asked for rankings (1–5) on both internal and external familial supports, including friend-

ships and help from community and professional sources.
(C) Factors: Peterson's measurement of the
perception variables was inventive. The
Holmes-Rahe Life Events Stress Checklist,
a standard scale of stressors, assigns a
number between 1 and 100 to each of 43
stressful changes; the numbers indicate relative severity of stress. Peterson presented
this scale with blank lines next to the other
57 numbers in the 1–100 interval. A sample
(*n*-105) of mothers of handicapped children
with developmental delays was asked to
place their experience of their children's
handicaps on the scale in the blank line, with
the number indicating the perceived severity
of this stress relative to the stressful events
on the Holmes-Rahe. This index was then
available to Peterson for use in his multivariate analyses.
(X) Factor: The outcome variable (X) was
characterized by using standard instruments
measuring marital satisfaction (Locke-Wal-

lace) and health of the mother (Hopkin's
Symptom Checklist).

Peterson's schema is shown in Figure 1. His
research found the stressor (A), when interacting with B and C factors, to be correlated with
the outcome (X) at .37 (p < .01). This finding
was expected on the basis of Hill's model. It is
noteworthy for the present review that Peterson's significant findings would *not* have been
detected if the two buffering factors had not
been taken into account. Indeed, when he removed (B) and (C) variables from the analysis,
the correlation between the stressor (A) and the
outcome (X) was reduced to −.02.

Wikler (1986)

In the second study, the ABCX model enabled
the author to explore whether the stressor (A),
mental retardation, may have a different impact on families at different points across the
life cycle. Transition periods for the developmentally disabled child were identified as they

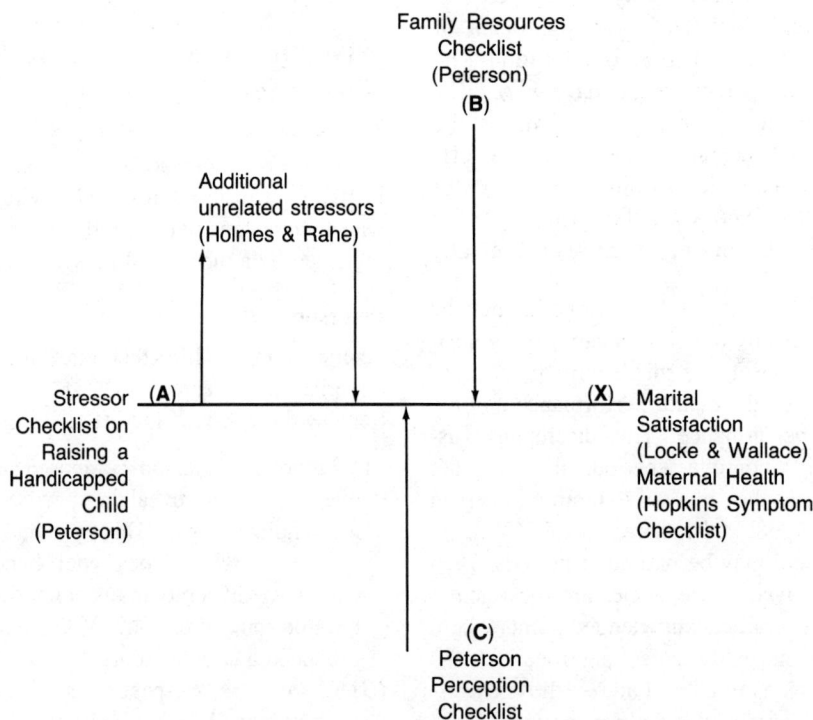

Figure 1.   Schema of Peterson's (1981) research.

related to their normal age-related developmental milestones (Wikler, 1981; Wikler et al., 1981). Transition periods were hypothesized to be more stressful to families than nontransition periods with *all other things being equal*. The "other things" in this instance are the family resources (B) and family perception (C) factors. By identifying those factors using a checklist and allowing for their variability, it was possible to detect and measure the impact of the complex stressor consisting of mental retardation *plus* transition points (see Figure 2).

The (B) and (C) factors were assessed through a 20-item checklist, with 10 items for family resources and 10 for the family perception factors previously identified in the literature as correlated with increased family problems attendant to the presence of a mentally retarded child. Each item was equally weighted with a 0–1 value. These were added together to provide individual family scores (Laten & Wikler, 1978; Wikler & Laten, in preparation).

The (X) factor, family distress, was operationalized using Holroyd's Questionnaire for Resources in Stress (QRS). As previously mentioned, the QRS, which was developed as 15 face-valid scales, has been used to differentiate types of stresses faced by mothers of children with various handicaps (Holroyd & McArthur, 1976), as a dependent variable indicating maternal coping (Friedrich, 1979), and as a measure of stress levels of families related to various types of burdens of care (Beckman, 1983).

The stressor (A) was transitions in families with mentally retarded children. The periodicity of stresses associated with the presence of a retarded child who was experiencing the onset of puberty (ages 11–15) or the onset of adulthood (ages 20–21) was explored in this study. Families with a child of these ages were contrasted with families of a mentally retarded child who was *not* in a transitional period (i.e., ages 7–10, 16–19, and 22–25).

Checklist scores, measuring B and C factors, were collected for the families, as were Holmes and Rahe scores (stressors unrelated to mental retardation). These B and C factors were significantly correlated to QRS and explained more variation than did transition status. The checklist and Holmes and Rahe scores of families in transition were compared to those of families not in transition. In comparing transition versus nontransition families, there were no significant differences; the two factors that

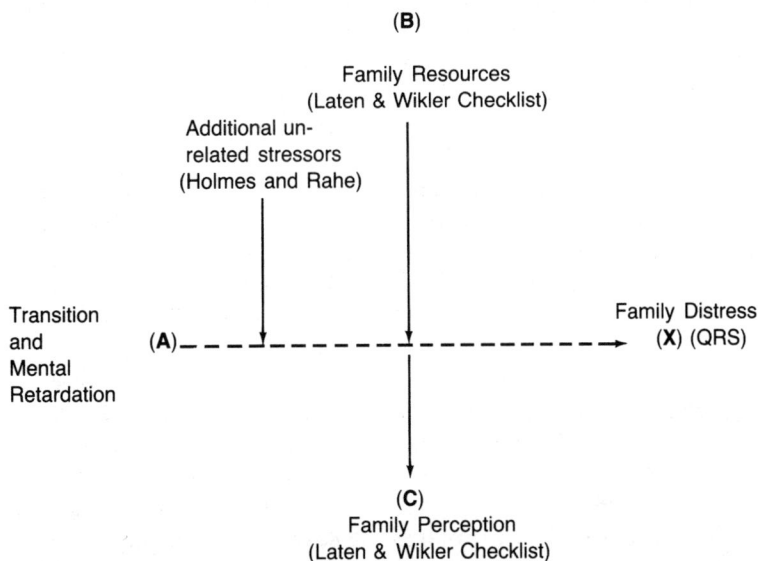

Figure 2. Schema of Wikler's (1986) research.

theoretically had a potential mediating influence did not seem to be affected by the age of the mentally retarded child in this sample.

Because the B and C factors did not vary (nor did the additional non-mental-retardation-related stressors), the relationship between transition and nontransition families could be directly tested. T-tests of transition and nontransition families' QRS scores showed a significant difference of $p < .001$ at T_1. Testing the same families at T_2, 2 years later (which placed most of them into different categories) showed a significant difference of $p < .05$, with the buffering factors still constant. Transitions (A) appeared to be related to more stress (X) than nontransitions (Wikler, 1986).

EXPLORING THE SUBJECTIVE C FACTOR

If it is true, as the above discussion suggests, that consideration of the B and C factors is indispensable for an understanding of the effect on families of having a retarded child, it is also true that these factors are quite difficult to investigate. The C factor, in particular, is elusive, as it is situated within the subjective realm of each family member. Its inaccessibility to the researcher may account for the lack of attention it has been given in studies.

Both studies reported in the previous section made a point of collecting data on the subjective factor; the Peterson study in particular displayed a willingness to use novel instruments in the pursuit. It is clear, however, that much more remains to be done in this area. A single numerical value, even if assigned by the family member himself or herself, cannot indicate the hugely complex web of beliefs, attitudes, morals, and intrapsychic conflicts and stratagems that make up the individual's perception of the stress. Such an index only reflects one person's perspective in any case and does not tell us anything about the collective experience of the stressor in the family group, which although it is ultimately the sum of the individual experi-

ences, is still given its character by their interaction and collective management. Researchers and policy-makers would find it easier if these subjective factors were merely private affairs and had no social impact. Yet, this is certainly not the case: Outcomes vary greatly from family to family, even as the objective character of the stressor and the extent of family resources are held constant. The details of family perception, considered both in individuals and in the group, probably ultimately make the difference between the families who continue to maintain their child at home and those that choose to institutionalize.

This section presents the results of one attempt by investigators to explore these subjective factors in detail, using techniques fashioned specifically for this purpose. The papers reporting this effort begin to supply some of the understanding of family perceptions that may provide a basis for further research and evaluation of interventions (Pollner & Wikler, 1977, 1985; Wikler, 1976, 1980).

These studies report intensive investigation into a single case history. Though the "n" could hardly be lower, the sample has provided and continues to yield a vast wealth of data. The study used the investigative concepts and techniques of ethomethodology, a development within academic sociology first formulated by Professor Harold Garfinkel of University of California-Los Angeles.

The case material is bizarre. A family of five (father, mother, teenage son and daughter, and a 6-year-old daughter) appeared in a psychiatric clinic to seek treatment for what was called "malingering" behavior by their young child Mary. Mary's particular offense, for which professional care was sought, lay in "acting retarded" in public. The family assured the clinicians that Mary was a bright, articulate 6-year-old at home.

Clinical observation and testing quickly revealed that Mary had the mental functioning of an infant, unable to recognize even her own name. The clinician's first assumption was that one or more family members were simply hallucinating Mary's "normal" behavior, but on examination, no evidence of psychosis was found. Nor was any ruse a likely explanation. Mary's family simply *perceived* a profoundly retarded child as normal.

This case thus provides an outlandish illustration of the thesis that family perceptions color their experience of the child's mental retardation. Its extreme nature makes it far removed from the ordinary case, but at the same time provided a laboratory for investigating the subjective factor. Accordingly, the investigators endeavored to study the family's perception in detail. The object of investigation was not the cause of the family's (mis)perception, but its structure and management; in particular, to explain precisely how a nonhallucinating, intelligent family could maintain the belief in Mary's normality in the face of daily—indeed constant—disconfirming evidence.

The data for the study consisted of 15 hours of videotapes of interactions between Mary and various members of her family. The truth— that is, how they interacted—emerged very slowly, requiring dozens, even hundreds of replays. By the end, the investigators came to realize that the family's perception was a product of highly skilled, although unconscious, stage-managing and coordination among the family members: an unconscious but purposive conspiracy, in effect, to make Mary seem competent to themselves.

The family members' stratagems were identified and sorted by means of the microobservation permitted by videotape. Two examples provide the flavor of the delusion's structure:

1. "Benevolent double-bind": The family members regularly issued commands to Mary that at the time of occurrence (or of first viewing on tape) she seemed—*in the eyes of family members and outsiders alike*—to obey. This sequence was evidence to all in favor of the (delusional) hypothesis that Mary was indeed normal. In fact, these commands turned out to order behavior that Mary could not physically avoid, given her trajectory at the instant of command. Some of these commands were disjunctive ("Mary, do X or

do Y!") and thus covered all the physical possibilities.

2. "Conversations" between Mary and two or more family members were eerily normal in initial appearance. Even though Mary's utterances, when they occurred, sounded to outsiders like random grunts and noises, the family members seemed to have a common understanding of what Mary just "said." This again lent support, for each interlocutor, to the thesis of Mary's normality: Mary was indeed talking, even if no one outside the family could understand her. In fact, the family members had developed a highly successful practice of "repeating" the content of Mary's utterances in their next statements ("Oh, so you want a raincoat, do you?"), thus providing clues for each other on the content of the supposed speech act from the nonspeaking child.

Thus did the family members stage manage, for their *own* consumption, Mary's pseudocompetence. The studies reported here developed a catalog of over two dozen of these strategies, each aimed at maintaining and reinforcing a series of perceptions of the child's mental capacity that, however wildly at variance with reality, were enormously powerful in shaping the family's response to the stressor.

The obvious and pitiful distress of this family naturally prompts the question, "Why?"; these studies, however, asked "How?" The findings, although relying on observation, rather than experiment, provide a set of clues to family reactions to stress that might otherwise have been missed. These may be useful in further research of this sort. The investigators' working hypothesis—indeed, the motivation for undertaking the research—is that the structure and means of maintenance of perceptions of a child's retardation are every bit as powerful in shaping family reactions when the perceptions are accurate as they are when the perceptions are delusions. Although the ordinary family's perceptions may be realistic, they are still colored in many hues and given selective attention and emphasis. It is only by detailed attention to the parents' and siblings' personal account of the child's retardation that we can fully comprehend the process of accommodation to the stressor.

SUMMARY

In this chapter, a theoretical model has been used in assessing and reviewing the research currently being conducted in the field of stress on families of children with mental retardation. Hill's ABCX family crisis theory was described, in which the stressor event (A) interacts with the family resources (B), which interact with the familial perception (C), which results in some level of family dysfunction (X). Several points have been made in this review that should be mentioned as a focus for future research.

First, although we cannot expect research on family stress to look at all these variables simultaneously, we should expect the community of researchers in this field to aim at gradually placing the results of many studies together as pieces of a large puzzle. This sort of commitment has been lacking.

Second, we are only beginning to develop reliable measures and other tools for the assessment of both family resources and family perceptions. Although several of the studies reported an examination of multiple components of family resources, they did so each in their own way, and there is no way of comparing their results. Efforts should be undertaken to operationalize these family resources in the form of validated instruments and then to put those instruments in general use. We are very far, however, from developing instruments or even concepts that can be confidently employed in the study of family perceptions. As the research reported in the previous section indicated, our first step must be to identify what it is the instruments should measure. Family members perceive a great number of items related to their subjective processing of the retarded person's personality, performance, and relationships with others. We need to learn which of these perceptions most powerfully influences the reaction of the fami-

ly to the stress, and we must achieve an understanding of the sources of these perceptions and of their strength, duration, malleability, and other characteristics.

Third, we do not have a clear idea of what is considered successful family functioning;— that is, what would be considered an acceptable level of adaptation or accommodation,— nor what is to count as an indicator of family crisis and family stress (defining X). This vagueness plagues the field of family research in general, as well as the specific area of families of children with mental retardation. This problem may be sidestepped by focusing on the degree of change in the level of family functioning after the introduction of the stressor. To this end, several researchers have turned to the use of a single outcome measure of family functioning (i.e., the QRS, Holroyd, 1976; or QRS-R, Friedrich, Greenberg, & Crnic, 1983). Doing so enhances the possibility of comparing findings across studies, although it does not identify a threshold of "adequate" functioning.

Fourth, we have barely begun to examine the processes that affect families over time as they attempt to accommodate to the demands of caring for a mentally retarded member. Whereas the stages of reactions to the initial diagnosis of the disability in the child are extensively described (see Blacher, 1984), the impact of accumulated stresses resulting from the chronicity of the caregiving burdens and effects of these stresses on family dynamics are seldom addressed. Deinstitutionalization, which imposes these burdens on the home, makes this set of issues particularly important.

Fifth, we do not have a clear picture of the stages involved in the process of family adaptation. Each life-cycle stage of the offspring with mental retardation probably produces distinctive stressors to parents who are themselves at different ages at each stage. There may be regular patterns of interaction at respective life-cycle stages, and these data could have clinical utility.

Sixth, we are lacking the longitudinal and prospectively designed studies that would give us a picture of the same families' adaptation across time. Because families stabilize and adapt at different levels and with different arrangements, it would be useful if we had a better picture of these options.

A historic shift in national policy has occurred, based on few data, which is premised on the belief that family life is better for the mentally retarded person than institutional life. The new policy seems to carry a moral message as well. The family should shelter and nurture the mentally retarded child, even if doing so is perceived as a burden and regardless of whether the family might have been inclined to resolve this conflict of interests by giving the child over to an institution.

Yet, we know little about families of persons with mental retardation: Why do some families adjust to the stress much better than others; why can some families be predicted to buckle under the impact of stress, and what might be done to ameliorate this impact?

Without this information, we cannot know what is best for the child or whether the burden

of his or her care is being fairly placed; and worst of all, we cannot determine what ought to be done to improve the lot of both the child and the family. This last problem is an urgent one, for if families have responsibilities newly imposed on them, surely they have a right to the means required to discharge them successfully.

In this review of research, it seems clear that there should be more attention paid to direct observation of minute details of family life (see Goode, 1984). Survey research correlating the child's mental retardation with a single family outcome measure tells us little about the process of adaptation over time. The family's experience of this stressor determines the family outcome: How the child's condition is perceived by family and others, attitudes toward that condition, feelings of helplessness or of empowerment;—all can be familial resources permitting successful accommodation. It is only through attention to these details of family life, suitably integrated into a theoretical framework, that we can make progress in our research and in national policy.

REFERENCES

Adams, B. N. (1968). *Kinship in an urban setting*. Chicago: Markham.

Adams, B. N. (1975). *The family: A sociological interpretation*. Chicago: Rand-McNally.

Altman, B. M. (1981). Studies of attitudes toward the handicapped: The need for a new direction, *Social Problems, 28*(3), 321–337.

Anderson, V. H., Schlottman, R. S., & Weiner, B. J. (1975). Predictions of parent involvement with institutionalized retarded children. *American Journal of Mental Deficiency, 6,* 705–710.

Barsch, H. (1968). *Parents of the handicapped child*. Springfield, IL: Charles C Thomas.

Barsch, E. T., Moore, J. A., & Hamerlynck, L. A. (1983). The foster extended family: A support network for handicapped foster children. *Child Welfare, 4,* (LXII).

Bates, M. *Survey Report on State Family Support Programs*. (1984) Unpublished report. Madison, WI. State of Wisconsin Health and Social Services.

Beavers, W. B. (1982). Healthy, midrange, and severely dysfunctional families. In F. Walsh (Ed.), *Normal family processes*. New York: The Guilford Press.

Beck, A. T. (1967). *Depression*. New York: Harper and Row.

Beckman, P. (1983). Influence of selected child characteristics on stress in families of handicapped infants. *American Journal of Mental Deficiency, 88,* 150–56.

Begab, M. J., Haywood, H. C., & Garber, H. L. (1983). *Psychosocial influences in retarded performance: Is-

sues and theories of development (Vol. 1)*. (NICHD-Mental Retardation Research Centers Series). Baltimore, University Park Press.

Berger, M. (1984). Social network interventions for families that have a handicapped child. In J. Hansen (Ed.), *Families with handicapped members: The family therapy collections* (pp. 127–137). Rockville, MD: Aspen Publication.

Berger, M., & Foster, M. (1976). Family-level interventions for retarded children: A multivariate approach to issues and strategies. *Multivariate Experimental Clinical Research, 2,* 1–21.

Berger, M., & Fowlkes, M. (1980). The family intervention project: A family network model for serving young handicapped children, *Young Children, 34,* 22–32.

Birenbaum, A. (1971). The mentally retarded child in the home and the family cycle. *Journal of Health and Social Behavior, 12,* 55–65.

Blacher, J. (1984). Sequential stages of parental adjustment to the birth of a child with handicaps: Fact or artifact? *Mental Retardation, 22,* 55–68.

Blackard, M. K., & Barsh, E. T. (1982). Parents' and professionals' perceptions of the handicapped child's impact on the family. *The Journal of the Association for the Severely Handicapped, 7,* 62–70.

Boss, P. (1986). Family stress: Perception and context. In M. B. Sussman & S. Steinmetz (Eds.), *Handbook on marriage and the family*. New York: Plenum Publishing Corp.

Bott, E. (1957). *Family and Social Network.* London: Tavistock Publications, Inc.

Bruhn, J. G., & Philips, B. U. (1984). Measuring social support: A synthesis of current approaches, *Journal of Behavioral Medicine, 7*(2), 151–169.

Bruininks, R. H., & Krantz, G. C. (Eds.). (1979) *Family care of developmentally disabled members: Conference proceedings.* Minneapolis: University of Minnesota.

Burnett, D. J., Tymchuck, A. J., & Smith, S. (1974, June). Self-concept of mothers of mentally retarded children and mothers of "clinical" children. Paper presented at American Association of Mental Deficiency, Toronto.

Burr, W. F. (1973). *Theory construction and the sociology of the family.* New York: Wiley.

Burr, W., Hill, F., Nye, F., & Reiss, I. (Eds.). (1979). *Contemporary theories about the family: Vol. 1. Research based theories.* New York: The Free Press.

Carver, J., & Carver, N. (1972). *The family of the retarded child.* Syracuse, NY: Syracuse University Press.

Chigier, E. (1972). *Down's syndrome.* Lexington, MA: D. C. Heath.

Cobb, S. (1976). Social support as a moderator of life stress. *Psychosomatic Medicine, 38,* 300–314.

Cook, J. J. (1963). Dimensional analysis of child-rearing attitudes of parents of handicapped children. *American Journal of Mental Deficiency, 68,* 354–361.

Crnic, K. A., Friedrich, W. N., & Greenberg, M. T. (1983). Adaptation of families with mentally retarded children: A model of stress, coping and family ecology. *American Journal of Mental Deficiency, 88,* 125–138.

Culver, M. (1967). Intergenerational social mobility among families with a severely mentally retarded child. Unpublished doctoral dissertation, University of Illinois.

Cummings, S. T. (1976). The impact of the child's deficiency on the father: A study of fathers of mentally retarded and chronically ill children. *American Journal of Orthopsychiatry, 46,* 246–255.

Cummings, S. T., Bayley, H. C., & Rie, H. E. (1966). Effects of the child's deficiency on the mother: A study of mothers of mentally retarded, chronically ill, and neurotic children, *American Journal of Orthopsychiatry, 36,* 595–608.

Darling, R. (1981). *Families against society: A study of reactions to children with birth defects.* Beverly Hills: Sage Publications.

Davis, M., & MacKay, D. (1973). Mentally subnormal children and their families, *The Lancet,* October 27, 5.

De Shazer, S. & Lipchik, E. (1984). Frames and reframing. In J. C. Hansen & E. I. Coppersmith (Eds.), *Families with handicapped members: The family therapy collections* (pp. 88–97). Rockville, MD: Aspen Publication.

Dingman, H. F., Eyman, R. K., & Windle, C. D. (1963). An investigation of some child rearing attitudes of mothers of retarded children, *American Journal of Mental Deficiency, 67,* 899–908.

Downey, K. (1963). Parental interest in the institutionalized severely mentally retarded child, *Social Problems, 11,* 185–193.

Dohrenwend, B. S., & Dohrenwend, B. P. (Eds.). (1974). *Stressful life events: Their nature and effect.* New York: Wiley.

Dudley, J. R. (1983). *Living with stigma: The plight of the people who we label mentally retarded.* Springfield, IL: Charles C Thomas.

Dunlap, W. R., & Hollingsworth, J. S. (1977). How does a handicapped child affect the family? Implications for practitioners. *The Family Coordinator, 7,* 286–293.

Dunlap, W., & Hollingsworth, R. (1976). Services for families of the developmentally disabled. *Social Work, 5,* 220–223.

Duvall, F. M. (1957). *Family development.* Philadelphia: Lippincott.

Earhart, E., & Sporakowski, M. J. (Eds.). (1984). *The family with handicapped members,* [special issue]. *Family Relations, 33,* (1).

Edgerton, R. B. (1970). Mental Retardation in Non-western societies: Toward a cross-cultural perspective on incompetence. In H. C. Haywood (Ed.), *Social-cultural aspects of mental retardation* (pp. 523–559). New York: Appleton-Century-Crofts.

Egeland, B., Breitenbucher, M., & Rosenberg, D. (1980). Prospective study of the significance of life stress in the etiology of child abuse. *Journal of Consulting and Clinical Psychology, 48*(2).

Ell, K. (1984). Note on research—social networks, social support and health status: A review. *Social Service Review, 3,* 133–149.

Erickson, M. T. (1968). MMPI comparisons between parents of young emotionally disturbed children and mentally retarded children. *Journal of Consulting Clinical Psychology, 32,* 701–706.

Farber, B. (1959). Effects of a severely retarded child on family integration. *Monographs of the Society for Research in Child Development, 24* (No. 2).

Farber, B. (1960). Perceptions of crisis and related variables in the impact of a retarded child on the mother. *Journal of Health and Social Behavior, 1,* 108–118.

Farber, B. (1964). *Family organization and interaction.* San Francisco: Chandler.

Farber, B. (1968). *Mental Retardation: Its Social Context and Social Consequences.* New York: Houghton-Griffin.

Farber, B. (1975). Family adaptations to severely mentally retarded children. In M. Begab & S. Richardson (Eds.), *The mentally retarded and society: A social science perspective.* Baltimore: University Park Press.

Farber, B. (1979, August). Sociological ambivalence and family care: The individual proposes and society disposes. In R. H. Bruininks & G. Krantz (Eds.), *Family care of developmentally disabled members conference proceedings.* Minneapolis: Department of Psychoeducational Studies, University of Minnesota.

Farber, B., & Jenne, W. C. (1963). Family organization and parent-child communication: Parents and siblings of a retarded child, *Monographs of the Society for Research in Child Development, 28*(7, Serial No. 91).

Farber, B., Jenne, W., & Toigo, R. (1960). Family crisis and the decision to institutionalize the retarded child. *Council for Exceptional Children, Research Monograph Series A, No. 1.*

Featherstone, H. (1981). *A Difference in the Family: Living with a Disabled Child.* New York: Penguin Books.

Friedrich, W. N. (1979). Predictors of the coping behavior of mothers of handicapped children, *Journal of Consulting and Clinical Psychology, 47,* 1140–1141.

Friedrich, W. N., & Friedrich, W. I. (1981). Comparison of psychological assets of parents with a handicapped child and their normal controls. *American Journal of Mental Deficiency, 85,* 551–553.

Friedrich, W. N., Greenberg, M. T., & Crnic, K. A. (1983). A short form of the questionnaire on resources and stress. *American Journal of Mental Deficiency, 88,* 41–48.

Gallagher, J. J., Beckman, P., & Cross, A. H. (1983). Families of handicapped children: Sources of stress and its amelioration, *Exceptional Children, 50,* 10–19.

Garfield, S. L. and Helper, M. M. (1962). Parental attitudes and socioeconomic status, *Journal of Clinical Psychology, 18,* 171–175.

Gath, A. (1973). The school-age siblings of mongol children. *British Journal of Psychiatry, 123,* 161–167.

Gath, A. (1974). Sibling reactions to mental handicap: A comparison of the brothers and sisters of mongol children. *Journal of Child Psychology and Psychiatry, 15,* 187–198.

Golan, N. (1981). *Passing through transitions: A guide for practitioners.* New York: The Free Press.

Goode, D. (1984). Presentation practices of a family with a deaf-blind, retarded daughter. *Family Relations, 33,* 173–185.

Gorelick, M. C., & Sandhy, M. (1967). Parent perception of retarded child's intelligence. *Personnel and Guidance Journal, 46,* 382–384.

Graliker, B., Koch, R., & Henderson, R. (1962). A study of factors influencing placement of retarded children in a state residential institution. *American Journal of Mental Deficiency, 66,* 838–842.

Grossman, F. K. (1972). *Brothers and Sisters of Retarded Children: An Exploratory Study.* Syracuse, NY: Syracuse University Press.

Gumz, E. J., & Gubrium, J. (1972). Comparative parental perceptions of a mentally retarded child. *American Journal of Mental Deficiency, 77,* 178–180.

Hansen, J. C., & Coppersmith, E. I. (Ed.). (1984). *The family therapy collections: Families with handicapped members.* Rockville, MD: Aspen Systems Corporation.

Harris, S. L. (1983). *Families of the developmentally disabled: A guide to behavioral intervention.* New York: Pergamon Press.

Harris, S. L. (1982). A family systems approach to behavioral training with parents of autistic children. *Child and Family Behavior Therapy, 4,* 21–35.

Haywood, H. C. (Ed.) (1970). *Social-cultural aspects of mental retardation.* New York: Appleton-Century-Crofts.

Hill, R. (1949). *Families Under Stress.* New York: Harper & Row.

Hill, R. (1958). Generic features of families under stress, *Social Case work, 49,* 139–150.

Hill, R. (1973). *Family life cycle: Critical role transitions.* Paper presented at Thirteenth International Family Research Seminar, Paris.

Hill, R., & Rodgers, R. (1964). The developmental approach. In H. Christensen (Ed.), *Handbook of marriage and the family.* Chicago: Rand McNally.

Hobb, N. (1976). *The futures of children.* San Francisco: Jossey Bass.

Holmes, T., & Rahe, R. (1967). The social readjustment rating scale. *Journal of Psychosomatic Research, 11,* 213–218.

Holroyd, J. (1974). The questionnaire on resources and stress: An instrument to measure family response to a handicapped family member. *Journal of Community Psychology, 2,* 92–94.

Holroyd, J., & McArthur, D. (1976). Mental retardation and stress of the parents: A contrast between Down's Syndrome and childhood autism. *American Journal of Mental Deficiency, 80,* (4), 431–436.

Holroyd, J., Brown, N., Wikler, L., & Simmons, J. (1975). Stress in families of institutionalized vs. non-institutionalized autistic children. *Journal of Community Consulting Psychology, 3*(1), 26–31.

Holt, K. S. (1958). The influence of the retarded child upon family limitations. *Journal of Mental Deficiency Research, 2,* 28–34.

Humphrey, R., & Jacobsen, R. B. (1979). Families in crisis: Research and theory in child mental retardation. *Social Casework, 60,* 597–601.

Jacobs, J. (1974). *The search for help: A study of the retarded child in the community.* New York: Brunner/Mazel.

Justice, R. S., O'Connor, G., & Warren, N. (1971). Problems reported by parents of mentally retarded children: Who helps? *American Journal of Mental Deficiency, 75,* 685–691.

Kanner, L. (1957). *Child Psychiatry* (3rd ed.) Springfield, IL: Charles C Thomas.

Kazak, A. E., & Marvin, R. S. (1984). Differences, difficulties and adaptation: Stress and social networks in families with a handicapped child. *Family Relations, 33,* 67–79.

Korn, S. J., Chess, S., & Fernandez, P. (1978) The impact of children's physical handicaps on marital quality and family interaction. In R. M. Lerner and G. B. Spanier (Eds.), *Child influence on marital and family interaction: A life span development.* New York: Academic Press.

Krause, E. B., & Ciccone, J. (1982). Special needs of low-income mothers of developmentally delayed children. *American Journal of Mental Deficiency, 87,* 26–33.

Laten, S. & Wikler, L. (1978). The systematic application of social sciences findings to assessment of a family with a mentally retarded member. Paper presented at American Association of Mental Deficiency, Denver, CO.

Legaay, & Keough, B. (1966). Impact of mental retardation on family life. *American Journal of Nursing, 66,* 1062–1065.

Levinson, R. (1975). *Family Crisis and Adaptation: Coping with a mentally retarded child.* Doctoral dissertation, University of Wisconsin, Madison, WI.

Lewis, J. M., Beavers, W. R., Gossett, J. T., & Phillips, V. (1976). *No single thread: Psychological health in family systems.* New York: Brunner/Mazel.

Lin, N., & Ensel, W. M. (1984). Depression-mobility and its social etiology: The role of life events and social support. *Journal of Health and Social Behavior, 25,* 176–188.

Locke, H. J., & Wallace, K. M. (1959). Short marital and adjustment tests: Their reliability and validity. *Marriage and Family Living, 21,* 251–255.

Longo, Di. C., & Bond, L. (1984). Families of the handicapped child: Research and practice. *Family Relations, 33,* 57–66.

Marshall, N. R., Hegrenes, J. R., & Goldstein, S. (1973). Verbal interactions: Mothers and their retarded children vs. mothers and their normal children. *American Journal of Mental Deficiency, 77,* 415–419.

Mattessich, P., & Hill, R. (in press). Family development and life cycle research and theory revisited. In M. Sussman and S. Steinmetz (Eds.), *Handbook of marriage and the family*. New York: Plenum Press.

McAllister, R., Butler, E., & Lei, T. J. (1973). Patterns of social interaction among families of behaviorally retarded children, *Journal of Marriage and the Family, 35*, 93–100.

McCubbin, H., Joy, C., Cauble, E., Comeau, J., Patterson, J., & Needle, R. (1980). Family stress and coping: A decade review, *Journal of Marriage and the Family, 42*(4), 855–870.

McCubbin, H., & Patterson, J. (1983). Family stress adaptation to crises: A double ABCX model of family behavior. In H. McCubbin, M. Sussman, & J. Patterson (Eds.), *Social stresses and the family: Advances and developments in family stress theory and research* (pp. 7–37). New York: The Haworth Press.

Mederer, H., & Hill, R. (1983). Critical transitions over the family life span: Theory and research. In H. I. McCubbin, M. B. Sussman, and J. Patterson (Eds.), *Social stress and the family: Advances and developments in family stress theory and research*. (pp. 39–60). New York: The Haworth Press.

Mercer, J. R. (1966). Patterns of family crisis related to reacceptance of the retarded. *American Journal of Mental Deficiency, 71*, 19–32.

Meyerowitz, H. D., & Farber, B. (1966). Family background of educable mentally retarded children. In B. Farber (Ed.), *Kinship and family organization*. New York: Wiley.

Miller, W. H., & Keirn, W. C. (1978). Personality measurement in parents of retarded and emotionally disturbed children: A replication. *Journal of Clinical Psychology, 34*, 686–690.

Moroney, R. *Families, social services, and social policy: The issue of shared responsibility*. DHHS Publication No. (ADM) 80-846). Washington, DC: National Institute of Mental Health, Studies in Social Change, U.S. Department of Health and Human Services.

National Association for Retarded Citizens (1975)

Nihira, K., Meyers, C. E., & Mink, I. T. (1980). Home environment, family adjustment and the development of mentally retarded children. *Applied Research in Mental Retardation, 1*, 5–24.

O'Connor, G. (1983). Social support of mentally retarded persons. *Mental Retardation, 21*, 187–196.

Olshansky, S. (1962). Chronic sorrow: A response to having a mentally defective child. *Social Casework, 43*, 190–192.

Peterson, H., & Lippa, S. (1978, May). *Life cycle crisis encountered by families of developmentally disabled children. Implications and recommendations for practice*. Paper presented at the annual meeting of the American Association on Mental Deficiency, Denver, CO.

Pollner, M., & Wikler, L. (1977). Cognitive enterprise in a case of *folie a famille*. In H. G. Soeffner (Ed.), *Interpretative verfahren in den sozial-und textwissenschaften*. Stuttgart, Germany: J. B. Metzlersche Verlagsbuchhandlung.

Pollner, N., & Wikler, L. (1985). The social construction of unreality: A case study of a family's attribution of competence to a severely retarded child. *Family Process, 24*, 241–257.

Price-Bonham, S., & Addison, S. (1978). Families and mentally retarded children: Emphasis on the father. *The Family Coordinator, 7*, 221–230.

Ramey, C. T., & Finkelstein, N. W. (1981). Psychosocial mental retardation: A biological and social coalescence. In M. J. Begab, H. C. Haywood, and H. L. Garber (Eds.), *Psychosocial influences in retarded performance: Vol. I. Issues and theories in development*, NICHD Mental Retardation Series. Baltimore: University Park Press.

Ricci, C. S. (1970). Analysis of child rearing attitudes of mothers of retarded, emotionally disturbed, and normal children. *American Journal of Mental Deficiency, 74*, 756–761.

Roesel, R., & Lawlis, G. F. (1983). Divorce in families of genetically handicapped/mentally retarded individuals. *American Journal of Family Therapy, 11*(1), 45–50.

Routh, D. K. (1970). MMPI responses of parents as a function of mental retardation of the child. *American Journal of Mental Deficiency, 75*, 376–377.

Rutter, M. (1975). *Helping troubled children*. New York: Plenum Publishing Corp.

Saenger, G. (1960). *Factors influencing the institutionalization of mentally retarded individuals in New York City*. Albany, NY: Interdepartmental Health Resources Board.

Schilling, R. F., Gilchrist, L., & Schinke, S. P. (1984). Coping and social support in families of developmentally disabled children. *Family Relations, 33*, 47–57.

Schonnel, F. J., & Watts, B. H. (1956). A first survey of the effects of a subnormal child on the family unit. *American Journal of Mental Deficiency, 61*, 210–219.

Schreiber M., & Fealey, M. (1965). Siblings of the retarded: A guided group experience. *Children, 12*, 221–225.

Schufeit, L. J., & Wurster, S. R. (1976). Frequency of divorce among parents of handicapped children. *Resources in Education, 4*, 71–78.

Seitz, S., & Geske, D. (1977). Mothers and trainees: Judgments of children, some effects of labelling. *American Journal of Mental Deficiency, 81*, 362–370.

Slater, M. A., & Mitchell, P. (Eds.). (1984). *Family support services: A parent professional partnership*. Stillwater, OK: National Clearinghouse of Rehabilitation Training Materials.

Stevenson, O. (1954). The first treasured possession. *Psychoanalytic Study of the Child, 9*, 199–217.

Stone, N. M. (1967). Family factors in willingness to place the mongoloid child. *American Journal of Mental Deficiency, 72*, 16–20.

Suelzle, M., & Keenan, V. (1981). Changes in family support networks over the life cycle of mentally retarded persons. *American Journal of Mental Deficiency, 86*, 267–274.

Tallman, I. (1965). Spousal role differentiation and the socialization of severely retarded children. *Journal of Marriage and the Family, 27*, 37–42.

Turnbull, H. R., & Turnbull, A. P. (1982). Parent involvement in the education of handicapped children: A critique. *Mental Retardation, 20*(3), 115–122.

Vadasy, P. F., Fewell, R. R., Meyer, D. J., & Schell, G. (1984). Siblings of handicapped children: A developmental perspective on family interactions. *Family Relations, 33*(1), 155–168.

Vincent, E. (1983). Use of support networks by parents of mentally handicapped children. Unpublished report, Madison, WI.

Waisbren, S. (1980). Parents' reactions after the birth of a developmentally disabled child. *American Journal of Mental Deficiency, 84,* 345–351.

Watzlawick, P., Weakland, J., & Fisch, R. (1974). *Change.* New York: Norton.

Waskowitz, C. H. (1959) The parents of retarded children speak for themselves. *Journal of Pediatrics, 54,* 319–329.

Wasow, M., & Wikler, L. (1983). Professionals's attitudes towards the person with severe mental retardation vs. chronic mental illness: An interesting twist for parents, *Family Therapy, X*(3), 299–307.

Weller, L., Chanan, C., Cohen, B., & Rahman, D. (1974). Social variables in perception and acceptance of retardation. *American Journal of Mental Deficiency, 79,* 274–278.

Wikler, L. (1976). *Delusions of competence: A sociobehavioral study of the maintenance of a deviant belief system in a family with a retarded child.* Unpublished doctoral dissertation, University of California-Irvine.

Wikler, L. (1979, May). *A neglected population: Needs of the single parent of a mentally retarded child.* Paper presented at American Association on Mental Deficiency, Miami, FL.

Wikler, L. (1980) Folie a familie: A family therapist's perspective. *Family Process, 9,* 257–268.

Wikler, L. (1981). Chronic stresses in families of mentally retarded children. *Family Relations, 30,* 281–288.

Wikler, L. (1986). Periodic stresses in families of children with mental retardation. *American Journal of Mental Deficiency,* May.

Wikler, L., Haack, J., & Intagliata, J. (1984). Bearing the burden alone? Helping divorced mothers of children with developmental disabilities. In J. C. Hansen & E. I. Coppersmith (Eds.), *Families with handicapped members: The family therapy collections* (pp. 44–62). Rockville, MD: Aspen Publications.

Wikler, L., Stevenson, P., & Seitz, S. (1984). Reducing the visibility of mental retardation by parent training. Paper presented at American Association of Mental Deficiency Annual Convention, Minneapolis, MN.

Wikler, L., Wasow, M., & Hatfield, E. (1981). Chronic sorrow revisited: Attitudes of parents and professionals about adjustment to mental retardation. *American Journal of Orthopsychiatry, 51*(1), 63–70.

Wikler, L., Wasow, M., & Hatfield, E. (1983). Seeking strengths in families of developmentally disabled children. *Social Work, 7,* 314–315.

Wikler, L., & Laten, S. (in preparation). *Predicting stress in families of mentally retarded children: A screening tool.*

Zuk, G. H. (1959). Autistic distortions in parents of retarded children. *Journal of Consulting Psychology, 23,* 171–179.

Zuk, G. H., Miller, R. L., Barham, J. B., & Kling, F. (1961). Maternal acceptance of retarded children: A questionnaire study of attitudes and religious background. *Child Development, 32,* 525–540.

Chapter

11

Contextual Issues in the Study of Sibling Socialization

Gene H. Brody and Zolinda Stoneman

IN RECENT YEARS, there has been an increased interest in families with mentally retarded children. Most of the research on interactions within these families, however, has focused on one family dyad, the mother and the handicapped child. The focus of this chapter is on another aspect within the family, the siblings.

It has been estimated that there are 1,700,000 mentally retarded children in the United States (Hobbs, 1975). Many of these children live in families that also contain nonhandicapped brothers and sisters. It is important from both developmental and social policy perspectives to understand more about relationships between mentally retarded children and their siblings. Little is actually known, however, about the developmental outcomes for either the nonhandicapped or the handicapped sibling when they are reared together at home (cf. Brody & Stoneman, 1983a). This void is surprising in light of data that show that by 1 year of age children spend as much time in interaction with their siblings as with their

mothers, and far more time than with their fathers (Lawson & Ingleby, 1974). Herein lies the crux of the developmental and social policy issues: How are nonhandicapped and mentally retarded children affected by growing up in the same household?

The presence of a mentally retarded child in the home can be expected to place great demands, in terms of time and sheer physical energy, on parents and other family members. Such demands affect not only the sibling relationship but other aspects of family functioning as well; these in turn reciprocally influence the sibling relationship. Clearly, the research community must provide scientifically sound information for policy-makers and families, so that the deinstitutionalization of children results in positive developmental outcomes for all family members.

The purpose of this chapter is to present a road map to aid researchers in the study of sibling socialization in families with a retarded child. To do this, the authors first attempt to glean from the social development

The preparation of this paper was supported in part by the National Institute of Child Health and Human Development grant no. HD 16817-01A1 and grant no. HD 06016, and March of Dimes grant no. 12-120.

and sibling literatures some clues suggesting the influence of siblings on one another's development. Then, the authors present an argument for the importance of contextual considerations in the study of sibling relations. Data are presented from several studies of sibling relations undertaken by the authors' research group that were designed to chronicle how contextual parameters influence sibling interactions. The chapter concludes with a discussion of the implications of this research for the study of interactions between children and their mentally retarded siblings.

DIRECT AND INDIRECT INFLUENCES

Interactions between mentally retarded children and their siblings can be conceptualized as having both direct and indirect influences on development. The roles that siblings assume when interacting with each other, such as teacher, playmate, or caregiver, and the developmental consequences of assuming these roles constitute the direct impact of having a retarded sibling. The retarded sibling is directly influenced by receiving feedback from the nonhandicapped sibling, as well as by observing the behavior of his or her sibling in a variety of settings. From a direct-effects perspective, one can think about sibling interactions involving a mentally retarded child as being similar to "in-home mainstreaming." Ongoing family activities provide opportunities for the retarded sibling to imitate and practice roles performed by an older or younger sibling, as well as for the normal sibling to expand his or her own repertoire to include such important roles as caregiver, teacher, and manager.

Hartup (1978) has suggested that mainstreaming is an attempt to determine the most desirable social context for the education of both handicapped and nonhandicapped children. This comment referred to classroom mainstreaming within the school system, but it could apply to the home as well. The opportunities afforded by a family-based, mainstreamed environment would seem to be *potentially* advantageous both to the retarded and

normal child, much as preschool mainstreaming has been argued to hold benefits for handicapped and nonhandicapped children alike (Bricker, 1978; Bricker & Bricker, 1971a, 1972).

As appealing as the results of the direct effects studies are, they tell only part of the story concerning occurrences in sibling socialization. Another set of influences are best described as indirect effects because they refer to the effect of sets of circumstances on the interactions of family members with one another. For example, the presence of a mentally retarded sibling in a family could have a marked effect on the socialization of a nonhandicapped sibling. The mentally retarded sibling may cause the parents to experience stress and fatigue, thereby affecting the parents' socialization practices and the quality of their relationship with the nonhandicapped child.

Indirect effects of membership in a sibling pair in which one child is retarded have been the focus of much speculation, but little research. The research that does exist yields confusing and often contradictory findings. Farber (1963) found that girls with a retarded sibling at home spend large amounts of time caring for that sibling and thus spend less time with peers. Other researchers, however, have failed to find disruptions in the nonhandicapped child's interactions with peers. Caldwell and Guze (1960) and Cleveland and Miller (1977) found that siblings of retarded children reported having numerous friends, often inviting them to their home to visit.

A common thread throughout the literature on retarded children and their siblings is the finding that the attitudes of these sibling pairs toward one another mirror the attitudes and adjustments of the parents toward the retarded child (Caldwell & Guze, 1960; Graliker, Fishler, & Koch, 1962; Grossman, 1972; Wolfensberger, 1967). Thus, parents have an indirect influence on the interactions between retarded children and their brothers and sisters. We know little, however, about how this parental influence occurs. For instance, do parents actively structure the roles that their children assume with each other, such as instructing the nonhandicapped child to teach his or her retarded sibling, or is this information communicated in a more subtle fashion?

SEARCHING FOR CLUES:
THE PEER AND SIBLING LITERATURES

In this section, aspects of the peer relations and sibling relations literatures are examined for clues to the direct and indirect influences of a retarded child and a normal sibling on one another's development. Siblings can be thought of as similar, but not equivalent to, different-age peers. Obviously, siblings have strong emotional feelings and attachments that are not considered characteristic of peers; however, they do share with different-age peers the need to adapt to one another's competencies in order to interact in a functional manner. As with sibling interactions, mixed-age interactions have been found to be characterized by asymmetrical rather than symmetrical relationships. Cross-cultural observations indicate that helping and sympathy are frequently directed by older children toward younger children, whereas assistance seeking and other dependent behaviors are most commonly directed to older children by younger children. Interactions among age-mates are characterized by more sociable and aggressive acts than are present among children who differ by a year or two (Whiting & Whiting, 1975).

Several studies now indicate that older children attempt to accommodate their behavior to the perceived cognitive and social needs of younger peers. For example, 4-year-olds use shorter and less complex utterances when they talk to 2-year-olds than when they talk to other 4-year-olds (Shatz & Gelman, 1973). Four-year-olds also make adjustments in their conversations with 2-year-olds according to individual differences in a younger child; for example, longer utterances and more complex syntactic structures are directed toward responsive 2-year old companions than toward less responsive ones (Masur, 1978). Another study demonstrated that even 3-year-olds use more mature communications with 5-year-olds than

with other 3-year-olds (Lougee, Grueneich, & Hartup, 1977).

Other researchers have examined social learning processes and have found that children prefer to imitate age-mates and older peer models, displaying little imitation of younger peer models (Brody & Stoneman, 1981b). In a subsequent study Brody and Stoneman (in press) found that second-grade children were willing to imitate the behavior of a younger peer if the younger peer model was as competent on the behavioral dimension as the average second grader. Moreover, second graders were unwilling to imitate the behavior of an age-mate described as functioning at the kindergarten level. These findings imply that children are most likely to be influenced by those models whom they consider competent on the issue in question. Similarly, reciprocal imitation appears to occur more frequently during children's interactions with same-age or older peers than with younger children (Thelen & Kirkland, 1976), and children are more likely to accept direction from older children than younger children (Allen & Feldman, 1976).

The peer relations literature also addresses the issue of similarity among relationships involving same-sex and opposite-sex sibling pairs. Jacklin and Maccoby (1978) studied 3-year-old children who were not well acquainted with one another. More social behavior, both positive and negative, was directed toward same-sex partners than toward opposite-sex partners, with few differences found between boy-boy and girl-girl dyads. Similar results were obtained in another study of well-acquainted children (Langlois, Gottfried, & Seay, 1973). These studies lead us to expect more social interaction in same-sex sibling pairs than in opposite-sex sibling pairs.

Taken together, the above results provide substantial support for the "in-home mainstreaming" notion introduced earlier. Older children systematically accommodate their behavior to the competencies of the younger child, and there is even some evidence that the younger child attempts to engage in more mature behavior in the presence of a more competent playmate. It is also interesting to note that competence, more than age, appears to govern children's willingness to imitate the behavior of a peer model. Again, the implications of these results for sibling pairs in which the older sibling is mentally retarded are encouraging.

Sibling Interactions

Most of what is known about sibling socialization can be found in studies of family constellation effects. A number of family constellation variables have been studied as possible influences on various aspects of children's development, including birth order, family size, the size of the spacing interval between children, and the sex of the older and younger siblings. Typically, family constellation data have been collected from college students in a group testing context. The psychological variables suspected of being influenced by family constellation parameters range from psychiatric deviations to intellectual performance.

The persistence of interest in the effects of family constellation variables can hardly be attributed to conclusive insights born of these labors. The number of firm conclusions that can be drawn are small; however, as independent variables, family constellation parameters have an attractive quality or, more accurately, an apparent simplicity that is actually quite deceptive. Schooler's (1972) cynical suggestion that investigators are unable "to resist the temptation of taking a cheap bet on a long shot by collecting birth order data on their subjects as they pursue studies more central to their interests (p. 174)" may come close to the truth.

The attractive simplicity mentioned above refers to the use of family constellation parameters as proxies for socialization processes. Family constellation, as are many parameters with which developmentalists are concerned, is a summary variable. Thus, instead of sampling socialization processes, a great deal of energy has been devoted to examining persons whose social experiences within the family were presumed to be different because of their birth order, spacing, gender, or so forth. It is fair to say that findings on the relationship between family constellation parameters and developmental outcome measures, such as intellectual attainment, have been inconsistent and that most of this body of research has not been grounded in theory. Where relationships have been described, the functional psychological variables underlying these associations remain a matter of speculation. The authors agree with Sutton-Smith (1983) that only after a rich foundation of research has been completed describing the day-to-day interactions and environments experienced by siblings can the "variables worthy of quantifiable attention" for predictive research be selected and operationalized.

In the last few years, researchers have recognized the limitation of the extant research base underlying the study of sibling relationships. Several different research teams have become involved in describing the form that sibling relationships take. The aforementioned mixed-age peer relations literature predicts that sibling relationships will be marked by asymmetries in roles and behaviors. Older siblings will be expected to assume dominant roles associated with caregiving, nurturing, and teaching, whereas younger siblings will be expected to assume complementary roles. Presumably, these differences will be related to the allocation of status to children as a function of age by both parents and by children themselves (e.g., Eisenstadt, 1956; Moore, 1969; Sutton-Smith & Rosenbaum, 1970). This allocation of status to older siblings is most likely mediated by the relative cognitive and behavioral competencies of the two siblings.

The peer relations literature also predicts higher rates of interaction for same-sex than for opposite-sex siblings. The reasons for such differences among peers are not clear. If such differences are also found among siblings, they could result from mediation by differences in the self-selected activities that provide the context against which interactions occur. Same-sex children share a wider variety of mutually enjoyed play activities than do opposite-sex children.

In reviewing the small number of studies that have observed sibling-sibling interactions, it becomes apparent that the peer relations literature serves as a useful heuristic device for understanding sibling relationships. Lamb (1978a, 1978b) observed 24 infants and their preschool-age siblings in a laboratory playroom in the presence of their parents. He found that both the infants and their older siblings preferred to interact with their parents than with one another. Young siblings appeared to monitor and model the behavior of their older siblings, whereas older siblings were more likely to offer toys and vocalize to their younger siblings. Lamb (1978b) observed the same siblings in the same laboratory context 6 months after the first observation. The younger and older siblings assumed similar roles to the ones assumed 6 months earlier. The infants monitored and imitated the older siblings, and the older siblings directed the attention of their younger siblings toward objects in the environment. Samuels (1980) also studied sibling interactions between infants and their older siblings, finding results very similar to those cited above. Sibling presence was shown to increase infant locomotor and object exploration. Taken together, these studies suggest that the presence of an older preschool-age sibling facilitates locomotor exploration and mastery of the object environment.

Abramovitch and her colleagues (Abramovitch, Corter, & Lando, 1979; Abramovitch, Corter, & Pepler, 1980) explored the actual patterns of sibling interactions in their homes. The younger siblings averaged 20 months of age, and the older siblings averaged 51 months. During the course of the naturalistic interactions, older siblings initiated agonistic and prosocial acts more often than their younger siblings. Younger siblings imitated their older siblings more often. These results parallel the aforementioned research and reveal consistent asymmetries in the behaviors and roles assumed by infants and their preschool-age siblings.

Other researchers, notably Dunn and Kendrick (1982) and Stewart (1983), have demonstrated the strong affective bonds that exist between preschool children and their infant siblings. The naturalistic observations of Dunn and Kendrick demonstrated that infants missed the elder sibling in his or her absence and used the older sibling as a source of comfort. Stewart demonstrated that over half of the older siblings in his laboratory experiment attempted to reassure and comfort their younger siblings in the absence of their mothers.

Interactions among school-age siblings have also been shown to be characterized by asymmetries. Observations of siblings while playing a board game (Brody, Stoneman, & MacKinnon, 1982; Stoneman, Brody, & MacKinnon, 1984), as well as during free-ranging self-selected activities (Brody, Stoneman, & MacKinnon, 1985; Stoneman, Brody, & MacKinnon, in press) have revealed clear asymmetries in the roles assumed by older and younger siblings. Older siblings assumed teacher, manager, and helper roles when playing with their brothers and sisters, whereas the younger siblings assumed the complementary learner, managee, and helpee roles. These results are not as straightforward as they appear at first glance as they are qualified by a number of contextual parameters that are discussed in a subsequent section.

To date, little of the sibling interaction literature has focused on processes. In those studies where process information is available, the data bear a striking similarity to the mixed-age peer literature. Infants apparently engage in a considerable amount of imitation of their older preschool-age siblings, who in turn appear not to imitate their younger siblings (Dunn & Kendrick, 1982; Lamb, 1978a, 1978b; Pepler, Abramovitch, & Corter, 1981). There is also some evidence that preschool-age older siblings attempt to accommodate their speech to the linguistic levels of their 1-year-old brothers or sisters (Dunn & Kendrick, 1982). Thus, in many respects sibling relationships resemble mixed-age peer relationships. This similarity ceases, however, when affective relationships are considered. Interactions between different-age peers have generally been found to be affectively neutral. Sibling interactions, on the other hand, are best characterized as an admixture of emotional responses that can quickly range from warm to hostile and back again (Dunn & Kendrick, 1982).

Finally, sibling interactions occur against the backdrop of relationships within the immediate and extended family. The quality of the sibling relationship has been found to be related to the quality of each child's relationship to his or her mother. For example, Dunn (1983) reports

> . . . in families with a particularly intense and playful relationship between mother and first-born girls, before and immediately after the birth of the sibling, not only was the behavior of the elder sibling relatively hostile to the younger over the next year but by 14 months the younger sibling was also particularly negative to the older.

The recognition that sibling relations are indirectly influenced by the quality of the mother-child relationship has important implications for the study of sibling relationships in which one sibling is mentally retarded. For as was indicated earlier, the attitudes of the normal sibling toward the retarded sibling appear to mirror the mother's attitudes. One of the important messages in these findings is that the study of sibling socialization must take into account the context in which sibling relationships are embedded.

CONTEXTUAL INFLUENCES
ON SIBLING RELATIONSHIPS

The present section describes a series of studies undertaken by the authors' research team to examine contextual influences on sibling interaction patterns. The motivation for engaging in this research program can be traced to the authors' perusal of the extant research. The literature primarily dealt with very young children who were observed in widely different settings—laboratory playrooms, livingrooms, backyards—and with different behavior coding systems. A series of studies on sibling interactions was then initiated, employing a common behavioral coding system. Sibling interactions were viewed as tied to properties of the interactional context in which they took place. This approach carries with it two important policy-related implications. First, evaluations of children's behavior in general, and sibling behavior in particular, requires disciplined and cautious interpretation. Second, decision

making in the absence of *data* about specific children in particular contexts is all but ruled out.

A contextual approach to sibling relationships assumes that the perceptions, attitudes, and behaviors of siblings cannot be understood without examining the contexts in which they occur. A context may be a physical setting or an activity, the presence or absence of specific persons, or a combination of settings and persons. Siblings are viewed as both adapting to existing contexts and contributing to the creation of new contexts through their own thoughts and actions.

In the following section, the authors present the results of several studies that were designed to address the following contextual issues: 1) How are sibling interaction patterns different from peer and parent-child interaction patterns? 2) How do person parameters, such as age, gender composition, maternal-rearing practices, and socioeconomic status, influence sibling interactions? 3) What kinds of activities do siblings self-select, and do sibling interactions vary as a function of different activities? 4) Does the behavior that siblings direct to one another change when the interactional context includes either a friend or parent?

A common behavioral coding system was employed in the descriptions of studies that follow. From the larger coding system, six roles and two classes of behavior are discussed here. The six roles are teacher, learner, manager, managee, helper, and helpee. The amount of prosocial and agonistic behavior that siblings direct to one another is also described. The particular roles were selected for observation because they relate directly to roles widely ascribed to siblings (Weisner & Gallimore, 1977); namely, serving as a socialization agent by directing behavior (manager role) and promoting cognitive growth (teacher role), as well as caregiving (helper role). Compliance with managing, teaching, and helping attempts by one sibling represented the acceptance of the complementary managee, learner, and helpee roles.

A description of the studies can be found in Table 1. Each study is assigned a letter, A through G. In subsequent tables, studies are referred to by the letter with which they are associated in Table 1.

Other Social Agents

Sibling relations occur in the midst of an interconnected social network that includes other family members, friends, relatives, and others. The sibling subsystem is only one of several that exist in many families. Other subsystems include the mother-child, the father-child, and the spouse subsystem. For children, the peer subsystem is another important source of influence. There is a suggestion in the literature that each of these subsystems is unique, with its own roles and patterns of behavior (Brody & Stoneman, 1983a; Hartup, 1980; Lewis, Feiring, & Weinraub, 1981). The authors' research focused on sibling relations as contrasted with peer relations, mother-child relations, and father-child relations. Table 2 presents a summary of results for these studies.

Studies A, B, and C made comparisons between sibling and peer subsystems, as well as examined interactions during triadic groupings involving both subsystems. Interactions were found to be more egalitarian when peers played together, whereas role asymmetries were more evident during sibling interactions. Older siblings assumed more dominant manager and teacher roles relative to their younger brothers and sisters. These findings suggest that sibling and peer relationships represent different types of interaction or qualitatively different "interaction systems." Bronfenbrenner (1979), among others, has argued that development is facilitated through interactions with persons who occupy a variety of roles. In learning and practicing a role, the child learns not only his or her own role but also the complementary roles. Theoretically, the role asymmetries displayed by the older siblings while part of two different "interaction systems" would be advantageous to development. These children have the opportunity to practice dominant roles with their siblings, as well as egalitarian roles with their friends.

Additionally, Study C found that the older siblings' friends complied with younger sib-

lings' management attempts proportionally more often than did the older sibling. This finding is consistent with other studies that have found that family members treat each other differently (more negatively) than do nonfamily members (Birchler, Weiss, & Vincent, 1975; Halverson & Waldrop, 1970; Ryder, 1968). It is plausible that the older sibling's friend and the younger sibling interact infrequently; therefore, the friend probably complies with the younger sibling's requests in order to be polite.

The second study (Study H) focused on comparisons between the sibling subsystem and the mother-child subsystem. Cicirelli (1976) compared the helping behavior of mothers and older siblings on a problem-solving task. Mothers gave younger siblings more explanations and feedback than did older siblings, whereas younger siblings responded to mothers with more help-seeking and accepting behaviors and fewer independence behaviors than they did to their older siblings. The behavior of both mothers and older siblings was also related to gender composition of the sibling dyad. Baskett and Johnson (1982) examined the interactions between younger siblings and their parents, as well as between younger siblings and their older sisters and brothers, during self-selected activities. A greater number and variety of child behaviors occurred in child-parent interactions compared with sibling interactions. Additionally, parent-child interactions were more positive in nature, whereas sibling interactions were more negative. Undesirable behaviors directed toward parents, such as whines and tantrums, seemed to be designed to attract parental attention, whereas undesirable behaviors directed toward siblings tended to be more overtly aggressive.

The authors' findings indicate that mothers assume helping, teaching, and managing roles and emit more prosocial behavior toward younger siblings than do older brothers and sisters. Sibling interactions were also found to be more negative than mother-child interactions. These findings are similar to those reported above. Additionally, the authors found that younger siblings assume teacher and manager roles with their mothers more frequently

Table 1. Description of studies

Study	Subjects	Age of younger sibling	Age of older sibling	Gender composition	Socioeconomic status	Activity	Persons observed	Grouping
A Role asymmetries	22 sibling pairs	4.5–7.0 years	8–10 years	$\frac{1}{2}$ males $\frac{1}{2}$ females	Upper-middle	Board game	Siblings and older sibling's friend	Sibling dyad, peer dyad, triad
B Naturalistic observations	22 sibling pairs	4.5–7.0 years	8–10 years	$\frac{1}{2}$ males $\frac{1}{2}$ females	Upper-middle	Self-selected	Siblings and older sibling's friend	Sibling dyad, peer dyad, triad
C Reciprocal roles	16 sibling pairs	4.5–7.0 years	8–10 years	$\frac{1}{2}$ males $\frac{1}{2}$ females	Upper-middle	Self selected	Siblings and older sibling's friend	Sibling dyad, peer dyad, triad
D Developmental changes	36 sibling pairs	Older group: 4.5–6.5 Younger group: 2.5–4.5	Older group: 7–9 Younger group: 4.5–6.5	$\frac{1}{2}$ males $\frac{1}{2}$ females	Upper-middle	Self-selected	Siblings	Sibling dyad
E Cross-gender comparisons	40 sibling pairs	4.5–6.5 years	7–9 years	10 male-male 10 female-female 10 male-female 10 female-male	Upper-middle	Board game Self-selected	Siblings	Sibling dyad
F Television context	13 sibling pairs	3.0–4.5 years	4.0–6.0 years	Males	Upper-middle	Television viewing	Siblings Mothers, fathers	Mother, father, quad
G Maternal-rearing practices and social context	24 sibling pairs and their mothers	4.5–7.0 years	8–10 years	$\frac{1}{2}$ males $\frac{1}{2}$ females	Working class Upper-middle	Television viewing Legos, board game	Siblings Mother	Sibling dyad Sibling and mother triad
H Mother preschool sibling observations	18 sibling pairs	2.5–4.5 years	4.5–6.5 years	$\frac{1}{2}$ males $\frac{1}{2}$ females	Upper-middle	Self-selected	Siblings Mother	Mother-younger sibling dyad Older sibling-younger sibling dyad

Table 2. Interactions among siblings and other social agents

Subsystem comparisons	Study	Selected findings
Sibling vs. peer	A,B,C	1. Older sibling assumes teaching and managing roles more during dyadic interactions with younger sibling than during dyadic interaction with a friend.
		2. Peer interactions are characterized by greater use of the symmetrical playmate role than are sibling interactions.
		3. Older sibling is the target of management more often during peer interactions than during sibling interactions.
		4. Male older siblings direct more negative behavior toward peers than they direct toward siblings.
		5. Managing attempts by younger siblings are complied with more often by the older sibling's friend than by the older sibling during triadic interaction.
Sibling vs. mother	H	1. Mothers assume helping and teaching roles more often than do older siblings during dyadic interactions with the younger sibling.
		2. Mothers emit more explicit directives, implicit directives, and prosocial behavior during dyadic interactions with the younger sibling than do older siblings when they interact with younger siblings.
		3. Older siblings direct more agonistic behavior toward younger siblings than do mothers.
		4. Younger siblings direct more information-seeking questions, teaching, and prosocial behavior toward mothers during dyadic interactions than they do during dyadic interactions with their older siblings.
		5. Siblings engage in more social conversation with each other than do mothers interacting with younger siblings.

than they do with their older siblings. Thus, it appears that, in interactions with mothers, younger siblings may have more of an opportunity to practice dominant roles than they do in interactions with older sisters and brothers, at least during certain activities. It is possible that older siblings actively discourage younger siblings from taking dominant roles, whereas mothers may be more relaxed and comfortable with their relative power in relation to the young child. As such, mothers may allow the younger siblings to "teach" them and "direct" their behavior, at least in play-oriented situations.

Activity

A discussion of the contextual importance of activities to the study of sibling relations must take into account both the self-selection of different activities by various sibling pairs and the functional relationships between certain activities and sibling behavior. Each of these is

considered in turn. Table 3 summarizes the results of the authors' studies that have addressed these questions.

Siblings help shape their own environments by choosing to participate in certain activities and not in others, as well as by selecting certain toys and games for play and ignoring others. In Study B, the patterns of activities selected by peers and siblings provided some insight into the ways in which children accommodate their activities to the competencies of other children in their presence. Girls and boys both displayed these accommodation processes, but their form differed by gender. Boys engaged in fewer competitive activities with their younger brothers than they did with their peers, whereas girls utilized doll play as a means of involving children of differing competencies in the same activity. When older siblings and peers did not select activities that accommodated the competencies of the younger siblings, the younger siblings tended to leave the group and play by

Table 3. Activities and sibling interactions

Activity dimension	Study	Selected findings
Self-selected activities	B	1. Boys playing with friends engage in more competitive physical activities than boys playing with their younger sibling. 2. Boys play with toys more often with their younger sibling than their friends. 3. Girls play ritualized children's games more often with their younger sibling than with their friends. 4. Girls play with dolls more frequently in triad with friend and younger sibling than in either dyadic interactions with sibling or friend. 5. Female siblings play indoors more frequently than male siblings. 6. Female siblings play with dolls more than male siblings, whereas male siblings engage in more competitive activity than female siblings.
Sibling interaction as a function of television viewing, a board game, and a construction task	G	1. Older siblings engaged in more helping, teaching, and agonistic behavior while playing the board game than during play with the construction task and television viewing. 2. The construction task occasioned more information-seeking and observing the younger siblings' behavior than did television viewing or play with the board game. 3. Younger siblings engaged in more managing, teaching, and information-seeking during the construction task and board game than during television viewing. 4. The construction task occasioned more helping and observing of the older siblings' behavior than did either the board game or television viewing. 5. The board game occasioned more agonistic behavior from younger siblings than did the construction task or television viewing.
Sibling interaction during three television programs	F	1. Siblings attended more to one another during the evening news than during the Muppets. 2. Siblings attended more to one another during the Muppets than during cartoons. 3. Children verbalized more to their siblings during the evening news than during the Muppets or cartoons. 4. Siblings asked more questions during the evening news than they did during the Muppets. 5. Siblings asked more questions during the Muppets than they did during cartoons. 6. Siblings responded to their father's questions proportionally less during cartoons than during either the Muppets or the evening news. 7. Siblings complied with proportionally more maternal managing attempts during the news than they did during cartoons.

themselves. For example, if the older brother and his friend began playing a competitive game beyond the skill level of the younger brother, the younger child would often leave. Female peers tended to select activities in which the younger sisters could participate with greater frequency than did male peers.

Thus, it appears that children respond to their perceptions of the cognitive and behavioral competencies of their siblings and friends by agreeing to engage in different activities depending on the relative competencies of the social agent in their presence. It further appears that sibling gender constellations exert an influence on children's activity selections. This finding supports Parke's (1978) suggestion that siblings and peers often serve as mediators of the environment through the selection of physical objects, as well as through the use of toys as mediators in social interaction.

The literature suggests that differences in activity selections are related to differences in behavior. In their classic study, Quilitch and Risley (1973) demonstrated that certain play materials elicited social play among preschool children, whereas other materials elicited isolate play. Other studies have found that certain play activities are associated with anti-social/aggressive play in children (Feshbach, 1956; Turner & Goldsmith, 1976), as well as different activity levels (Cohen, Hulls, & Paige, 1978). Cohen et al. (1978) suggest a probable interaction between the preference for different activities by children with certain characteristics and the propensity for certain activities to elicit specific patterns of behavior. In terms of their research on activity level, it is plausible that very active children would choose to play with large motor toys, rather than puzzles, whereas at the same time, large motor toys elicit much more active play from most children than do puzzles.

In Study G the authors examined the roles and behaviors of working-class and upper-middle class sibling pairs during three activities: play with Legos (a construction toy), play with a board game, and television viewing. Play with Legos was selected as a relatively unstructured activity that allowed the children to be as creative or innovative as they wished when they played. The board game ("Trouble," from Gilbert Industries), on the other hand, was much more structured, with rules for appropriate play. The board game also introduced a competitive spirit to the sibling play by having a winner and a loser. Television viewing was included as a very popular activity that tends to focus attention away from interaction toward the television set itself. Past research by the authors (Brody, Stoneman, & Sanders, 1980) found television viewing to reduce dramatically family interac-

tions (especially for children and fathers) when compared to family play.

As expected, In Study G the types of activities made available to the siblings influenced their role relationships and behavior. Television viewing generally reduced the number of sibling exchanges. The nature of sibling interactions during the board game and construction task followed closely the predictions that were derived from the work of Quilitch and Risley (1973). The construction task, which does not require the cooperation of two persons, occasioned more passive interaction patterns; more observing and information seeking characterized the interactions. The board game, as expected, occasioned more managing, teaching, and helping by the other sibling and more agonistic behavior in both siblings.

Thus, the findings of Study G strongly suggest that patterns of sibling interaction are directly related to the activities in which the siblings are engaged. In Study G, television viewing was associated with very low levels of interaction between siblings. It is highly unlikely, however, that all types of television programs would affect family interactions identically. Specific television programs may be more or less interesting to any given family member and that level of interest should affect the person's interactions with other family members. Study F was designed to examine the relationship between program salience and family interaction.

Three television programs were selected to represent three separate family television-viewing contexts. The evening national news was selected to represent programs with low child interest and high adult interest. Cartoons were selected as programs with high child interest and low adult interest, and the "Muppet" show was selected as a program of interest to both adults and children. As expected, family interaction patterns varied across the three programs. Siblings interacted the least and evidenced the lowest levels of contingent responsiveness to their parents during the cartoon show, the program with highest salience for children. Similarly, siblings interacted the most and evidenced the highest levels of contingent responsiveness during the evening news. These findings supported a model proposed by the authors to explain the influence of television viewing on family interactions (Brody & Stoneman, 1983b). The results suggested that the salience of television programming is an important contextual variable that influences sibling interactions and the sequential exchanges between siblings and other family members.

Person Parameters

Despite the fact that siblings share at least 50% of a common gene pool, they often behave very differently (Scarr & Grajek, 1982). To explain these differences, behavior geneticists have recommended that researchers examine the direct influence of siblings on one another, differential treatment by parents, and self-selection by siblings of different environments within the home. In turn, the authors' focus has been to examine the interaction among siblings and the selection of environments that siblings choose when they interact with one another. Table 4 summarizes the results of the studies that have addressed these questions.

There is ample suggestion in the literature that same-sex sibling interactional contexts should be different from opposite-sex sibling contexts. The results of these studies, however, have not always been consistent. One group of researchers has predicted that children in same-sex sibling pairs should be the most stereotypically sex-typed, whereas children from cross-sex sibling pairs should be more androgynous. These predictions were derived from a social learning perspective. Findings from several studies have supported this position (Bigner, 1972; Brim, 1956; Lamke, Bell, & Murphy, 1980; Rosenberg & Sutton-Smith, 1964, 1968). Others have argued that sibling modeling occurs infrequently and that, in the majority of instances, same-sex siblings become dissimilar on dimensions such as sex-typing in order to avoid comparison and competition (Schachter, 1982). This latter position predicts that same-sex siblings deiden-

tify (become different) more than opposite-sex siblings, because of the heightened rivalry that accompanies the closeness in desires and interests that occur for children of the same gender. In this framework, then, siblings would be expected to develop dissimilar interests and characteristics in order to decrease competition and unfavorable social comparisons. This theoretical orientation posits processes similar to those posed by Leventhal's (1970) comparison-prevention strategy and by Tesser's (1980) self-esteem maintenance model. Studies by Grotevant (1978), Leventhal (1970), and Schachter (1982) provide empirical support for this position.

In an attempt to reconcile these two positions, Sutton-Smith (1983) suggested that different processes may be active during different developmental periods or that differences in the dependent measures are responsible for the inconsistent results. He went on to suggest that the research direction of choice on the question of sibling sex-role effects, as well as for the field of sibling research in general, should be to provide descriptive information of actual siblings interacting in specific contexts. In line with this suggestion, study E had as its primary purpose the description of same-sex and cross-sex sibling interactions.

The results of study E (Stoneman, Brody, & MacKinnon, in press) implied that sibling gender composition creates interactional contexts that may have both direct and indirect effects. For example, the ecology of younger male siblings' rooms varied according to the sex of the older sibling. Boys with older brothers had more masculine items and decorations in their room than did boys with older sisters. Similarly, boys with older brothers engaged in a greater proportion of male sex-typed activities, as well as proportionally fewer cross-sex activities, when playing with their siblings than did boys with older sisters. This pattern of engaging in own-sex stereotyped activities carried over into times when the younger brother played alone.

Girls with older brothers engaged in more opposite sex-typed activities than girls with older sisters, both during times when the older

Table 4. Contributions of person parameters to sibling interactions

Person parameters	Study	Selected findings
Gender composition	E	1. During interactive play, boys with older brothers engaged in more own-sex activities than did boys with older sisters.
		2. Boys with older sisters took part in more opposite-sex activities than did boys with older brothers.
		3. During solitary play, boys with older brothers again engaged in more own-sex activities than boys with older sisters.
		4. Girls with older brothers engaged in more opposite-sex activities during play with their siblings than did girls with older sisters.
		5. Younger male siblings with older brothers had more male items in their rooms than did younger boys with older sisters.
		6. Male siblings engaged in more solitary activity than any other sibling gender combination.
		7. Male siblings spent less time as playmates than any other sibling gender combination.
		8. Older girls taught their younger sisters more frequently than older siblings in any other group.
		9. Older girls managed their siblings more often than did older brothers.
		10. Sibling pairs in which the older child was female exhibited greater role asymmetries than did pairs containing an older male child.
		11. Older sister/younger brother pairs had the most positive verbals, older brother/younger sister pairs were the next highest, whereas both groups of same-sex pairs emitted the fewest positive verbals.
		12. Female pairs emitted the most positive physicals, while male pairs emitted the least.
Age X gender	D	1. School-age female siblings directed more prosocial behavior toward one another than male school-age siblings or male and female preschool-age siblings.
		2. Preschool-age male siblings directed more negative behavior toward one another than preschool-age female siblings or male and female school-age siblings.
		3. Preschool-age female siblings spent more time in solitary play than preschool-age male siblings, whereas school-age male siblings spent more time in solitary play than school-age female siblings.
		4. Older school-age female siblings assumed the teacher role more often than older male school-age siblings or older male and female preschool-age siblings.
		5. Younger school-age females comply more often with teaching attempts than younger school-age males or younger preschool-age males and females.

and younger siblings were playing together and during times when they were playing alone. Thus, the gender of the older siblings not only affected the activities in which younger boys and girls engaged while playing with their siblings, but also carried over into times when the younger siblings were playing by themselves.

Female sibling pairs engaged in more teaching and managing of one another than any of the other gender combinations. The sibling literature has revealed a consistent tendency for female siblings to assume the teacher role with younger siblings (Cicirelli, 1973; Minnett, Vandell, & Santrock, 1983). Whether these results are due to normative sex-role related expectations or to girls' self-selection of activities that are more likely to occasion teaching is not yet known.

Differences emerged in the affect that siblings directed to one another across the four sibling groups. Female sibling pairs managed each other most frequently, and these same siblings resisted proportionally more managing attempts than male pairs or older female/younger male pairs. Older girls with younger brothers emitted the most positive verbals, whereas same-sex pairs emitted the fewest. These results are in line with both Shachter's and Tesser's theories, which predict increased friction between siblings who are more similar. The only affective finding not consistent with this pattern was the frequency of positive physicals in same-sex sibling pairs. It is plausible that gender-related cultural norms for positive physical contact, which sanction such contact for females and discourage it for males, may be responsible for this difference.

Study D (Brody et al., 1985) was initiated to determine whether sibling interactional contexts change as siblings develop and acquire new competencies. To date, different behavioral coding systems have been employed in studies that have observed interactions between preschool-age siblings and school-age siblings. In addition to examining the role relationships that characterized sibling interactions in two age groups, the authors sought to examine whether the amount of prosocial and agonistic behaviors that siblings direct to one another changed with the age and gender of the siblings.

Many of the role asymmetries that have been observed in studies of school-age sibling pairs were also observed in studies of preschool-age sibling pairs. More specifically, older siblings in school-age and preschool-age sibling pairs assumed the manager and helper roles more often than their younger siblings who, in turn, assumed the managee and helpee roles more often than their older brothers and sisters.

Several of the role asymmetries and behavioral differences found in previous studies with either preschool-age or school-age sibling pairs were found to be specific to one age group. For example, preschool-age male siblings directed more agonistic behavior toward one another, and school-age female siblings directed more prosocial behavior toward one another. Both of these results replicate findings from studies that observed either pre-

school-age siblings or school-age siblings (Abramovitch et al., 1979, 1980; Brody et al., 1982; Stoneman et al., 1984).

The authors also found that preschool-age females siblings played with each other less than preschool-age male siblings, whereas school-age female siblings played with each other more than school-age male siblings. The latter finding replicates previous research (Stoneman et al., 1984). One of the reasons that female siblings appear to interact with one another more as they develop, whereas male siblings appear to do just the opposite, may have to do with the willingness of the older female sibling to accommodate her behavior to the competencies of her younger sister. Data from the Stoneman et al. study suggested that school-age female siblings displayed a willingness to interact around activities that were interesting and appropriate for the competencies of both the older and younger siblings, whereas older male school-aged siblings chose to engage in competitive activities. Anecdotal reports suggested that younger male siblings would often find such contexts frustrating and would withdraw after a short period of time.

Older female school-age siblings assumed the teacher role more often than any sibling group x gender x person combination. Similarly, younger school-age female siblings accepted teaching attempts from their older sisters more often than their male counterparts, thus spending more time in the learner role than any sibling group x gender x person combination. These results corroborate previous research that was conducted in structured laboratory contexts (Cicirelli, 1973, 1975). There are several plausible explanations for these findings. One possibility is that female siblings are responding to normative expectations about sibling role relationships that are socialized by parents and other social agents. Parents may place more emphasis on teaching caregiving behaviors to older female children. A second possibility that appears to fit better with the available evidence (cf. Scarr & Grajek, 1982) argues that the temperament and interpersonal propensities of female siblings make them more likely to self-select caregiving roles that are presented to them by their home environments. That is, male and female siblings may choose roles and behavior related to aspects of their genotypes. In addition, the roles and behaviors they choose to perform with their siblings would be related to the behavior of their younger siblings. To the extent that younger sisters are more socially engaging and attentive than younger brothers, one would expect them to receive more instructional interactions from older siblings.

Cross-System Influences

Studies D and E described sibling interaction patterns and their relation to age, gender, and ordinal position; however, they did not focus on the sibling relationship as influenced by events that transpire within the family system. The purpose of Study G was to examine the relations between maternal child-rearing practices and sibling interaction patterns. A transactional or systems approach to socialization (cf. Belsky, 1981) suggests that events that occur in the parent-child subsystem would have implications for the sibling subsystem. From this perspective, rearing practices would be expected to influence directly the behavior of each child and influence indirectly the behavior of siblings with one another.

The child-rearing literature is consistent in demonstrating that children whose parents are consistent, promote curiosity, are not too restrictive, and employ inductive rather than fear-based disciplinary practices are most likely to develop optimally (Belsky, 1981; Brody & Shaffer, 1982; Parke, 1978). On the basis of this literature the authors hypothesized that supportive, nonpunitive parenting practices would be related to supportive, nonpunitive sibling interactions. In addition, the authors speculated that the extent to which mothers reported they enjoyed the parental role and the extent to which mothers valued having an identity separate from the maternal role would be related to sibling behavior. It was hypothesized that, in families where the mothers enjoyed the maternal role, siblings would direct more prosocial and less agonistic behavior toward one another. In families where the mothers valued maintaining an identity separate from the maternal role, older siblings would be more accustomed to assuming caregiving functions and therefore would be more likely to display guidance and caregiving behaviors while interacting with their younger siblings. Table 5 summarizes the findings of Study G on the effects of maternal child-rearing practices.

Maternal child-rearing practices proved to be good predictors of sibling interaction patterns. These data provide additional support for Belsky's (1981) contention that events—in this case, rearing practices—that occur within one family subsystem (parent-child) have implications for other subsystems within the family. To date, most studies of sibling interaction patterns have focused almost exclusively on sibling interpersonal behavior without considering the fact that siblings are part of a complex family system. The correlational data suggest that more attention should be focused on the contribution of rearing practices and attitudes to the development of sibling relationships.

Roles that are widely ascribed to older siblings—namely, serving as a socialization agent by directing behavior (manager role) and caregiving (helper role) —were positively related to maternal child-rearing practices that encouraged curiosity and openness and to the mother's valuing a separate life from her children. The performance of these roles was negatively related to maternal inconsistency and anxiety induction. These findings are interesting as they demonstrate that rearing practices that have been found to relate to the development of competencies in individual children are also related to the assumption of important roles by older siblings when interacting with their younger brothers and sisters. These data also suggest that older siblings may take on more socialization functions when their mothers have activities that they value outside the family. These results have implications for older siblings in families where the mother is employed full-time and in single-parent families where role demands likely necessitate older siblings' assuming more caregiving responsibilities.

Table 5.   Cross-system influences

Study		Selected findings
G	1.	Maternal encouragement of curiosity and openness to experience positively related to the amount of managing behaviors the older sibling directed toward his or her brother or sister.
	2.	The extent to which mothers reported they valued having lives separate from their children was related to the amount the older siblings helped and managed their younger siblings.
	3.	When mothers reported that they enjoyed being a parent, older siblings directed more prosocial behavior to their younger siblings.
	4.	When mothers reported they frequently used nonpunitive child-rearing practices, older siblings directed less agonistic behavior to their younger siblings.
	5.	Frequent use of anxiety induction by mothers was negatively related to the amount the older siblings helped and managed.
	6.	Maternal inconsistency was negatively related to the amount that older siblings helped and engaged in information-seeking behaviors.
	7.	When mothers highly valued having separate lives from their children, younger siblings directed more prosocial behavior and less teaching and information-seeking behaviors toward their older siblings.
	8.	Frequent use of guilt induction was negatively related to the amounts of prosocial behavior that younger siblings directed to their older brothers and sisters.

Maternal use of nonpunitive control techniques and enjoyment of her maternal role were related respectively to less agonistic behavior and more prosocial behavior. The relationship involving the use of nonpunitive control techniques is consistent with other findings in the child-rearing literature (Brody & Shaffer, 1982). These data suggest that some of the child-rearing correlates of prosocial behavior also facilitate the development of prosocial behavior among siblings. It also follows that mothers who enjoy being parents are more likely to display prosocial values and behavior for their children to emulate in their absence.

The best predictor of the younger sibling's behavior was the mother's desire to have a separate life from her children. This attitude was positively related to the amount of prosocial behavior directed toward the older sibling and negatively related to teaching and information-seeking behaviors. The authors suspect that this pattern of relationships may be related in the following manner to the amount of status given older siblings when they assume added caregiving responsibilities. Mothers who delegate some caregiving responsibilities to older siblings place the older child in a position that enables him or her to dispense valued resources to the younger sibling. It is therefore in the younger sibling's best interest to behave in a prosocial manner toward the older sibling and to assume dominant roles, such as teacher, less often. At this stage of the research program, the authors do not know how individual differences in status assigned by parents to older siblings affect sibling interactions. It is a process, however, that seems worthy of further study.

Sibling Interactions in Different Social Groupings

Sibling interactions take place in the presence and absence of other persons. For example, siblings can direct behavior toward one another either alone, in the presence of one of the siblings' friends, or in the presence of their parents. Thus, one of the goals of the authors' research program has been to ascertain the effect of the presence of peers and parents on the quantity and quality of siblings' behavior toward one another. Again, the basic premise that served to guide this research was that the impact of the addition of a third person to a sibling dyad will vary according to who the person is (peer or parent) and the nature of the activity around which the group is interacting. Table 6 summarizes the results of our studies that addressed this research issue.

Table 6. Sibling interactions in different social groupings

Social grouping comparisons	Study	Finding
Sibling dyad vs. triad with older sibling's friend	A,B,C	1. Older sibling assumes teaching and managing roles less in triadic interactions with friend than in dyadic interactions with younger sibling.
		2. Older sibling assumes the playmate role more in triadic interactions with friend than in dyadic interactions with younger sibling.
		3. The older sibling directs less teaching, managing, and play behaviors toward the younger sibling in the triad than in dyadic interactions.
		4. Young male siblings spend more time engaged in solitary play in the triadic interaction involving the older sibling's friend than in dyadic interactions with the older sibling.
		5. Younger siblings behavior is more prosocial in the triad than in the dyad.
		6. Older siblings receive more managing attempts in the triad than in the dyad.
		7. Older and younger siblings complied with managing attempts more often in triadic than in dyadic interactions.
Sibling dyad vs. triad with mother	G	1. Older siblings directed less helping, teaching, implicit and explicit directives, and positive and negative behaviors in triadic interactions with the mother than in dyadic sibling interactions.
		2. The above differences for helping, implicit directives, explicit directives, and teaching were most pronounced during the playing of a board game, intermediate during a construction task, and nonexistent during television viewing.
		3. The younger sibling directed less helping, positive behavior, negative behavior, explicit directives, and implicit directives during triadic interactions involving the mother.
		4. The above changes for helping and implicit directives were most pronounced for a construction task, whereas the differences for negative behavior and explicit directives were most pronounced for a board game. Differences for television were nonexistent.

Two different groups of studies suggest that sibling interactions change as a function of the social context. First, studies by social psychologists of small group behavior indicate that dyadic interactions have several unique properties that seldom appear in triadic interactions (see Weick & Penner, 1966). Specifically, dyadic interactions are characterized by more individual participation than are interactions among groups of three or more. Second, several recent studies of interactions between parents and children have found similar results (e.g., Brody & Stoneman, 1981a; Clarke-Stewart, 1978; Lamb, 1978a,b; Parke & O'Leary, 1976; Stoneman & Brody, 1981). Thus, increases in the number of persons in a group cause behavior and attention to be directed less toward any one group member.

The results from studies A, B, and C demonstrated that older siblings directed propor-tionally fewer teaching, managing, and play-mate role behaviors toward their younger siblings when their friends were present. In the presence of a friend, then, the older siblings distributed their behavior between the younger sibling and the friend, thereby reducing the amount of interaction with each.

It was also interesting to note that younger male siblings found themselves as the "odd man out" in the triadic context. As was noted earlier, younger males spent more time in solitary play in the triadic context than did younger female siblings. Presumably this difference is influenced by the willingness of female friends to select activities that are cognitively and motorically appropriate for the younger sibling.

Sibling interactions also changed as a function of the presence or absence of their mothers and fathers (Study G). Siblings generally decreased the amount and type of behavior they directed to one another when the sibling dyad became a triad with a parent. It is important to note, however, that these changes were more pronounced in some contexts than in others. For example, in comparing the sibling dyad with a triad containing the mother, it was found that older siblings relinquish more of their guidance, helping, and teaching functions during a board game than during a construction task and television viewing. The explanation for this difference lies in the demands of the board game. To play the game, the older siblings had to monitor and provide the younger sibling with assistance, whereas the construction task required little more than coordinating fantasy themes and work allocation.

The younger siblings' behavior in the dyad and in the trial containing the mother also varied as a function of the task. Decreases in helping and implicit directives were the most pronounced for the construction task, whereas dyadic to triadic decreases in the use of negative behavior and explicit directives were more common for the board game. The nature of the two activities probably account for some of these differences. The relative competencies of the siblings were more similar on the construction task than on the board game. This allowed the younger sibling to assume more of a helping role in the former dyadic context. The competitive nature of the board game probably accounts for the greater use of negative behavior and explicit directives by the siblings in the dyadic contact. Apparently, the use of these behaviors is reduced in the presence of the mother.

SUMMARY AND IMPLICATIONS

As more researchers study family interactions involving a mentally retarded child, the need increases to abstract from the literature on nonhandicapped children and their families those research strategies that yield meaningful findings. This chapter has focused on contextual variables in observational research. In the preceding sections, the authors at-

tempted to demonstrate that a sensitivity to contextual differences in behavior—specifically in sibling behavior—is important in designing research. Research using other methodologies, such as self-report instruments, must also take into account the importance of contextual influences. For example, asking a sibling if he or she is embarassed by a handicapped sibling is too vague. Embarrassed in what situations? Embarrassed when which other people are present?

The findings presented in this chapter, as well as other findings in the literature, suggest that characteristics of the sibling pairs, such as gender composition, age, and ordinal position, are important determinants of behavior. Too often, in research with handicapped children and their siblings, these important characteristics are ignored. This is understandable from a practical viewpoint because locating sibling pairs who fit a particular narrow range of personal and demographic characteristics can be frustrating and difficult. This is particularly true when the researcher is focusing on sibling pairs in which one child has a particular handicapping condition. The solution to this problem involves cooperation between researchers and programs, so that sufficient numbers of sibling pairs can be located, rather than being satisfied with research on heterogeneous groups of siblings and families. Such research yields only confusing and uninterpretable findings if such variables as gender, age, ordinal position, and race are ignored or confounded across groups.

The sibling subsystem appears to be unique, having different behavioral norms and relationship patterns than the peer group, mother-child, or father-child interactions. As such, siblings must be studied in their own right, rather than attempting to generalize findings from peers or other groups to describe sibling relations.

Two important contextual factors, activities in which the siblings participate and the presence of other persons during sibling interactions, have a powerful influence on sibling behavior. As such, sibling interactions must be studied across a wide range of ecologically valid activities in order to gain a genuine understanding of sibling behavior. Similarly, siblings interact with each other when they are alone, as well as when they are in the presence of peers, mothers, fathers, other relatives, and numerous other persons. However, studying the sibling dyad alone, with no other social agents present, will give a distorted picture of the day-to-day patterns of sibling interactions.

The authors' research program has concentrated on children from two-child families. Obviously, many children live in families in which they have more than one sibling. In addition, patterns of sibling interactions in families from different cultural and ethnic subgroups, as well as from a wider variety of social classes and from urban and rural areas, should be studied.

The literature on nonhandicapped siblings has much to teach us concerning methodologi-cal strategies. Contextual variables are important and must be included in any study of interactions between handicapped children and their siblings. Unless we incorporate research findings from the study of typical siblings into our research on sibling pairs including a handicapped child, we will fail to gather the information that we are seeking. Sibling pairs that include an atypical child are, first and foremost, brothers and sisters; these children should be expected to be more similar to typical sibling pairs than they are different. Thus, research on handicapped siblings is a natural extension of the research on typical siblings, rather than a new field of study. As such, this research will progress most quickly by building on the extant knowledge base concerning the development and interactions of nonhandicapped siblings and their families.

REFERENCES

Abramovitch, R., Corter, C., & Lando, B. (1979). Sibling interaction in the home. *Child Development, 50,* 997–1033.

Abramovitch, R., Corter, C., & Pepler, D. J. (1980). Observations of mixed-sex sibling dyads. *Child Development, 51,* 1268–1271.

Allen, V. L., & Feldman, R. S. (1976). Studies on the role of tutor. In V. L. Allen (Ed.), *Children as teachers* (pp. 97–111). New York: Academic Press.

Baskett, L. M., & Johnson, S. M. (1982). The young child's interactions with parents versus siblings: A behavioral analysis. *Child Development, 53,* 643–650.

Belsky, J. (1981). Early human experience: A family perspective. *Developmental Psychology, 17,* 3–23.

Bigner, J. J. (1972). Sibling influence on sex-role preference of young children. *Journal of Genetic Psychology, 121,* 271–282.

Birchler, G., Weiss, R., & Vincent, J. (1975). Multimethod analysis of social reinforcement exchange between maritally distressed and nondistressed spouse and stranger dyads. *Journal of Personality and Social Psychology, 31,* 349–360.

Borduin, C. M., & Henggeler, S. W. (1981). Social class, experimental setting, and task characteristics as determinants of mother-child interaction. *Developmental Psychology, 17,* 209–214.

Bricker, D. D. (1978). A rationale for the integration of handicapped and nonhandicapped preschool children. In M. J. Guralnick (Ed.), *Early intervention and the integration of handicapped and nonhandicapped children* (pp. 97–113). Baltimore, MD: University Park Press.

Bricker, D. D., & Bricker, W. A. (1971). Toddler research and intervention report: Year 1. *IMRID Behavioral Science Monograph 20.* Nashville, TN: Institute on Mental Retardation and Intellectual Development.

Bricker, D. D., & Bricker, W. A. (1971). Toddler research and intervention report: Year 2. *IMRID Behavioral Science Monograph 20.* Nashville, TN: Institute on Mental Retardation and Intellectual Development.

Brim, O. J. (1956). Family structure and sex role learning by children: A further analysis of the Helen Koch's data. *Sociometry, 21,* 1–16.

Brody, G. H., & Shaffer, D. (1982). Contributions of parents and peers to children's moral socialization. *Developmental Review, 2,* 31–75.

Brody, G. H., & Stoneman, Z. (1981a). Parental nonverbal behavior within the family context. *Family Relations, 33,* 187–191.

Brody, G. H., & Stoneman, Z. (1981b). Selective imitation of same-age, older, and younger peer models. *Child Development, 52,* 717–720.

Brody, G. H., & Stoneman, Z. (1983a). Children with atypical siblings: Socialization outcomes and clinical participation. In B. B. Lahey & A. Kazdin (Eds.), *Advances in clinical child psychology* (Vol. 6, pp. 285–326). New York: Plenum.

Brody, G. H., & Stoneman, Z. (1983b). The influence of television viewing on family interactions: A contextualist framework. *Journal of Family Issues, 4,* 329–348.

Brody, G. H., & Stoneman, Z. (in press). A comparison of status and competence hypotheses. *Genetic Psychology.*

Brody, G. H., Stoneman, Z., & MacKinnon, C. (1982). Role asymmetries in interaction among school-age children, their younger siblings, and their friends. *Child Development, 53,* 1364–1370.

Brody, G. H., Stoneman, Z., & MacKinnon, C. (1985). Developmental changes in sibling role relationships and behavior. *Developmental Psychology, 21,* 124–129.

Brody, G. H., Stoneman, Z., & Sanders, A. K. (1980). Effects of television viewing on family interactions: An observational study. *Family Relations, 29,* 216–220.

Bronfenbrenner, U. (1979). *The ecology of human development*. Cambridge, MA: Harvard University Press.

Caldwell, B. M., & Guze, S. B. (1960). A study of the adjustment of parents and siblings of institutionalized and noninstitutionalized retarded children. *Journal of Mental Deficiency, 64*, 845–861.

Cicirelli, V. G. (1973). Effects of sibling structure and interaction on children's categorization style. *Developmental Psychology, 9*, 132–139.

Cicirelli, V. G. (1975). Effects of mother and older sibling on the problem solving behavior of the younger child. *Developmental Psychology, 11*, 749–756.

Cicirelli, V. G. (1976). Mother-child and sibling-sibling interactions on a problem-solving task. *Child Development, 47*, 588–596.

Clarke-Stewart, K. A. (1978). And daddy makes three: The father's impact on mother and young child. *Child Development, 49*, 466–478.

Cleveland, D. W., & Miller, N. (1977). Attitudes of life commitments of older siblings of mentally retarded adults: An exploratory study. *Mental Retardation, 15*, 38–41.

Cohen, A. S., Hulls, J., & Paige, R. (1978). The influence of context on activity level of young children. *Journal of Genetic Psychology, 132*, 165–175.

Dunn, J. (1983). Sibling relationships in early childhood. *Childhood Development, 54*, 787–811.

Dunn, J., & Kendrick, C. (1982). *Siblings: Love, envy, and understanding*. Cambridge, MA: Harvard University Press.

Eisenstadt, S. N. (1956). *From generation to generation*. New York: Free Press of Glencoe.

Farber, B. (1963). Interactions with retarded siblings and life goals of children. *Marriage and Family Living, 25*, 96–98.

Farber, B., & Jenne, W. C. (1963). Family organization and parent-child communication: Parents and siblings of a retarded child. *Monographs of the Society for Research in Child Development, 28*(7).

Feshbach, S. (1956). The catharsis hypothesis and some consequences of interaction with aggressive and neutral play objects. *Journal of Personality, 24*, 449–462.

Graliker, B. V., Fishler, K., & Koch, R. (1962). Teenage reaction to a mentally retarded sibling. *American Journal of Mental Deficiency, 66*, 838–843.

Grossman, F. K. (1972). *Brothers and sisters of retarded children*. Syracuse, NY: Syracuse University Press.

Grotevant, H. D. (1978). Sibling constellations and sex-typing of interests in adolescence. *Child Development, 49*, 540–542.

Halverson, C. F., & Waldrop, M. R. (1970). Maternal behavior toward own and other preschool children: The problem of "ownness." *Child Development, 41*, 839–845.

Hartup, W. W. (1978). Peer interaction and the process of socialization. In M. J. Guralnick (Ed.), *Early intervention and the integration of handicapped and nonhandicapped children*. Baltimore: University Park Press.

Hartup, W. W. (1980). Two social worlds: Family relations and peer relations. In M. Rutter (Ed.), *Scientific foundations of developmental psychiatry* (pp. 215–235). London: Heineman.

Hobbs, N. *The futures of children*. (1975). San Francisco: Jossey-Bass.

Jacklin, C. N., & Maccoby, E. E. (1978). Social behavior at thirty-three months in same-sex and mixed-sex dyads. *Child Development, 49*, 557–569.

Lamb, M. E. (1978a). The development of sibling relations in infancy: A short-term longitudinal study. *Child Development, 49*, 1189–1196.

Lamb, M. E. (1978b). Interactions between 18-month-olds and their preschool-aged siblings. *Child Development, 49*, 51–59.

Lamb, M. E. (1978). The development of sibling relations in infancy: A short-term longitudinal study. *Child Development, 49*, 1189–1196 (b).

Lamke, L. K., Bell, N. J., & Murphy, C. (1980). Sibling constellation and androgynous sex role development. *The Journal of Psychology, 105*, 139–144.

Langlois, J. H., Gottfried, N. W., & Seay, B. (1973). The influences of sex of peer on the social behavior of preschool children. *Developmental Psychology, 8*, 93–98.

Lawson, A., & Ingleby, J. D. (1974). Daily routines of preschool children: Effects of age, birth order, sex, social class, and developmental correlates. *Psychological Medicine, 4*, 399–415.

Leventhal, G. S. (1970). Influence of brothers and sisters on sex role behavior. *Journal of Personality and Social Psychology, 16*, 452–465.

Lewis, M., Feiring, C., & Weinraub, M. (1981). The father as a member of the child's social network. In M. Lamb (Ed.), *The role of the father in child development* (pp. 189–217). New York: Wiley.

Lougee, M. D., Grueneich, R., & Hartup, W. (1977). Social interaction in same-and mixed-age dyads of preschool children. *Child Development, 48*, 1353–1361.

Masur, E. F. (1978). Preschool boys' speech modifications: The effect of listener's linguistic levels and conversational responsiveness. *Child Development, 49*, 924–927.

Minnett, A. M., Vandell, D. L., & Santrock, J. W. (1983). The effects of sibling status on sibling interaction: Influence of birth order, age spacing, sex of child, and sex of sibling. *Child Development, 54*, 1064–1072.

Moore, W. E. (1969). Social structure and behavior. In G. Lindzey & E. Aronson (Eds.), *The handbook of social psychology* (2d ed.) (pp. 217–286). Reading, MA: Addison-Wesley.

Parke, R. D. (1978). Children's home environments: Social and cognitive effects. In I. Altman and J. F. Wohlwill (Eds.), *Children and the environment* (pp. 114–132). New York: Plenum Publishing.

Parke, R. D., & O'Leary, S. (1976). Father-mother-infant interaction in the newborn period: Some findings, some observations, and some unresolved issues. In M. K. Riegel & J. Meacham (Eds.), *The developing individual in a changing world* (Vol. II, pp. 51–74). The Hague: Mouton.

Parke, R. D., & Tinsley, B. R. (1981). The father's role in infancy: Determinants of involvement in caregiving and play. In M. Lamb (Ed.), *The role of the father in child development* (pp. 113–140). New York: Wiley.

Pepler, D. J., Abramovitch, R., & Corter, C. (1981). Sibling interaction in the home: A longitudinal study. *Child Development, 52*, 1344–1347.

Quilitch, H. R., & Risley, T. R. (1973). The effects of play materials on social play. *Journal of Applied Behavior Analysis, 6*, 573–578.

Rosenberg, B. G., & Sutton-Smith, B. (1964). Ordinal position and sex role identification. *Genetic Psychology Monographs, 70,* 297–328.

Rosenberg, B. G., & Sutton-Smith, B. (1968). Family interaction effects on masculinity-femininity. *Journal of Personality and Social Psychology, 8,* 117–120.

Ryder, R. G. (1968). Husband-wife dyads versus married strangers. *Family Process, 7,* 233–238.

Samuels, H. R. (1980). The effect of older sibling on infant locomotor exploration of a new environment. *Child Development, 51,* 607–609.

Scarr, S., & Grajek, S. (1982). Similarities and differences among siblings. In M. E. Lamb & B. Sutton-Smith (Eds.), *Sibling relationships: Their nature and significance across the lifespan* (pp. 284–311). Hillsdale, NJ: Lawrence Erlbaum.

Schachter, F. F. (1982). Sibling deidentification and split-parent identification. In M. E. Lamb & B. Sutton-Smith (Eds.), *Sibling relationships: Their nature and significance across the lifespan* (pp. 170–203). Hillsdale, NJ: Lawrence Erlbaum.

Schooler, C. (1972). Birth order effects: Not here, not now. *Psychological Bulletin, 78,* 161–175.

Shatz, M., & Gelman, R. (1973). The development of communication skills: Modifications in the speech of young children as a function of listener. *Monographs of the Society for Research in Child Development, 35*(5).

Stewart, R. B. (1983). Sibling attachment relationships: Child input interactions in the Strange Situation. *Developmental Psychology, 19,* 192–199.

Stoneman, Z., & Brody, G. H. (1981). Two's company, three makes a difference: An examination of mothers' and fathers' speech to their young children. *Child Development, 52,* 705–707.

Stoneman, Z., Brody, G. H., & MacKinnon, C. E. (1984). Naturalistic observations of children's roles and activities while playing with their siblings and friends. *Child Development, 55,* 617–621.

Stoneman, Z., Brody, G. H., & MacKinnon, C. (in press). Same-sex and cross-sex siblings: Gender stereotypes, activity choices, roles, and behavior. *Sex Roles.*

Sutton-Smith, B. (1983). Birth order and sibling status effects. In M. E. Lamb & B. Sutton-Smith (Eds.), *Sibling relationships.* Hillsdale, NJ: Lawrence J. Erlbaum Associates.

Sutton-Smith, B., & Rosenbaum, B. G. (1970). *The sibling.* New York: Holt.

Tesser, A. (1980). Self-esteem maintenance in family dynamics. *Journal of Personality and Social Psychology, 39,* 77–91.

Thelen, M. H., & Kirkland, K. D. (1976). On status and being imitated. *Journal of Personality and Social Psychology, 33,* 691–697.

Turner, C. W., & Goldsmith, D. (1976). Effects of toy guns and airplanes on children's antisocial free play behavior. *Journal of Experimental Child Psychology, 21,* 303–315.

Weick, K. E., & Penner, D. D. (1966). Triads: A laboratory analogue. *Organizational Behavior and Human Performance, 1,* 199–211.

Weisner, T. S., & Gallimore, R. (1977). My brother's keeper: Child and sibling caretaking. *Current Anthropology, 48,* 1250–1254.

Whiting, B. B., & Whiting, J. W. M. (1975). *Children of six cultures.* Cambridge, MA: Harvard University Press.

Wolfensberger, W. (1967). Counseling the parents of the retarded. In A. A. Baumeister (Ed.), *Mental retardation* (pp. 217–240). Chicago: Alpine Publishing Co.

Zegiob, L., & Forehand, R. (1975). Maternal interactive behavior as a function of race, socioeconomic status, and sex of child. *Child Development, 46,* 564–568.

Zussman, J. V. (1978). Relationship of demographic factors to parental discipline techniques. *Developmental Psychology, 14,* 685–686.

Chapter

12

Behavioral Parent Training Research

Contributions to an
Ecological Analysis of Families of Handicapped Children

Ann P. Kaiser and James J. Fox

ALMOST SINCE ITS INCEPTION as a scientific and clinical approach, applied behavior analysis has included a focus on the treatment of children in the context of their families (cf. O'Dell, 1974; Wolf, Risley, & Mees, 1964). Although siblings and other relatives have occasionally acted as intervention agents, parents have most often been the focus of training and research efforts. Such a focus on parent training and parent-based intervention studies seems justified on the basis of both logical and empirical considerations. First, it seems more efficient to teach parents to modify their child's problem behavior than to rely on direct intervention by professional personnel because there are far fewer such personnel than families in need of treatment.

Second, a behavioral perspective strongly emphasizes that inappropriate child behavior is at least partly a function of the way that significant others, such as parents, respond to that child. Consequently, whether or not the original cause of the child's behavioral excesses or deficits is social or biological, a behavioral perspective virtually requires that positive child development be accomplished by teaching the parent(s) to change the current manner in which they respond to or interact with their child (Gordon & Davidson, 1981; O'Dell, 1974; Tharp & Wetzel, 1969).

Finally, as is described more fully in later sections of this chapter, the empirical evidence too supports the efficacy of behavioral parent training (BPT). That is, there is an increasingly well-defined scientific data base attesting to measureable, reliable, and replicable changes in parent and child behavior as a function of training parents in the application of learning theory-based procedures (Gordon & Davidson, 1981; O'Dell, 1974). Currently, BPT is widely recognized as an effective intervention strategy for modifying behaviors of and teaching new skills to handicapped children (Heward, Dardig, & Rossett, 1979). Such training is available through public schools, early intervention programs, mental health agencies, private clinicians, and workshops and classes offered by various community agencies. Considering the ready availability of these training procedures and the apparently strong empirical basis for their use, a chapter describing BPT may seem unwarranted. In fact, quite the opposite is true.

For all its scientific and clinical progress, BPT has to a considerable extent existed outside the mainstream of clinical and developmental analyses of family functioning. Although there have been relatively frequent experimental applications of BPT with families of handicapped children, most of these studies are reported alongside other applications of behavioral principles, rather than integrated with studies of families of handicapped children. Results derived from different research paradigms are often isolated from each other. Such separateness is no longer justifiable either from a clinical viewpoint or from a scientific one. The existing dualistic state of affairs represents an unfortunate rift in research on the ecology of the mentally retarded child and his or her family. The general premise of the discussion that follows is that there is both a clinical and scientific need for an ecological perspective in research with such families and that BPT research should make a contribution to the ecological perspective.

From an applied viewpoint, the problems of handicapped children and their families are particularly pressing ones. Families of handicapped children are often families in stress (Gallagher, Beckman, & Cross, 1983), needing interventions to maintain the basic functions of the family unit. The timing, content, and mode of presentation of BPT may be critical to sustaining those functions. Further, BPT may best be offered in combination with other treatments (e.g., counseling, liaison services, educational intervention for the child). Currently, it is not a question of choosing BPT over other possible interventions, but rather of placing parent training in the context of family needs and maximizing its effectiveness in meeting those needs. Demonstrating the durable and generalized effects of parent training on the functioning of the family system and investigating the application of BPT in combination with other treatments in order to discover more effective intervention packages are pressing applied research problems.

There is also a more basic scientific argument for integrating behavior analytic studies of families into the broader scope of research on families with handicapped children. Behavior analysis provides a particularly rigorous scientific paradigm for investigating interactions within families. Given the current emphasis on family ecology (see other chapters in this volume) and the limited development of an ecological method, the addition and integration of behavior analytic research methods with other strategies for investigating family interactions seem particularly timely. The critical need for an observational data base describing the interactions of handicapped children with their family members is readily apparent from an examination of the existing literature on families with handicapped children. The gap between proposals for an ecological theory of family functioning (Gabel & Kotsch, 1981; Salzinger, Antrobus, & Glick, 1980) and a data base that supports such theory is considerable. Bridging that gap will require evidence emerging from a strong experimental paradigm, in addition to descriptive data generated on the basis of a theory of ecological effects. As is discussed later, there is sufficient overlap in perspective between behavioral research and the emerging ecological view of family functioning to permit data generated within the behavioral paradigm to serve the dual purpose of supporting an ecological perspective on families of mentally retarded children and a behavioral analysis for parent-child interactions.

This chapter is divided into two sections. The first describes and discusses the existing parent training technology in relation to applied issues in clinical treatment of families with handicapped children. Included in this section is a brief review of BPT literature and a discussion of key applied research issues. The second section focuses on the contributions made by the behavioral research paradigm to the study of family ecology. An overview of the emerging ecological perspective on families is offered with a discussion of its theoretical basis. Ecological and behavior analytic methods are compared, and studies by Wahler and Patterson are reviewed with an emphasis on their dual contributions to behavioral and ecological perspectives in family interaction. The second section concludes with a discussion of experiments that would contribute to a data base for understanding family interactions.

BEHAVIORAL PARENT TRAINING: ISSUES IN APPLIED RESEARCH

Behavioral parent training (BPT) is a triadic intervention model (Tharp & Wetzel, 1969) in which the professional helping agent trains parents to change their behavior in order to effect change in their child's behavior. Parents are trained to apply basic behavior modification procedures, such as reinforcement, extinction or planned ignoring, time out, fading, and shaping, contingent on their child's behavior, in order to increase desired behaviors and decrease undesirable or deviant behaviors. Parents may be trained specifically to teach new skills, such as self-help skills or language, in addition to being taught to manage the child's ongoing behaviors. Conceptually, BPT can be distinguished from other theoretical approaches in that the parent is educated in the application of learning theory, its principles and procedures, and in the deliberate modification of parent-child interactions (Lilly, 1974). BPT is distinct in its direct (as opposed to indirect) modification of parent-child interactions and in its use of the parent, rather than the professional, as the primary intervention agent.

BPT is conducted in a variety of formats. Parents may be taught initially to observe their child's behavior and to collect systematic data on the frequency or duration of problem behaviors. Principles of behavior modification are introduced through reading materials (manuals, books, handouts), lectures or didactic interchanges, videotaped examples, and/or role playing. Parents may be observed as they use the techniques, and feedback about their per-

formance and the child's behavior may be provided by the parent trainer. Actual training of parents may be done by a consultant who advises parents in conjunction with their reading of related materials or by a trainer who visits the family at home and provides intensive coaching during the parents' applications of the behavioral procedures. Training may also vary in breadth; parents may be taught to modify only one particular behavior—toilet training, for example—or to apply behavioral procedures to a range of behaviors. Parents may be trained singly or in groups. Frequently, even in clinical or educational applications of parent training, data are collected on the parent's use of the trained techniques and on the child's target behaviors. In sum, all BPT programs share the common goal of teaching parents to alter their behavior in order to modify their children's behavior; however, the means by which parents are trained to change their behavior can vary considerably.

Despite the many apparent variations in the implementation of BPT, the immediate outcomes reported in research evaluations of these procedures generally have been positive. In particular, it has been demonstrated that: 1) parents can acquire and demonstrate proficiency in learning behavioral principles and specific theory-based procedures; 2) following training, parents can accurately apply these principles and procedures in interactions with their children; and 3) child behavior can be reliably changed through parents' applications of behavioral procedures (see for example, Baker, 1980; Forehand & King, 1977; Peed, Roberts, & Forehand, 1977; Watson & Bassinger, 1974).

Although the overall reported results of experimental applications of parent training have been positive, it should be noted that BPT is a developing area of applied research with its own set of practical constraints. Individual studies have been methodologically unsophisticated. Frequently the analyses of effects of training have been limited in terms of the number of behaviors treated, settings, or time periods over which behavior change has been evaluated. Of special concern have been

the measurement of independent variables—
that is, frequency and consistency of parents'
application of behavioral procedures—quality
of child behavior data, and adequacy of the
experimental designs used to evaluate treatment outcomes. Magnitude of change in parent
and in child behavior and the generalizability
of the results of sample families to the larger
population have also been questioned. Reviews of the BPT have discussed these methodological concerns in detail (Franks, 1982;
Gordon & Davidson, 1981; Johnson & Katz,
1973; O'Dell, 1974). Although there is cause
for judicious evaluation of the reported outcomes, in general, BPT research has been
shown to be effective in modifying a diverse
range of child behaviors (Gordon & Davidson,
1981; Watson & Bassinger, 1974).

BEHAVIORAL PARENT TRAINING
FOR PARENTS OF
MENTALLY RETARDED CHILDREN

Parents of mentally retarded and other handicapped children have been the frequent recipients of BPT in research and clinical settings.
Handicapped children frequently present behavioral and learning problems that benefit
from parent-based interventions. In some
cases, the presenting behavioral problems are
so severely disruptive that parent training is a
critical intervention for the entire family. In
comparison to the extensive literature on BPT
with oppositional and disruptive children,
there are relatively few research studies that
specifically have addressed BPT with parents
of mentally retarded children. However, the
procedures, methods, and results of studies
with families of mentally retarded children
have been quite similar to those reported in
studies involving families of nonretarded children. Applications of BPT with this population
have varied along the lines described previously, but again generally positive results
have been reported. (See Baker, 1976 for a
more complete review of parent training studies with handicapped children.)

Parents have been trained successfully to
modify a diverse set of their retarded children's

behavior problems and to teach adaptive skills,
including chewing and other feeding skills
(Butterfield & Parson, 1973; Rose, 1974);
motor imitation (Freeman & Thompson,
1973); self-help skills (Rose, 1974; Watson &
Bassinger, 1974); appropriate play behaviors
and social interaction with the parent (Mash &
Terdal, 1973); articulation and vocabulary
skills (Heifetz, 1977; Rose, 1974; Watson &
Bassinger, 1974); self- and other-directed aggression (Rose, 1974); and compliance and
other parent-identified behavior problems
(Heifetz, 1977; Rose, 1974; Tavormina, 1975;
Tavormina, Hampson, & Luscomb, 1976).

Although the results reported in studies with
families of mentally retarded children are typically positive, these studies share many of the
same procedural limitations and methodological problems found in research with nonhandicapped children and their parents. For example, among the relatively small number of
studies specifically investigating training with
parents of mentally retarded children, there are
only a few that have analyzed the effects of
various training formats on parent performance. Two studies have assessed parent mastery of behavioral principles and actual application of these principles with their child
(Heifetz, 1977; Watson & Bassinger, 1974);
one reported that parent verbal mastery of principles and procedures did not immediately
transfer to accurate performance in naturalistic
interactions (Watson & Bassinger, 1974). In a
frequently cited study comparing the use of
three different training procedures (instructional manual only, manual plus consultant
phone calls, and manual plus direct training by
the consultant), Baker et al. (1980) reported
positive changes in parent and child behaviors
and maintenance of these gains over a 14-
month period for all three training procedures.
These results were based on parent reports collected in telephone interviews. In light of Tavormina's (1975) finding that parents' *ratings* of
their child's behavior were more favorable
after training, but that parent frequency *counts*
of target behaviors did not differ significantly,
Baker et al.'s findings should be interpreted
cautiously.

Mentally retarded children often present problems that are topographically quite similar to those presented by normally developing but behaviorally deviant children (e.g., Rose, 1974). Thus, the finding that general BPT procedures produce similar positive results when applied by parents of mentally retarded children is not surprising. However, there are some notable differences in the overall prognosis for mentally retarded children that should be considered in relation to BPT. The most pressing issues in parent training research are generalization and durability of effects. These issues are especially critical for interventions with families of mentally retarded children. The behavioral and learning deficits associated with retardation are chronic ones. Although parents of oppositional children may "solve" their child's behavior problems through relatively procedurally limited or short-term interventions, parents of retarded children are likely to have continuing, long-term needs for behavioral techniques to manage their children's behavior. Even when disruptive or problem social behaviors are brought under control, the need for training in new skills continues throughout the time these children live with their parents. Although research has verified that behavioral procedures applied by parents produce short-term changes in child behavior, few studies have thoroughly analyzed the generalized and long-term effects of BPT with parents of mentally retarded handicapped children or with behavior problem children (Baker, 1976, 1980; O'Dell, 1974; Lutzker, McGimsey, McRae, & Campbell, 1983).

Research describing generalization across settings and maintenance of parent training with mentally retarded children is especially sparse. Both positive and negative outcomes have been reported. The conflicting findings may be the result of the methods used to determine generalization. For example, Rose (1974) reported that interviews with parents 3–6 months after termination of group BPT indicated that 21 of 27 moderately to severely retarded children were maintaining all their behavioral gains. Most parents claimed to be continuing to use behavioral procedures, but none

were monitoring their child's behavior as they had done during treatment. Baker et al. (1980) interviewed parents who had been trained in one of several different parent training formats and found that, with the exception of one group trained by reading an instructional text and receiving telephone consultation from a trainer, parents maintained their knowledge of principles and procedures, that they continued to apply informally the learned procedures, and that their children's adaptive behavior gains were maintained. Interestingly, other data from that study, based on an independent assessment of parents' mastery of teaching behaviors, indicated that mastery reported in the follow-up phase may have accounted for relatively little of the variance in parents' actual teaching behaviors.

These follow-up reports paint a rather positive picture of maintenance of training. However, their findings should be interpreted with caution. First, empirical investigations of initial parent training effects with families of mentally retarded children are relatively few, and follow-up data are even fewer. Second, the type of data in these studies—parent interviews and parent-generated ratings or recordings of their own and their children's behaviors—typically suggest more positive results than do direct observations by a trained observer (Koegel, Schriebman, Britten, Burke, & O'Neill, 1982; Tavormina, 1975). Third, follow-up data are based on the sample of families successfully completing training. In addition to those parents who do not maintain trained behaviors, there are parents who drop out of training and those who fail to show initial training success. For example, Rose (1974) reported that, of 33 families recruited for training, 3 dropped out of the program, another 3 failed to successfully modify their children's behavior, and 6 of the remaining 27 families did not maintain the trained behaviors. In sum, 12 families or 36% of his sample did not show any long-term positive gains from the training program. Finally, there is the question of quality of behavior during the maintenance phase. Baker et al. (1980) reported that 86% of their families continued to perform "some scorable teaching efforts" during the follow-up phase. This general description does not provide a basis for determining if the maintained behavior was sufficient to support continued child behavior gains, although Baker et al. reported that children maintained skills learned during the intervention phase of the study. Level of behavior during the maintenance phase is an especially important issue in families of handicapped children because of the chronic nature of the children's learning and behavioral deficits. For families with long-term needs for child management and teaching skills, appropriate criteria for maintenance may be continued, frequent, and generative application of the newly trained skills. However, in the behavior analysis literature in general, there are no systematic analyses defining criteria for sufficient generalization and maintenance (Warren, Rogers-Warren, Baer, & Guess, 1980).

The reasons why some families do not initially acquire or fail to maintain newly learned skills are unclear. Personal skill deficits, situational variables beyond the training procedures, and child characteristics may affect outcomes. Rose (1974) described parents who did not successfully intervene in their retarded child's behavior as appearing "uncommitted to change and unskilled . . . only incidentally involved in monitoring, and arranging contingencies" (p. 138). Furthermore, Rose indicated that these parents "never completed contracts; but were either changing the responses to be observed or ineffectively implementing unauthorized procedures" (Rose, 1974, pp. 138–139). Baker et al. (1980) asked parents about 24 possible obstacles to continued home programming for their retarded child. Lack of time to do training was the most highly rated inhibiting factor. Lack of support from spouse, limited materials for teaching, inability to find appropriate reinforcers, and lack of confidence were also cited frequently. Baker (1980) found that parents who performed little or no teaching during follow-up were characterized by more severely disruptive life events (death, divorce, illness in the family) and more time constraints (lack of time, daily interruptions). Although

Baker's explanations are tentative ones based on correlational data, it appears that parents' initial and continued success in applying behavioral procedures may be influenced considerably by conditions external to the teaching situation and parent-child dyadic interactions. Further support for this premise is provided by Wahler (1980) in his study of insular mothers with behavior disordered children. (Wahler's findings are discussed more extensively in a later section of this chapter.)

If Baker's data accurately describe the characteristics of parents who are having or will have difficulty continuing to apply behavior management skills, parents of handicapped children may be especially unlikely to maintain their newly trained skills. Often the demands on parents' time are increased by the needs of the handicapped child. These children may exhibit a greater number and greater diversity of behaviors requiring systematic management. Because of their learning deficits, they may respond more slowly to the parents' applications of contingencies. Parents of handicapped children may need to persist in the absence of natural reinforcers for their efforts (i.e., rapid change in child behavior). In addition, families of handicapped children may be stressed by conditions related to the handicapped child's health, limited financial resources, and continuing demand for parent involvement in a range of advocacy and educational activities. Although many of these demands are quite similar to those experienced in any family with young children, the number of demands and the length of time that such demands continue may particularly characterize families of handicapped children (De-Meyer & Goldberg, 1983; Holroyd & Mac-Arthur, 1976).

On the other hand, there is some evidence to indicate that effective BPT may ameliorate some of the stress that parents of handicapped children typically experience. Koegel et al. (1982) report findings from a study comparing clinic-based and parent-based treatment for autistic children. Although both types of treatment were successful in reducing inappropriate child behaviors and increasing skill acquisition, parents who served as trainers for their children reported a significant increase in family leisure-time activities after the intervention phase. The reasons for this increase are not immediately obvious. One possible interpretation is that parents generalized their behavioral skills across settings. Another is that they promoted their children's generalization across settings and thus were able to manage their children better in leisure-time settings. Alternatively, time saved by sound child management in other settings may have allowed families more free time for leisure activities. Another study (Burden, 1980) has reported decreases in parent stress levels as ascertained from parent reports following training.

Typically, the case for parent training has been made on the basis of child needs. It has been argued that parents, as persons who spend a considerable amount of time each day with their handicapped child in a variety of settings, are the ideal trainers for their children. Parents could teach skills in naturalistic contexts and could apply the intervention procedures intensively throughout the day. This argument, although sound, fails to recognize the importance of behavior management skills to the parents and other family members. If the findings related to stress and increased leisure time are replicable ones, there may be some basis for suggesting that parent training is a supportive intervention for both children and parents.

The critical applied research and clinical issues that arise from reviewing the existing research on parent training in families of mentally retarded children are readily apparent:

1. A more complete analysis of generalization across settings and child behaviors is needed to determine the extent to which BPT affects parent-child interaction outside the immediate training contexts.
2. An analysis of maintenance that addresses the quality of behavior management skills used by parents following intervention is needed. Measures of frequency, of generalization across settings and child responses, and correctness of parental im-

plementation of procedures periodically for at least 1 year after training would provide a basis for judging the quality of skills maintained.
3. Comparisons of long-term maintenance resulting from various training formats are needed. Teaching procedures that previously have been shown to facilitate generalization (e.g., multiple exemplar training, use of self-control strategies to mediate behavior, training across contexts) should be incorporated into these across-format comparisons.
4. For families whose characteristics suggest that they may be at-risk for completing training or for generalizing newly learned skills, experimental analysis of intervention "packages" that include social support or time management procedures should be undertaken.
5. The same methodological issues that merit careful attention in BPT research with families of normally developing but behaviorally disordered children are of continuing concern in research with families of handicapped children. Better specification of independent and dependent variables is needed. In particular, descriptions of training procedures and parents' actual application of the trained behavior management skills are lacking in the literature.
6. Finally, there is a need to address the effects of parent training on parent and sibling interactions with the mentally retarded child and on the activities and interactions of the family in general. Replications of the studies reporting increases in leisure time and reduction in reported stress levels following BPT are in order.

BEHAVIORAL RESEARCH PARADIGMS AND AN ECOLOGICAL PERSPECTIVE

During the past two decades the concept of an ecological perspective on human behavior has become increasingly accepted by researchers. This perspective is based on the examination of behavior in its systemic or environmental contexts. In psychology, "ecology" has come to refer to: 1) the environmental contexts for behavior, 2) the interdependent relationships among persons or behaviors within a system, 3) the patterns of interaction resulting from the direct and indirect interactions of system components with one another, and 4) the interactions resulting from the intersection of two or more systems.

An ecological perspective is not a unified theory of human behavior. Rather, it is an emphasis on behavior in context with a broader psychological theory. Ecological perspectives have arisen in at least three different theoretical orientations: the transactional-ecological model of behavior presented by Lewin (1951); the environmental-ecological theory offered by Barker (1963) and Wright (1969); and, within the behavioral paradigm, the interbehavioral approach of Kantor (1959). Based on the ecological aspects of these orientations, more specific statements describing the tenets and potential benefits of adopting an ecological perspective have been made. For example, Bronfenbrenner (1977) presented an elegant argument for the analysis of the ecological contexts of behavior and proposed guidelines for studying behavior in its naturalistic contexts. Willems (1974) cautioned about potential side effects of behavioral change resulting from unanticipated interrelationship among behaviors in a system. Rogers-Warren, Warren, and their colleagues (1977) offered a model for integrating behavioral and ecological approaches in intervention.

Criteria for an Ecological Analysis

The following characteristics might be used to define the scientific application of an ecological perspective:

1. The analysis of the effects of two or more distinct physical environmental conditions on a specific behavior or pattern of behavior
2. The analysis of the bidirectional effects of two behaviors or patterns of behavior on each other
3. The analysis of multidirectional, primary,

and/or secondary effects of three or more behaviors or patterns of behavior on each other
4. The bi- or multidirectional analysis of two or more systems (standing patterns of multidirectional influences resulting from the interaction of three of more behaviors) as they intersect to produce patterns of behavior
5. Combinations of two or more of these analyses (e.g., an analysis of the bidirectional effects of mother and child behavior across two settings—home and pediatrician's office)

To date, most studies employing an ecological perspective have been of the first two types. For example, Barker and Wright (1954) and their colleagues have analysed the behavior patterns of persons in community, school, and hospital settings. In the field of mental retardation, studies by Landesman-Dwyer, Sackett, and Kleinman (1980) and by Hursh and House (1983) are examples of this type of ecological analysis.

Over the last 10 years, there has been a marked increase in the analysis of bidirectional or interactional influences in dyads, particularly in the fields of child development and child language (see discussions by Bond & Joffe, 1982; Sameroff & Chandler, 1975). Studies of caregiver-child interaction (cf. Clarke-Stewart, 1973; Wood, Bruner, & Ross, 1976) typify this application of an ecological perspective; however, only the most recent studies have analyzed systematically the mutual, sequential, or concurrent influences of the behaviors of both dyad members. Rarely, studies of triads (mother, father, child; mother, child, sibling) have been conducted with the intention of analyzing multidirectional influences (however, see Stoneman & Brody, this volume). Studies with mentally retarded children and their caregivers have followed a similar trend (cf. Petersen & Sherrod, 1982; Rondal, 1978).

The remaining three types of ecological analyses have been less frequent, largely because of the complex methodology required to carry out the analysis of multidirectional influences exerted by several persons or behaviors. The absence of testable models of multidirectional ecological influences has made interpretation of descriptive ecological data difficult, especially when individual relationships among variables are relatively weak in comparison to the main effects reported in typical unidirectional analysis. In general, the strong causal analysis models that set the standards for examining unidirectional and some bidirectional relationships are not easily applied in studying systems, and feasible, scientifically rigorous alternatives have not yet been developed.

Ecological Analyses of Families with Handicapped Children

The applicability of an ecological approach to studying families with mentally retarded children is widely recognized (see, for example, Chapters 3, 4, 5, and 14 in this volume). The pattern of ecological investigations with this population is similar to that seen in other areas. There is an apparent acceptance of the theoretical perspective, as judged by the frequent descriptions of families of handicapped children as systems (cf. Hobbs, 1980; Paul, 1981; Turnbull, Summers, & Brotherson, 1983). There are some descriptive studies of family characteristics and standing patterns of family behavior (cf. Mink, Nihira, & Meyers, 1982; Moos & Moos, 1976) based primarily on questionnaire or interview data. Observational studies of caregiver-child interaction in families with handicapped children are similar to those conducted with normally developing children and their caregivers constituting the primary observational data base (cf. Petersen & Sherrod, 1982b; Rondal, 1978). Finally, there is a small data base drawn from studies of applications of BPT with handicapped children discussed earlier.

Although the ecological perspective is recognized as a clinically useful viewpoint from which to treat families (Harris, 1982), a substantive scientific data base that maps critical, multidirectional influences in families of hand-

icapped children is lacking. Data describing complex interactions within families and the influences of such interactions on the development of the child and functioning of the family unit would not only be immediately useful in interventions with these families but would also have the longer-term benefit of contributing to the understanding of the impact of the mentally retarded child on the family and scientifically confirming the tenets of an ecological perspective. The current ecological perspective does not provide a model of analysis that facilitates rapid development of such a data base. One alternative is to return to the theories that have given rise to the ecological perspective and to consider how these paradigms might yield an ecological data base relevant to families of handicapped children.

An Ecological Perspective Derived from Behavioral Parent Training Studies

Returning to a behavioral model to study the ecology of families of handicapped children is an attractive alternative for several reasons: 1) Social learning theory is based on the effects of environment on behavior, a principle entirely consistent with an ecological perspective; 2) although bidirectional influences have been studied less frequently than unidirectional effects, there is a theoretical basis for the consideration of such effects (Skinner, 1953); and 3) within the behavioral model, there is an emphasis on observational data and a well-developed methodology for observationally based research. Further, studies of behavioral parent training (BPT) often are representative of an experimental paradigm that permits the examination of the influences of ecological variables in a rigorous scientific manner while maintaining the ecological validity of the analysis.

Bronfenbrenner (1977) suggests a set of guidelines for conducting an ecological experiment. Among his guidelines are those that potentially overlap with the behavioral research paradigm: 1) Allow for and document reciprocity in interactions; in particular, pay attention to the process of adaptation because it is central to human behavior; 2) study behavior under contrasting setting conditions; and 3) study behavior in its natural contexts, preferably through the application of the transforming experiment. Experimental studies of BPT are examinations of dyadic interactions. Typically, the primary data in these studies have been of measures of parent contingencies provided for their children and rates of child behavior. However, documentation of child contingencies for parent behavior and examination of the larger, systemic pattern of interaction between parent and child are possible within the typical observation system and have been done.

The parallel premises of BPT are: 1) changes in parent behavior result in changes in their children's behavior, and 2) the resultant changes in child behavior affect parent behavior, resulting in the continued use and generalization of the newly trained behavior management techniques. A modest expansion of data collection and analysis procedures would permit exploration of the latter assumption, which is especially critical to effective parent training, as well as providing a data base describing parent-handicapped child interactions under two contrasting conditions (pre- and posttraining).

Examining parent and child behavior under two contrasting conditions known or experimentally demonstrated to have differential effects allows an examination of secondary or broader ecological effects under these contrasting conditions. For example, when it is experimentally demonstrated that increases in parent contingent, positive attention produce increases in child vocalizations, it is possible to examine changes in other related child behaviors (vocalizations to siblings, smiling, gesturing, attention to adults) and in other related parent behaviors (attention to other children, positive attention to spouse, positive physical contact with the handicapped child).

Although focusing on a small set of behaviors under strictly contrasting conditions initially limits the ecological analysis, it ultimately makes it possible to map in a systematic and scientific fashion the interrelationships among classes of parent and child behaviors that contribute to the family ecology. The selection of focal behaviors and contrasting conditions provides a window on the family ecology. This window is an important organizing device for viewing the ecology because it provides a referent from which the system can be studied. Rather than viewing or mapping an entire ecological system, only the portions that directly relate to the set of focal behaviors are described. The contrasting experimental conditions allow examination of interrelationships and co-variations among the set of behaviors and members of their behavioral class. This type of behavioral analysis is an ecological compromise: It simplifies the view of the system, but does not totally eliminate the study of interactive effects. In making this arrangement or in selecting a behavioral design as the basis for studying the ecology, a compromise has been made for the sake of a clearer analysis. The resulting study of the ecology is not comprehensive, however, and caution must be used in interpreting the results as representing the system in its entirety.

Finally, applied behavior analytic studies of parent training are almost always conducted under naturalistic conditions and address everyday functional behaviors. Such studies vary in terms of the amount of data collected in nonlaboratory settings, but most investigations include some data collected in the home and almost all include data collected during naturalistic interactions (free play with child, mealtimes, and so forth).

In sum, experimental analyses of BPT may provide three critical conditions that will permit an ecological analysis of families within a behavioral framework:

1. An identified set of target behaviors that provide an organizing window on the family ecology
2. Contrasting ecological conditions known or demonstrated to produce differential effects on the target behaviors
3. Observational data that can be used in determining the effects of changes in the target behavior on other system variables postulated to be members of the same response class. Additionally, analyses of

BPT may permit documentation of the process of adaptation to new ecological conditions when continuous data are collected during the implementation of an intervention; measurement of the effects of changes in target behaviors in one system (community or school) on behavior within the family system; and expanded analysis of bi- or multidirectional interactions to include examinations of larger, standing patterns of behavior within the family.

SOME EXAMPLES OF ECOLOGICAL BEHAVIORAL PARENT TRAINING STUDIES

Although there are few studies that examine the ecologies of families with mentally retarded children through the experimental analysis of BPT, research from three different research groups has provided relevant examples of such analyses in families with disruptive, behavior-disordered children, or abused children. Recent work by Wahler, by Patterson, and by Lutzker and their colleagues is discussed below to highlight the contributions of BPT research to the developing ecological analyses of family interaction and to suggest how this model might be extended to the analysis of families with mentally retarded children.

Patterson: Cycles of Coercion in Mother-Child Dyads

Patterson and his colleagues are well known for their innovative analyses of family interactions in the context of a social learning model of intervention. Their recent research (cf. Patterson, 1980; Patterson & Fleischman, 1979; Patterson & Reid, 1973) and theoretical writings (Patterson, 1977, 1982) on coercive cycles in mother-child interaction present particularly useful examples of how analyses of intervention data yield descriptions of the functioning of family systems. These descriptions are of an ecological nature in that they: 1) describe bidirectional and, in some cases, multidirectional interactions within families; 2) consider multiple levels of the family system concurrently and relate the functioning of family

members at two or more levels of analysis; and 3) examine primary and secondary changes in individual behaviors and behavior patterns under contrasting ecological conditions.

Patterson's (1980) monograph provides a comprehensive description of his ecological analyses. In this report, he expands on his earlier work describing the interaction patterns that prevail in families with out-of-control children who are highly disruptive or abusive in their interactions with family members. The monograph results from a set of data accumulated over a period of 10 years and including about 150 families. The data are derived from detailed observational records of interactions of families with problem children and comparison families with normally developing children. Two types of comparisons are made: across-group comparisons of normal and problem families, and within-group comparisons before and after BPT to teach one or both parents child management skills as a means of altering the child's disruptive behavior.

The monograph focuses on coercive cycles that arise between mother and disruptive child. Patterson postulates a sequential progression in child coercive behavior and mother responses that leads to very high levels of coercive interactions. The bidirectional influences of mother and child behavior are analyzed individually and as a resulting behavioral pattern, the coercive cycle. Two family system influences are discussed: the limited role of father, resulting in increased mother-child contact, and the effects of mothers' limited skills in behavioral management of their child. One within-person ecological or response class analysis is offered based on data demonstrating a relationship between mothers' skill in managing their children's behavior and mothers' scores on the depression scales of the Minnesota Multiphasic Personality Inventory (MMPI). The latter analysis compares observational data and MMPI profiles collected before and after BPT. This comparison showed a positive change in measures of mother depression following interventions that increased their child management skills.

Patterson's data are not entirely sufficient to prove the sequential progression of events resulting in the coercive cycles he postulates (see commentary by Maccoby, 1980), and the relationships between family structure (in terms of time mothers and fathers spent engaged with the child) and development of the coercive cycle are based on a correlational analysis. However, the overall analysis conducted across three aspects of the family system and based on multiple data sources is convincing and useful from both applied and basic research perspectives.

As an ecological analysis, Patterson's work is not easily replicable because it is based on 10 years of data from multiple studies. However, it does present a prototype of ecological analysis that might be conducted on a more modest scale. The implications of his results are important for the clinical application of BPT because they suggest a linkage between child management skills and more general family functioning that has not been thoroughly explored. Families in which there is a high demand for mother management of the child (as a result of restricted father participation in child management) appear to be more vulnerable to the escalating cycle of child coercive behavior. Lack of child management skills in mothers' repertoires may be a second critical condition in the bidirectional interchanges between mother and child that, when combined with the child's high levels of disruptive behavior, contribute to the coercive cycle. In the perspective of the overall family system, it is the confluence and interaction of three factors—high rates of child disruptive behavior, unusually high levels of mother-child contact, and lack of child management skills—that produce the coercive cycles described by Patterson. The final test of this theory—prediction of coercive family interchanges on the basis of data indicating the presence of these three conditions—remains to be done.

Wahler: Insular Families

Wahler and his colleagues have contributed two types of ecological analyses conducted in the context of research on BPT: 1) research on co-variation of child behaviors and 2) research on the relationship between mothers' community contacts and their interactions with their disruptive children.

Wahler began his analysis of response co-variation in a series of studies in which solitary, productive play was an intervention target (Wahler & Fox, 1980; Wahler & Moore, 1975). In these studies, Wahler sought to demonstrate that interventions, in the form of parent-implemented contracts with their oppositional-aggressive children directed toward increasing solitary play, would result in concomitant changes in other child behaviors. These other child behaviors were postulated to be members of the same response class or within-person ecological system. Modification of the "keystone" behavior (i.e., solitary play) should promote increases in related positive and decreases in related negative behaviors. Although Wahler and colleagues did demonstrate that there were functional response classes within children's behavioral repertoires, the modification of the "keystone" behavior did not always result in the high levels of generalization and maintenance of behavior change that were considered indicative of truly effective behavioral interventions.

The limited generalization and maintenance obtained with some families prompted Wahler (Wahler, Leske, & Rogers, 1979) to analyze the characteristics of those families from a broader systems perspective. Typically, these families consisted of a single mother and her child or children living in poverty, with a relative lack of education. But most importantly, these families exhibited a particular pattern of interpersonal interactions outside the parent-child dyad. These "insular" parents reported that they experienced frequent and aversive interactions initiated by extended family members (own parents, in-laws, and so forth) and by helping/service agency personnel (e.g., protective service worker, mental health personnel, legal authorities). In comparison to a sample of middle-class families, insular families reported fewer friendship contacts and rated their contacts with family and service agency representatives more negatively.

Wahler (1980) analyzed the relationship between the aversive community contacts of 18 insular mothers and their acquisition and maintenance of child management skills. All mothers successfully implemented the management techniques; mother-child aversive interchanges were substantially reduced during training. Follow-up measures collected 8 months to 1 year after training, showed that problem interactions involving negative adult attention and child opposition had returned to their preintervention levels. Analyses of mother insularity measures collected throughout the study and the follow-up period showed an inverse relationship between mother-child aversive interactions and the frequency and valence of mothers' interactions with friends outside the home. In those sessions when mothers reported relatively more frequent and more positive friendship contacts, their interactions with their children were more positive. When mothers reported a low number of friendship contacts and many negative kinfolk or service agency contacts, interactions with their children were aversive.

Wahler's research constitutes a succession of ecological analyses. First, specific behavior-environment relationships were documented between children's oppositional behavior and parents' responses to those behaviors in bidirectional analysis of dyadic interaction before, during and after BPT. Next, the relationship of a keystone behavior, solitary play, to other positive and negative child behaviors was documented when solitary play was experimentally increased by altering parent contingencies for this behavior. Finally, following an analysis of characteristics of families who did and did not maintain changes resulting from BPT, the relationship between positive community contacts and parent-child interaction was demonstrated. Wahler's research program, although quite different from Patterson's, also provides a dual outcome: further documentation of the multiple effects of parent training and an ecological analysis of some aspects of

the family system related to parent-child interaction.

Lutzker: Multiple Interventions to Treat and Prevent Child Abuse

A more purposefully ecological analysis of family functioning has been undertaken by Lutzker and his colleagues in conjunction with BPT interventions. Lutzker (1984) began by assessing the family system at four levels: the parents' self-directed behavior, functioning within the parent-child dyad, interactions between parents, and the functioning of family members in the community (e.g., in regard to jobs, contacts with friends and social service agencies). Parents in Lutzker's studies were abusive or thought to be at risk for abusing their children. His data, which include both observational measures and family report measures, are by no means as comprehensive nor as thoroughly analyzed as those of Patterson or Wahler. Yet, his findings may offer another useful model for determining the ecological effects of behavioral interventions and for describing the functioning of the family system.

For example, Lutzker (1984) showed that, by intervening sequentially on several aspects of the family ecology (typically three or more aspects, including initiating BPT to improve parent-child interactions, marital counseling, and job counseling), abusive interactions can be greatly reduced. Initial studies of this type have not been as methodologically sound as is desirable, but they do offer some interesting results and a potential model for a more thorough investigation of multiple interventions.

Lutzker has also examined the relationship between some aspects of the physical environment and parent-child abusive interactions (Tertinger, Greene, & Lutzker, 1984). In this study of home safety, it was shown that safety hazards (e.g., exposed wires, access to dangerous substances, such as cleaning fluid, paint thinner, broken glass, exposed nails) in the home often set the occasion for abusive interchanges. A home with many safety hazards and certain standing patterns of interaction between parent and child was a higher-risk environment (in terms of the likelihood of abuse) than a home in which the interaction patterns were similar but there were few setting events that prompted reprimand-giving episodes.

Lutzker's data, as do those of Wahler and Patterson, suggest that families become dysfunctional as a result of the interaction of multiple aspects of the family system. Negative interchanges are most likely to be established as a standing pattern of behavior when both setting events and behavioral patterns of parents and children support these interchanges.

Taken together, the work of Patterson, Wahler, and Lutzker demonstrates that research investigating the effects of BPT might reasonably contribute to both the applied research base and the ecological analysis of family functioning. Although these studies provide a model for such research, it is not clear if their specific findings accurately describe the ecologies of families with handicapped children. Handicapped children may present other problem behaviors in addition to the disruptive or oppositional behaviors that typically prompt the initiation of parent training. Such differences in behavioral repertoires may be sufficient to alter the influences of parent behavior and other setting variables, resulting in a different pattern of behavior and/or ecological system than has been observed with normally developing, but disruptive children. The chronic nature of handicapped children's behavioral and learning deficits may affect parent-child interaction to produce patterns of interaction that are significantly different from those that form the basis for parent-child interaction in normally developing families. The existing observational data base on mother-handicapped child interactions suggests that this may be the case. (See Rogers-Warren & Warren, 1983, for a more complete discussion of this issue.)

RESEARCH ISSUES

Research in BPT with families of mentally retarded children should be designed to yield two general types of information: analyses of the effects of training on parents and children

and descriptions of the functioning of family systems. Both types of information are needed in order to understand the needs of this population of families and to formulate interventions that facilitate family functioning. In addition, future studies should consist of experimental tests of the predictions made on the basis of analyses of multiple effects and descriptions of family functioning. Ideally, investigations in all three areas should meet the criteria for ecological analyses discussed earlier. That is, the studies should include naturalistic observational data, allow for bi- or multidirectional analysis of behavior, provide comparison data from contrasting ecological conditions, and, if possible, describe multiple levels of the family system.

The first, and most general, ecological investigations of BPT might focus on the systemic effects of this training. Studies with oppositional children (see previous discussion of work by Wahler and Patterson) and with autistic children (Koegel et al., 1982) suggest that changes in the overall family system do occur as a result of such training, but further examination of the type, consistency, and strength of these effects is needed. In addition to determining if BPT results in generalization of the newly learned skills to untrained instances of child behavior and to conducting analyses of maintenance, investigations of this type might address multiple levels of the family system. For example, changes in the overall frequency of parent-child interaction and quality of these interactions might be monitored by observing the frequency of positive parent-child contact not associated with caregiving and parent perceptions of the child. Assessment of changes in development-facilitating behaviors, such as language teaching or promoting social interaction, would provide a secondary analysis of generalization, as well as measuring the impact of BPT on family interaction. Examination of changes in marital happiness and perceived burden of care might also be undertaken in this category of research.

In the context of generalization and maintenance, the preceding studies should determine the conditions under which BPT succeeds or fails to produce durable effects. Following the logic in the work of both Patterson and Wahler, analysis of the conditions contributing to failure to change or maintain changes permits an examination of critical differences in family ecology. On the basis of their work, it is likely that a confluence or interaction of setting conditions, child behavioral characteristics, and parent characteristics is associated with behavioral training failures. Specification of those conditions and the processes associated with them would serve the dual functions proposed for this area of research.

In addition to analysis of specific behavioral interventions (e.g., the effects of training parents to be teachers of their children; the effects of intervention into the family when the child is very young), there should be a third set of studies that tests the predictions made on the basis of data generated in the two classes of studies just described. Predictive studies are notably absent in all parent training research. In terms of ecological studies of parent training and family interaction, the current focus on exploratory descriptive and functional analyses seems quite appropriate. However, as the empirical base develops, it will become increasingly necessary to conduct hypothesis-testing, predictive studies. Such studies will allow us to evaluate the accuracy and utility of ecological theory and its components in a scientific account of human behavior. In all studies of BPT, there is an obvious need to focus on the real and pressing problems of families with handicapped children, to quantify the independent and dependent variables in reliable and valid ways, and to use measures that yield descriptions of several levels of the family system. In these regards, the work of Wahler, Patterson, and Luzker should provide useful models. Although the guidelines provided by Bronfenbrenner (1977) are potentially useful in undertaking new research in this area, it is his mentor Dearborn's advice that best fits behavioral ecological research: "If you want to understand something, try to change it" (cited in Bronfenbrenner, 1977, p.528).

REFERENCES

Baker, B. (1976). Parent involvement in programming for developmentally disabled children. In L. Lloyd (Ed.), *Communicatin assessment and intervention strategies* (pp. 691–733). Baltimore: University Park Press.

Baker, B. L. (1980). In S. Salzinger, J. Antrobus, & J. Glick (Eds.), *The ecosystem of the sick child: Implications for the classification and intervention for disturbed and mentally retarded children* (pp. 201–215). New York: Academic Press.

Baker, B., Heifetz, L., & Murphy, D. (1980). Behavioral training for parents of mentally retarded children: One-year follow-up. *American Journal of Mental Deficiency, 85,* 31–38.

Barker, R. G. (1963). *The stream of behavior.* New York: Appleton-Century-Crofts.

Barker, R. G., & Wright, H. F. (1954). *Midwest and its children: The psychological ecology of an American town.* Evanston, IL: Row, Peterson.

Bond, L. A., & Joffe, J. M. (Eds.). (1982). *Facilitating infant and early childhood development.* Hanover, NH: The University Press of New England.

Bronfenbrenner, U. (1977). Toward an experimental ecology of human development. *Journal of the American Psychological Association, 32,* 513–529.

Burden, R. L. (1980). Measuring the effects of stress on mothers of handicapped infants: Must depression always follow. *Child Health: Care and Development, 6,* 111–125.

Butterfield, W. H., & Parson, R. (1973). Modeling and shaping by parents to develop chewing behavior in their retarded child. *Journal of Behavior Therapy and Experimental Psychiatry, 4,* 285–287.

Clarke-Stewart, K. A. (1973). Interactions between mothers and their young children: Characteristics and consequences. *Monographs of the Society for Research on Child Development, 38.*

DeMeyer, M. K., & Goldberg, P. (1983). Family needs of the autistic adolescent. In E. Schopler & G. Mesibov (Eds.), *Autism in adolescents and adults* (pp. 225–250). New York: Plenum Publishing.

Forehand, R., & King, H. E. (1977). Non-compliant children: Effects of parent training on behavior and attitude change. *Behavior Modification, 1,* 93–108.

Franks, C. M. (1982). Behavior therapy with children and adolescents. In C. Franks, G. Wilson, P. Kendell, & K. Brownell (Eds.), *Annual review of behavior therapy theory and practice* (Vol. 8, pp. 273–304). New York: Guilford Press.

Freeman, S., & Thompson, C. (1973). Parent-child training for the mentally retarded. *Mental Retardation, 11,* 8–10.

Gabel, H., & Kotsch, L. S. (1981). Extended families and young handicapped children. *Topics in Early Childhood Special Education, 1,* 29–35.

Gallagher, J. J., Beckman, P., & Cross, A. H. (1983). Families of handicapped children: Sources of stress and its amelioration. *Exceptional Children, 50,* 10–18.

Gordon, S. B., & Davidson, N. (1981). Behavioral parent

training. In A. S. Gurman & D. P. Kniskern (Eds.), *Handbook of family therapy* (pp. 515–575). New York: Brunner/Mazel.

Harris, S. L. (1982). A family systems approach to behavioral training with parents of autistic children. *Child and Family Behavior Therapy, 4,* 21–35.

Heifetz, L. (1977). Behavioral parent training for parents of retarded children: Alternative formats based on instructional manuals. *American Journal of Mental Deficiency, 82,* 194–203.

Heward, W. L., Dardig, J. C., & Rossett, A. (1979). *Working with parents of handicapped children.* Columbus, OH: Charles E. Merrill Publishing Co.

Hobbs, N. (1980). An ecological oriented, service-based, system for the classification of handicapped children. In S. Salzinger, J. Antrobus, & J. Glick (Eds.), *The ecosystem of the "sick" kid: Implications for classification and intervention* (pp. 271–290). New York: Academic Press.

Holroyd, J., & MacArthur, D. (1976). Mental Retardation and stress on the parents: A contrast between Down's Syndrome and childhood autism. *American Journal of Mental Deficiency, 80,* 431–436.

Hursh, D. E., & House, D. J. (1983). Designing environments for handicapped students: The evaluation of a play unit. *Exceptional Children Quarterly, 4*(2), 54–66.

Johnson, C., & Katz, C. (1973). Using parents as change agents for their children: A review. *Journal of Child Psychology and Psychiatry, 14,* 131–200.

Kantor, J. R. (1959). *Interbehavioral psychology.* Granville, OH: Pricipia Press.

Koegel, R. L., Schreibman, L., Britten, K. R., Burke, J. C., & O'Neill, R. E. (1982). A comparison of parent training to direct child treatment. In R. L. Koegel, A. Rincover, & A. L. Egel (Eds.), *Educating and understanding autistic children* (pp. 260-281). San Diego, CA: College-Hill Press, Inc.

Landesman-Dwyer, S., Sackett, G. P., & Kleinman, J. S. (1980). Relationship of size to resident and staff behavior in small community residences. *American Journal of Mental Deficiency, 85,* 6–17.

Lewin, K. (1951). *Field theory in social science.* New York: Harper.

Lilly, D. L. (1974). Dimensions in parent programs: An overview. In J. Grim (Ed.), *Training parents to teach—four models. 1st chance for children* (Vol. 3, pp. 1–9). Chapel Hill, NC: Technical Assistance Development Systems.

Lutzker, J. R. (1984). Project 12-ways: Treating child abuse and neglect from an ecobehavioral perspective. In R. F. Dangel & R. A. Polster (Eds.), *Parent training: Foundations of research and practice* (pp. 260–297). New York: Guilford Press.

Lutzker, J. R., McGimsey, J. P., McRae, S., & Campbell, R. V. (1983). Behavioral parent training: There's so much more to do. *the Behavior Therapist, 6,* 110–112.

Maccoby, E. E. (1980). Commentary by Eleanor E. Maccoby. *Monographs of the Society for Research in Child Development, 45,* 56–64.

Mash, E., & Terdal, L. (1973). Modification of mother-child interactions: Playing with children. *Mental Retardation, 11,* 44–49.

Mink, I. T., Nihira, K., & Meyers, C. E. (1982). *Family typologies: Families with severely retarded and slow*

learning children. Unpublished manuscript, University of California, Neuropsychiatric Institute, Los Angeles.

Moos, R., & Moos, B. (1976). A typology of family social environments. *Family Process, 15,* 357–371.

O'Dell, S. (1974). Training parents in behavior modification: A review. *Psychological Bulletin, 81,* 418–433.

Patterson, G. (1977). Accelerating stimuli for two classes of coercive behaviors. *Journal of Abnormal Child Psychology, 5,* 334–350.

Patterson, G. R. (1980). Mothers: The unacknowledged victims. *Monographs of the Society for Research in Child Development, 45*(Serial No. 186).

Patterson, G. (1982). *Coercive family processes.* Eugene, OR: Castalia Publishing.

Patterson, G., & Fleischman, M. (1979). Maintenance of treatment effects: Some considerations concerning family systems and follow-up data. *Behavior Therapy, 10,* 168–185.

Patterson, G., & Reid, J. (1973). Intervention for families of aggressive boys: A replication study. *Behavior Research and Therapy, 11,* 383–394.

Paul, J. (Ed.). (1981). *Understanding and working with parents of children with special needs.* New York: Holt, Rinehart & Winston.

Peed, S., Roberts, M., & Forehand, R. (1977). Evaluation of the effectiveness of a standardized parent training program in altering the interaction of mothers with their non-compliant children. *Behavior Modification, 1,* 323–350.

Petersen, G. A., & Sherrod, K. B. (1982a). Maternal speech patterns: Their relationship to language development and language delay. *Journal of Mental Deficiency, 86,* 391–398.

Petersen, G. A., & Sherrod, K. B. (1982b). Relationship of maternal language to language development and language delay in children. *American Journal of Mental Deficiency, 86,* 391–398.

Rogers-Warren, A., & Warren, S. (1977). *Ecological perspectives in behavior analysis.* Baltimore, MD: University Park Press.

Rogers-Warren, A., & Warren, S. (1983). Facilitating early language and social development: Parents as teachers. In E. Goetz & K. Allen (Eds.), *Early childhood education: Special environmental and legal considerations* (pp. 69–89). Rockville, MD: Aspen Press.

Rondal, J. (1978). Maternal speech to normal and Down's Syndrome children matched for mean length of utterance. *American Association on Mental Deficiency Monographs* (No. 3).

Rose, S. (1974). Training parents in groups as behavior modifiers of their mentally retarded children. *Journal of Behavior Therapy and Experimental Psychiatry, 5,* 135–140.

Salzinger, S., Antrobus, J., & Glick, J. (1980). *The ecosystem of the "sick" child.* New York: Academic Press.

Sameroff, A. J., & Chandler, M. J. (1975). Reproductive risk and the continuum of caretaking causalty. In F. D. Horowitz (Ed.), *Review of child development research* (Vol. 4, pp. 187–244). Chicago: University of Chicago Press.

Skinner, B. F. (1953). *Science and human behavior.* New York: MacMillan.

Tavormina, J. (1975). Relative effectiveness of behavioral

and reflective group counseling with parents of mentally retarded children. *Journal of Consulting and Clinical Psychology, 43,* 22–31.

Tavormina, J., Hampson, R., Luscomb, R. (1976). Participant evaluations of the effectiveness of their parent counseling groups. *Mental Retardation, 14,* 8–9.

Tertinger, D. A., Greene, B. F., & Lutzker, J. R. (1984). Home safety: Development and validation of one component of an ecobehavioral treatment program for abused and neglected children. *Journal of Applied Behavior Analysis, 17,* 159–174.

Tharp, R. G., & Wetzel, R. J. (1969). *Behavior modification in the natural environment.* New York: Academic Press.

Turnbull, A. P., Summers, J. A., & Brotherson, M. J. (1983, September). *Family life cycle: Theoretical and empirical implications and directions for families with mentally retarded members.* Paper presented at the NIC-HD Conference on Research on Families with Retarded Children, Chapel Hill, NC.

Wahler, R. G. (1969). Oppositional children: A quest for parental reinforcement control. *Journal of Applied Behavior Analysis, 2,* 159–170.

Wahler, R. G. (1975). Some structural aspects of deviant child behavior. *Journal of Applied Behavior Analysis, 8,* 27–42.

Wahler, R. G. (1980). The insular mother: Her problems in parent-child treatment. *Journal of Applied Behavior Analysis, 13,* 207–219.

Wahler, R. G., & Fox, J. (1980). Solitary toy play and time-out: A family treatment package for children with aggressive and oppositional behavior. *Journal of Applied Behavior Analysis, 13,* 23–39.

Wahler, R. G., Leske, G., & Rogers, E. S. (1979). The insular family: A deviance support system for oppositional children. In L. A. Hamerlynck (Ed.), *Behavioral systems for the developmentally disabled: 1. School and family environments* (pp. 102–127). New York: Brunner/Mazel, Inc.

Wahler, R. G., & Moore, D. R. (1975, December). *School-home behavior change procedures in a "high risk community."* Paper presented in a AABT symposium Child behavior modification in the community: A progress update. San Francisco.

Warren, S., Rogers-Warren, A., Baer, D., & Guess, D. (1980). The assessment and facilitation of language generalization. In W. Sailor, B. Wilcox, & L. Brown (Eds.) *Methods of instruction for severely handicapped students,* Baltimore: Paul H. Brookes Publishing Co.

Watson, L., & Bassinger, J. (1974). Parent training technology: A potential service delivery system. *Mental Retardation, 12,* 3–10.

Willems, E. P. (1974). Behavioral technology and behavioral ecology. *Journal of Applied Behavior Analysis, 7,* 131–165.

Wolf, M., Risley, T., & Mees, H. (1964). Application of operant conditioning techniques to the behavior problems of an autistic child. *Behavior Research and Therapy, 3,* 305–312.

Wood, A. J., Bruner, J. S. (1976). The role of tutoring in problem-solving. *Journal of Child Psychology, 17,* 89–100.

Wood, D. J., Bruner, J. S., & Ross, G. (1976). The role of tutoring in problem solving. *Journal of Child Psychology and Psychiatry, 17*(2), 89–100.

Wright, H. F. (1969). *Children's behavior in communities differing in size. Parts 1, 2, 3, Supplement.* Lawrence, KS: University of Kansas, Department of Psychology.

Chapter

13

Patterns and Trends in Public Services to Families with a Mentally Retarded Member

Marty Wyngaarden Krauss

FAMILIES WITH A mentally retarded member face two enduring challenges: to marshal their own emotional, physical, and economic resources to maintain the family unit and to ensure that the mentally retarded member receives the best care and training possible. To a large extent, public policies and programs have been geared to the latter challenge. Families have received only sporadic public support in coping with the at times overwhelming task of adjusting family life and relationships to meet the responsibilities of care for the mentally retarded member.

Our knowledge of the effects on the family of having a handicapped child has been enriched by family members themselves. There is a substantial body of literature written by parents and siblings of handicapped persons that describes in vivid detail the ways in which family and personal lives are affected (Darling, 1979; Featherstone, 1980; Massie & Massie, 1975; Park, 1967; Turnbull & Turnbull, 1984). These portraits often provide startling accounts

of the insensitivity of professionals, the public, and society at large to the daily concerns and needs of families in providing care and love to a handicapped family member.

There is also a considerable amount of empirically based research showing the effects on families of having a mentally retarded child. Although comprehensive reviews of this research are available elsewhere (Blacher, 1984; Crnic, Friedrich, & Greenberg, 1983; Skrtic, Summers, Brotherson, & Turnbull, 1984), it has generally been characterized by the enumeration of negative outcomes for families (e.g., social isolation, physical and financial burdens, increased familial stress). Farber (Chapter 1) argues that these studies were based on the notion that the birth of a handicapped child precipitates a family crisis and that the purpose of the research undertaken was to determine the ways in which family life departed from the norms of a "healthy" family life. Further, research tended to define and justify areas of need for families with a handicapped member and to analyze the efficacy of various remediation strategies. Despite the advances that were made in the development of such strategies as parent training (Baker, 1984) and specialized social work practices (Dickerson, 1981; Dybwad, 1964), comparatively little was achieved in the development of family support services that focused on the family rather than on the handicapped child as the target of services (Dybwad, 1982).

There has been a renewed interest, however, on the part of social planners, researchers, and service providers in identifying, analyzing, and meeting the long-term needs of families with a mentally retarded member (Horejsi, 1979; Perlman & Giele, 1983). This interest has been fueled by the assumption that family support services will contribute to the prevention or delay of out-of-home placement of the mentally retarded family member. Strategies to achieve a reduction in the use of inappropriate out-of-home placement both to promote optimal individual development and to curb the costs of publicly supported residential programs have become a major public policy issue. Although the available research testing this assumption is limited and inconclusive (Seltzer & Krauss, 1984a; Sherman & Cocozza, 1984; Townsend & Flanagan, 1976; Zimmerman, 1984), the need to include variables measuring social and community support in studies on family adaptation processes and placement decision outcomes is widely acknowledged.

For example, Crnic et al. (1983), drawing on both the family systems and mental retardation literature, point out that internal family dynamics and coping mechanisms, mediated by the ecological system within which families interact and are acted on, may provide more salient explanations of the observed variability in family adaptation patterns. Their analysis includes a theoretical model that integrates the concepts of stress, coping, and ecological systems to guide future studies of family adaptation and functioning. Of particular interest for the present discussion is their inclusion of ecological factors (e.g., the external environments, such as schools, home, agencies, neighborhoods, workplaces, social networks) as predictor variables of family adjustment. Further, their conceptualization of the family as a system of interdependent members and functions appropriately recasts the focus of support services to the family as a unit, rather than to a single member of the family (e.g., the mother or the handicapped child).

Despite the centrality of the family in providing care for mentally retarded members, very little research has been conducted on the constellation of services needed by families to support or ensure their long-term caregiving capacity. Indeed, there is considerable public ambivalence regarding the appropriate relationship between the family and its caregiving functions, on the one hand, and the state and its power to support, supplement, or substitute for familial roles and responsibilities (Farber, 1979; Gelman, 1979; Steiner, 1981). The lack of consensus regarding the legitimacy and forms of family-oriented services has resulted in families, as a type of social services, being largely ignored in policy and program development (Moroney, 1983). Bruininks (1979) summarizes the situation as follows:

> Given the fact that most developmentally disabled people spend much of their lives with members of their natural families . . . it is surprising that so little attention has been given by units of government, agencies, and researchers to the needs of natural or surrogate families with developmentally disabled members . . . there is little in the published literature regarding the social, economic, or programmatic issues involved in providing care and opportunities for developmentally disabled people in family care settings. (p. 3)

The purpose of this chapter is to review current trends in the provision of support services to families with a mentally retarded member. It focuses on the general patterns of services available to families, with a specific emphasis on the balance (or imbalance) between services that support and those that supplant the natural family (Skarnulis, 1979). The chapter reviews the recent development of family support programs in the various states and concludes with recommendations for research that is needed to inform the policy-making and program-design process. The chapter thus concentrates on broader or macrolevel service delivery issues rather than on the determinants or outcomes of the relationships between individual families and service providers.

SERVICE NEEDS OF FAMILIES

Although the impact on families of having a mentally retarded child has been a subject of research for decades, it is only recently that comprehensive programs of family support have been conceptualized and/or promulgated. Evidence of the current activity in identifying, analyzing, and meeting the long-term needs of families may be seen in, for example, a national conference on family care of developmentally disabled members (Bruininks & Krantz, 1979), the establishment of a national clearinghouse for information on home-based services to children (Maybanks & Bryce, 1979), and the compilation of a nationwide resource guide on family support service (Michigan Association of Community Mental Health Boards, 1983).

These activities have analyzed and restated problems that are voiced by families with a mentally retarded member; namely, that support services are fragmented, lack coordination, have seemingly capricious eligibility criteria, and are not structured or organized in ways that reflect family preference or need (Berger & Foster, 1976). Indeed, much of the research conducted on service needs of families reports that parents are frequently unaware of services that may be available to them or their families and/or they are not receiving adequate support from the services that they are receiving (Gollay, Freedman, Wyngaarden, & Kurtz, 1978; Justice, O'Connor, & Warren, 1971). For example, Bruininks, Morreau, and Williams (1979) surveyed parents, policymakers, and state agency personnel in six states and found that nearly all respondents indicated family-related services to be both low in availability and quality.

An earlier study by the Minnesota Department of Welfare (Minnesota State Planning Agency, 1975) asked parents of developmentally disabled children which types of services were needed to maintain the child at home. The services were rank-ordered as follows: medical, supplemental income, home assistance, special school programs, respite care, social activities for the child, transportation for the child, home tutors, parent guidance, and day activity centers. In a similarly focused investigation, Dunlap (1976) surveyed 404 families of mentally retarded, cerebral palsied, or epileptic individuals in Alabama to determine services most useful or needed by the families. The responses indicated that financial assistance and educational services were the most needed services, followed by transportation, training, and medical services.

Although empirical studies on the services most needed by families are rather consistent in their findings, there are only a limited number of studies on the services utilized over time by families. Such investigations are needed for they reveal the variability in service needs across different stages in the mentally retarded child's development and in the family's progression through the life cycle (Turnbull, Summers, & Brotherson, Chapter 3, this volume). Suelzle and Keenan (1981) studied the utilization of personal and professional support networks of 330 parents over the life cycle of their mentally retarded children. Four distinct stages were posited: preschool (birth to 5 years old), elementary (6 to 12 years old), teenage (13 to 18 years old), and young adult (19 to 21 years old). They found that utilization of personal support networks (e.g., use of family members or friends as babysitters, parent support groups) declined over the life cycle, whereas utilization of health care professionals and school personnel increased over time. Differences were also found regarding parental perceptions of unmet service needs. Although the majority of parents of younger children perceived inadequate diagnostic services and living alternatives, parents of young adults perceived deficiencies in these services more acutely. Further, a U-shaped function was reported for unmet family support services (e.g., crisis lines, respite care, and counseling services). Unmet needs in these areas were reportedly high among parents of preschoolers and young adults, whereas parents of children in the middle two age groups were less likely to report unmet family support service needs.

Additional support for the variability in family needs over time is offered by Wikler (1981), who analyzed the types of periodic and predictable stresses that families of mentally retarded children experience. She noted, as have others (Berger & Foster, 1976), that professionals tend to concentrate on the needs of families primarily during the early years of their child's development, rather than on management issues that arise over time. Her analysis posits specific events and developmental milestones that can be expected to be accompanied by more pronounced stress for families. These events and milestones are thus occasions when more intensive and skilled parental support services may be especially crucial.

In an empirical investigation of the extent to which chronic versus time-bound stress is experienced, Wikler, Wasow, and Hatfield (1981) found that both parents and social workers indicated that increased stress is associated with developmental and crisis periods. There were differences in the accuracy of social workers' assessments of stressful periods, however. For example, professionals tended to overestimate the amount of stress experienced during the child's early years of development and underestimate the amount of stress that accompanied events during the young adulthood period.

Other recent studies have compared the amount of individual, marital, and parenting stress experienced by families with and without a handicapped child (Kazak & Marvin, 1984), the coping mechanisms developed by families with a handicapped or chronically ill child (Longo & Bond, 1984; McCubbin, McCubbin, Patterson, Cauble, Wilson & Warwick, 1983; Schilling, Gilchrist, & Schinke, 1984), and the characteristics of the social networks of such families (Friedrich & Friedrich, 1981; Kazak

& Marvin, 1984; Schilling & Schinke, 1983). The accumulating evidence suggests that an interactive model is needed for understanding the ways in which families are affected by a handicapped child and for analyzing the services needed by these families to maintain the family and to ensure their child's optimal development (Turnbull, Brotherson & Summers, 1985). As Crnic et al. (1983) note, "Family functioning cannot be considered simply as a response to a retarded child; rather, it is more meaningful to consider familial adaptation as a response to the child mediated by the coping resources available and influenced by the family's ecological environments" (p. 136).

SERVICE PROVIDED TO FAMILIES

Although the knowledge base is expanding regarding the needs of families, it is particularly sobering to consider the publicly supported services available to meet these needs. Virtually any analysis of the dominant characteristic of the service system currently in place to assist families with a mentally retarded member confirms the fact that the most concentrated effort is in support of out-of-home care (Gruber, 1978; Lakin, Bruininks, Doth, Hill & Hauber, 1982; MacEachron & Krauss, 1983; Moroney, 1983; Seltzer & Krauss, 1984b; Skarnulis, 1979). As Moroney notes (1979):

> Despite the rhetoric of choice and preferences for the disabled and their families, priority (resources) has been given to institutional care. And yet, the evidence is that most families favor home care over institutional care, that they actually are providing a supportive environment for their disabled members whether they are severely retarded children or elderly parents, and that they are doing so with little support from the organized health and welfare system. (pp. 68–69)

A brief review of current expenditures for services to mentally retarded persons and their families supports Moroney's conclusions. Braddock, Howes, and Hemp (1984) analyzed the distribution of federal, regional, and state funds for services to the mentally retarded and other developmentally disabled populations. Their findings for the cumulative federal reimbursements under the Intermediate Care Facilities for the Mentally Retarded (ICF/MR) program between FY 1977–1984 show that, of the $12.9 billion expended, 82% was for institutional programs and 18% for community-based residential programs. Comparisons of the total annual expenditures from all sources for institutional versus community services during this same period indicate that the amount spent for community-based services (which would include services to families) is less than 50% of that spent for institutional services for 5 of the 8 years included.

Moroney (1981) examined 31 federal programs sponsored by the (then) Department of Health, Education and Welfare in 1976 that could in principle be supportive to families with handicapped members. Of the $102.7 billion obligated by these programs, 71% were accounted for by various income maintenance programs, 25% by programs supporting medical services, and 4% for the provision of services. He notes (1981) that, "While services and financial support are provided to handicapped persons—the elderly, the sick and the disabled—their families are not the object of the policy or service. . . . These policies have tended to ignore the family with a handicapped member, just as they ignore families in general" (p. 226).

These conclusions are supported by other investigations that indicate that families of deinstitutionalized mentally retarded members receive far fewer support services and have more pronounced unmet service needs than other providers of care (Gollay et al., 1978), that families of mentally retarded children receiving public social services are more likely to have out-of-home placements recommended and implemented for their children than other families receiving social services (MacEachron & Krauss, 1983), and that the absence of community-based support services to families contributes to the decision to seek an out-of-home placement (Eyman, Dingman, & Sabagh, 1966; Sherman & Cocozza, 1984).

There are some powerful reasons offered for the absence of public services, programs, and policies designed to shore up families' internal and external resources to maintain their mentally retarded member at home. The factors reflect both societal ambivalance about the appropriate role of governmental bodies in family life and general political concerns about the fiscal feasibility of offering more targeted services to families. For example, Moroney (1979) cites five reasons for the emphasis on substitute services for families: 1) lack of sufficient resources to meet the demand for services; 2) lack of professional skill and knowledge about methods to support families; 3) perceptions that families are themselves part of the "problem," rather than social units to be supported; 4) a service tendency to focus on the individual, rather than the family, as the recipient of services; and 5) the technical ease of substituting for the family compared to developing a plan of shared responsibility. Tapper (1979) echoes several of these points in his analysis of the barriers to family subsidy programs. He adds, however, the perceived problem of parental accountability in the use of public funds and the notion that parents are less organized and thus less likely than the professional service-providing establishment to compete successfully for public monies.

Although these barriers or factors represent potent obstacles, the pattern of services to families is undergoing some fundamental changes. The development and implementation of formalized family support programs in various states across the country signals a sharp break with previous service and policy patterns of ignoring or in many ways subverting family-based care. The next section of this chapter considers the scope, characteristics, and benefits of these innovative, though limited, family support programs.

FAMILY SUPPORT PROGRAMS

A family support program has been defined as "a statewide initiative to provide systematic support to families with developmentally disabled members that is funded and monitored through the administrative auspices of the state" (Human Services Research Institute, 1984, p. 5). The development and implementation of family support programs marks a significant change in the states' approach to serving mentally retarded and other developmentally disabled persons because their focus is on supporting the natural families' efforts to care for their developmentally disabled member. In this sense, families are increasingly being seen as providers of the same type of social services that states have traditionally funded more formalized agencies to provide (Moroney, 1983).

Conceptualizations about the types of services that should be included in a model family support program have been offered by a number of policy analysts (Klerman, 1983; Moroney, 1979; Michigan Association of Community Mental Health Boards, 1983; Zimmerman, 1979). In general, the services that are identified provide instrumental or concrete support to the family, such as case management, respite care, financial assistance or subsidies, parent training, homemakers, and architectural modifications to the home.

Results from three national surveys of state-administered family support programs (Human Services Research Institute, 1984; Michigan Association of Community Mental Health Boards, 1983; New York State Office of Mental Retardation and Developmental Disabilities, 1984) illustrate the extent to which state supported community-based service systems are recognizing the critical role of the family in achieving two specific policy objectives. First, family support programs are intended to prevent or delay the premature or unnecessary out-of-home placement of the family's developmentally disabled member. The assumption is that, by assisting families to mediate the known stresses often accompanying in-home care, families will be better able to continue to keep the disabled member in the family unit. For example, providing periodic respite care services is expected to cushion the impact of the physical and emotional demands of round-the-clock care that many retarded persons require. The second and related objective of family support programs is to enhance the caregiving capacity of families. This objective reflects the belief that families provide the most

enduring, committed, and dependable source of care to its members and that, with specific and concrete assistance, families will provide the optimal environment in which the retarded member's development will be maximized.

The most comprehensive national survey of family support programs was conducted by the National Association of State Mental Retardation Program Directors and the Human Services Research Institute (HSRI) between November, 1983 and February, 1984 (Human Services Research Institute, 1984). The results show that 41 states currently operate a family support program. Of the nine states without a program (Illinois, Kansas, Mississippi, Missouri, New York, Oklahoma, South Dakota, West Virginia, and Wyoming), two states (Illinois and New York) have pilot family support programs, and two other states (Kansas and Missouri) offer local family support services as demonstration projects. In contrast, earlier national surveys indicated that only 21 states (Michigan Association of Community Mental Health Boards, 1983) or 17 states (New York Office of Mental Retardation and Developmental Disabilities, 1984) had such programs.

The HSRI survey documents the considerable variability in the states' programs in terms of services included, eligibility criteria, numbers of families served, and costs of the program. This variability may be due to each state developing programs that reflect its unique service needs and capabilities, or it may reflect the relative youth of the programs. Only seven states had family support programs during the 1970s, with the remaining states initiating their programs within the last 4 years. Thus, no single or core model has emerged from these efforts as the most effective or efficient system to achieve the twin objectives described earlier. (For detailed descriptions of family support programs, see Herman, 1983; Michigan Association of Community Mental Health Boards, 1983; Rosenau, 1983).

Although over 35 different types of services are offered among the 41 state programs, the most commonly offered services are respite care, case management, parent training, home adaptations, special equipment, and transportation. HSRI (1984) has categorized the program models as follows: 1) cash subsidy programs that provide money directly to families for the purchase of services and/or habilitation materials (11 states), 2) supportive programs that provide direct services to families from providers contracted by the state (24 states), and 3) combination programs that offer both cash subsidies and direct services (5 states). One obvious distinction that can be drawn among the three types of programs is the degree to which families take a primary role (as in cash subsidy programs) or a secondary role (as in supportive programs) in defining what services are needed and utilized. Research comparing the cost-effectiveness and family satisfaction with various program models is obviously needed to determine the relative advantages to both the state and the service recipients of the administrative options available for defining the services and/or mechanisms by which services are obtained.

The eligibility criteria that the states use for their family support programs indicate that the issue of the extent to which such programs should achieve vertical or horizontal equity is still unresolved. Vertical equity is achieved when programs are targeted toward those most in need of the services. Need may be determined on the basis of income, severity of the disability, or some measure of the vulnerability of the family to unmanageable stress that is likely to result in a request for a residential placement for the disabled family member. The underlying assumption of services that are organized along vertical equity principles is that resources should be placed at the disposal of those whose objective or inferred needs are greater than other persons or families. Horizontal equity refers to the principle that services or programs should be available to all members of a specified target group, regardless of additional criteria based on need or other arbitrary limitations. The underlying assumption of services organized along horizontal equity principles is that it is either impossible or undesirable to judge relative need and/or that all persons (or families) with a common characteristic (e.g., a men-

tally retarded member living at home) will have periodic or sustained needs for the services offered.

According to the data presented by HSRI (1984), all states have eligibility criteria for services, but there is considerable variability among these criteria. Of the 11 states with a cash subsidy program, 4 have no additional criteria beyond the family having a developmentally disabled or mentally retarded member living at home. In three states, there are age limitations, with the disabled member being either under 21 or 18. One state has an income restriction for the family, and one state targets its program to those families with a profoundly retarded family member living at home. Other criteria include families with a child returning from an institutional setting, families who are "needy" (not defined), or families for whom services are unavailable elsewhere.

Eligibility information was presented for only 7 of the 21 states with supportive family programs. Of these seven states, however, five had no additional criteria for program services beyond having a mentally retarded child at home. In two states there is an age criterion (0–6 years or under 22), and one of these states also imposes restrictions based on the child being either in an out-of-home placement or at risk of being placed outside the home.

Of the five states that offer both cash subsidies and supportive family services, only two had no additional criteria beyond having a mentally retarded person living at home. Other states impose such criteria as age (e.g., child under 18), severity of handicapping condition (e.g., severely disabled), and having a child recently institutionalized for over 90 days.

Although the data are not complete regarding eligibility criteria across the three types of programs, it may be suggested that programs that provide supportive services are more likely to be horizontally equitable (e.g., have the fewest eligibility criteria) and thus be targeted for the broadest range of families, and programs offering cash subsidies are the most vertically equitable (e.g., targeted to those most in need). Further research is needed to determine the most effective ways for states to manage such programs and to control the resources available to families. The above analysis suggests, however, that control is either exercised through eligibility criteria (vertical vs. horizontal equity) or through family-driven (cash subsidy programs) or state-determined (supportive services programs) systems. An important area for further investigation is the extent to which these administrative options available to the states meet the specific objectives to which the programs are directed.

The number of families served by family support programs varies widely from over 35,000 families in California (which offers supportive services) to 15 in South Carolina (which offers a cash subsidy program). This spread in state coverage cannot be explained solely on the basis of the state's eligibility criteria. For example, Louisiana has only 25 families receiving cash subsidies, and the program criteria do not include age or income restrictions. Important areas for further study are the factors that explain utilization of the available programs. It appears that factors other than specific program eligibility criteria operate to reduce the number of recipients, and these factors need to be uncovered.

As expected, the cost of family support programs varies, depending on the types of services offered and the number of families served. Pennsylvania spends over $3.4 million a year to serve over 11,500 families (for an average of approximately $295 per family), whereas South Carolina spends $23,000 a year for 15 families (for an average of approximately $1533 per family).

That almost all states either have a family support program or are on the verge of establishing the legislative authority to implement one is clearly a positive sign. Family care is emerging as a legitimate arena for public support and as a focus of social policy. However, support for family care has not achieved parity with the public support given to out-of-home care and is, indeed, lagging far behind. As HSRI (1984) concludes, "Our survey findings substantiate the observation that relative to available institutional and community based services, family support systems do not offer a comprehensive service array, lack continuity from state to state, and are grossly underfunded" (p. 34).

AN ALTERNATIVE MECHANISM FOR PROVIDING FAMILY SUPPORT SERVICES

Virtually all the family support programs developed in the 41 states are funded solely from local or state revenues. Recent changes in the federal policies regarding the use of Title XIX (Medicaid) funds for services to mentally retarded people are expected, however, to encourage states to finance some of the services typically included in family support programs from federal sources.

Section 2176 of the Omnibus Budget Reconciliation Act of 1981 (PL 97-35) authorized the waiver of statutory requirements of Title XIX to permit states to finance noninstitutional long-term care services for Medicaid-eligible individuals. The purpose of the waiver program is to remove the financial incentives for placement in Medicaid-reimburseable settings, such as ICFs/MR, of persons whose care can be more efficiently and appropriately provided in the home or other type of community-based service system. States must apply to the Health Care Financing Administration for authorization to waive existing Title XIX regulations and, as of February 15, 1983, 26 states had been granted such a waiver (Lakin, Greenberg, Schmitz, & Hill, 1984). Of these 26 states, 16 had included community-based services to mentally retarded persons among their specifically targeted populations.

The waiver program specifies seven core services that may be included in the states' community-based service plan: case management, homemaker services, home health aide services, personal care, adult day health services, habilitation services, and respite care. Except for adult day health services, these services are typically included in both conceptualizations about family support programs and in the programs currently provided in the 41 states. For the 16 states receiving waivers that targeted their alternative programs to mentally retarded persons, the most commonly included services were habilitation services (15 states), case management (13 states), respite care (12 states), homemaker services (7 states), personal care services (7 states), adult day health services (6 states), and home health aides (5 states) (Lakin et al., 1984).

It is not yet known how and if states currently operating family support programs will respond to the potential additional source of revenue for financing the specific services covered under the waiver program that are already a part of their family support program. The waiver program does represent, however, a possible mechanism for expanding family support programs (other than cash subsidy type programs), both in terms of the number of families eligible for services and the types of services offered.

CONCLUSIONS

This discussion of emerging patterns of services to families with a mentally retarded member suggests that both the resources and commitment needed to support more concretely the staggering amount of care provided by families are on the policy-making and program-development agenda for the future. The degree to which substantial changes in the service delivery systems will occur will depend in part on the conduct of more extensive research on the effects of family support programs.

Although some preliminary studies have been reported (Herman, 1983; Rosenau, 1983; Zimmerman, 1984), no longitudinal studies have been conducted that permit a more refined understanding of the utilization and effects of family support programs over time. The ultimate benefit of such programs cannot be judged adequately by cross-sectional studies because the basic premise of family support programs is that the services provided will contribute to increasing the long-term "staying power" of families. As noted earlier, research has documented that families'

needs vary with the age of their mentally retarded member (Suelzle & Keenan, 1981) and with specific developmental stages (Wikler, 1981). These findings suggest that there may be cyclical demands on family support services unique to each family. It is, therefore, critical that appropriate resources be devoted to investigating the fit between support services and family needs over the life cycle of family-based care.

Research also needs to be conducted on the factors contributing to the design of states' programs. As noted earlier, the variability in services included, eligibility criteria, and program resources suggests that states are using a wide range of administrative options to limit access to family support programs. This variation in program design features presents an unusually rich opportunity for large-scale research on the consequences of different types of programs on expected outcomes.

Basic issues with respect to effects of family support programs need to be investigated. For example, some types of family support services may be perceived as more critical to the maintenance of family well-being than others. Respite care, and especially home-based respite care, is a frequently expressed need by families (Upshur, 1982). Case management services are also noted as important for relieving individual family members of the responsibility for locating and coordinating varied services (MacEachron, this volume). Research needs to be conducted on the comparative value from a family's perspective of the range of services commonly subsumed under family support programs.

Another issue for research is to identify distinguishing characteristics among families that are associated with their need for and/or use of family support services. For example, families with well-developed and extensive informal support networks may be less dependent on publicly financed family support services (Kammeyer & Bolton, 1968). Alternatively, other variables, such as family size, marital status, geographic location, and/or level of the mentally retarded member's functioning, may be important predictors of use, in general, and of specific service needs, in particular. There are currently no published studies that address these questions. More tailored program development is seriously compromised until a more detailed analysis of the efficacy and impact of family support programs for specific types of families with a mentally retarded child is available.

It is clear from the discussion about the various eligibility criteria utilized by the 41 programs that there is an underlying assumption that some families "need" support programs more than other families. Research from the family systems and mental retardation fields have begun to address the basic question of why some families cope or adapt better to periodic or chronic stress than other families (McCubbin, 1979; McCubbin, Joy, Cauble, Comeau, Patterson & Needle, 1980; Olson & McCubbin, 1983; Wikler et al. 1981).

Both the conceptual models and their operationalizations that have been developed present important guidelines for research into the impact of family support programs on the families' capacities to meet the long-term demands of caring for a mentally retarded child. Recent research on the contribution of family functioning and coping mechanisms to specific child and family outcomes demonstrates that family typologies can be developed that may be equally useful in explaining variability in family outcomes for families served by family support programs (Mink, Meyers, & Nihira, 1984; Mink, Nihira, & Meyers, 1983). Thus, the development of family support programs represents a significant advance for both social policy considerations on publicly financed support for potentially vulnerable families and for research investigating the impact of external resources and services on family functioning.

REFERENCES

Baker, B. L. (1984). Intervention with families with young, severely handicapped children. In J. Blacher (Ed.), Severely handicapped young children and their families: Research in review (pp. 319–375). Orlando, FL: Academic Press.

Berger, M., & Foster, M. (1976). Family-level interventions for retarded children: A multivariate approach to issues and strategies. Multivariate Experimental Clinical Research, 2, 1–21.

Blacher, J. (Ed.) (1984). Severely handicapped young children and their families: Research in review. Orlando, FL: Academic Press.

Braddock, D., Howes, R., & Hemp, R. (1984). A summary of mental retardation and developmental disabilities expenditures in the United States: FY/1977–1984. (preliminary working data). (Public Policy Monograph Series No. 3). Chicago: Institute for the Study of Developmental Disabilities, The University of Illinois at Chicago.

Bruininks, R. H. (1979). The needs of families. In R. H. Bruininks & G. C. Krantz (Eds.), Family care of developmentally disabled members: Conference proceedings. Minneapolis: University of Minnesota.

Bruininks, R. H., & Krantz, G. C. (Eds.). (1979). Family care of developmentally disabled members: Conference preceedings. Minneapolis: University of Minnesota.

Bruininks, R. H., Morreau, L. E., & Williams, S. M. (1979). Issues and problems of deinstitutionalization in HEW region V (Project Report No. 2). Minneapolis: University of Minnesota.

Crnic, K. A., Friedrich, W. N., & Greenberg, M. T. (1983). Adaptation of families with mentally retarded children: A model of stress, coping, and family ecology. American Journal of Mental Deficiency, 88, 125–138.

Darling, R. B. (1979). Families against society: A study of reactions to children with birth defects. Beverly Hills: Sage Publications.

Dickerson, M. U. (1981). Social work practice with the mentally retarded. New York: The Free Press.

Dunlap, W. R. (1976). Services for families of the developmentally disabled. Social Work, 21, 220–223.

Dybwad, G. (1964). Group approaches in working with parents of the retarded: An overview. In G. Dybwad, Challenges in mental retardation (pp. 41–52). New York: Columbia University Press.

Dybwad, G. (1982). The rediscovery of the family. Canadian Journal of Mental Retardation, 32, 18–30.

Eyman, K., Dingman, F., & Sabagh, G. (1966). Association of characteristics of retarded patients and their families with speed of institutionalization. American Journal of Mental Deficiency, 71, 93–99.

Farber, B. (1979). Sociological ambivalence and family care. In R. H. Bruininks & G. C. Krantz, (Eds.), Family care of developmentally disabled members: Conference proceedings (pp. 27–36). Minneapolis: University of Minnesota.

Featherstone, H. (1980). A difference in the family. New York: Basic Books.

Friedrich, W. N., & Friedrich, W. L. (1981). Comparison of psycho-social assets of parents with a handicapped child and their normal controls. American Journal of Mental Deficiency, 85, 551–553.

Gelman, S. R. (1979). Governmental intrusiveness in the family: A continuing dilemma. Children and Youth Services Review, 1, 147–175.

Gollay, E., Freedman, R., Wyngaarden, M., & Kurtz, N. (1978). Coming back: The community experiences of deinstitutionalized mentally retarded people. Cambridge, MA: Abt Books.

Gruber, A. R. (1978). *Children in foster care*. New York: Human Science Press.

Herman, S. E. (1983). *Family support services: Report on meta-evaluation study*. Lansing, MI: Michigan Department of Mental Health.

Horejsi, C. R. (1979). Social and psychological factors in family care. In R. H. Bruininks & G. C. Krantz (Eds.), *Family care of developmentally disabled members: Conference proceedings* (pp. 13–24). Minneapolis: University of Minnesota.

Human Services Research Institute. (1984). *Supporting families with developmentally disabled members: review of the literature and results of a national survey*. Boston: Author.

Justice, R. S., O'Connor, G., & Warren, N. (1971). Problems reported by parents of mentally retarded children—Who helps? *American Journal of Mental Deficiency, 75*, 685–691.

Kammeyer, K., & Bolton, C. (1968). Community and family factors related to the use of a family service agency. *Journal of Marriage and the Family, 30*, 488–498.

Kazak, A. E., & Marvin, R. S. (1984). Differences, difficulties and adaptation: Stress and social networks in families with a handicapped child. *Family Relations, 33*, 67–77.

Klerman, L. V. (1983). Adolescent mothers and their children: Another population that requires family care. In R. Perlman (Ed.), *Family home care: Critical issues for services and policies* (pp. 111–128). New York: Haworth Press.

Lakin, K. C., Bruininks, R. H., Doth, O., Hill, B., & Hauber, F. (1982). *Sourcebook on long-term care for developmentally disabled people*. Minneapolis: University of Minnesota.

Lakin, K. C., Greenberg, J. N., Schmitz, M. P., & Hill, B. K. (1984). A comparison of Medicaid waiver applications for populations that are mentally retarded and elderly/disabled. *Mental Retardation, 22*, 182–192.

Longo, O. C., & Bond, L. (1984). Families of the handicapped child: Research and practice. *Family Relations, 33*, 57–65.

MacEachron, A. E., & Krauss, M. W. (1983). A national survey of handicapped children receiving public social services: Prevalence rates and service patterns in 1977. *Children and Youth Services Review, 3*, 117–134.

Massie, R., & Massie, S. (1975). *Journey*. New York: Alfred A. Knopf.

Maybanks, S., & Bryce, M. (Eds.) (1979). *Home-based services for children and families*. Springfield, IL: Charles C Thomas.

McCubbin, H. I. (1979). Integrating coping behavior in family stress theory. *Journal of Marriage and the Family, 41*, 237–244.

McCubbin, H. I., Joy, C. B., Cauble, A. E., Comeau, J. K., Patterson, J. M., & Needle, R. H. (1980). Family stress and coping: A decade review. *Journal of Marriage and the Family, 42*, 855–871.

McCubbin, H. I., McCubbin, M. A., Patterson, J. M., Cauble, A. E., Wilson, L. R., & Warwick, W. (1983). CHIP—Coping health inventory for parents: An assessment of parental coping patterns in the care of the chronically ill child. *Journal of Marriage and the Family, 45*, 359–370.

Michigan Association of Community Mental Health Boards. (1983). *Family support services: A nationwide*

resource guide. Lansing, MI: Michigan State Planning Council for Developmental Disabilities, Michigan Department of Mental Health.

Mink, I. T., Meyers, C. E., & Nihira, K. (1984). Taxonomy of family life styles: II. Homes with slow-learning children. *American Journal of Mental Deficiency, 89*, 111–123.

Mink, I. T., Nihira, K. & Meyers, C. E. (1983). Taxonomy of family life styles: I. Homes with TMR children. *American Journal of Mental Deficiency, 87*, 484–497.

Minnesota State Planning Agency. (1975). *CAIR: Community Alternatives and Institutional Reform*. St. Paul, MN: Author.

Moroney, R. M. (1979). Allocation of resources for family care. In R. H. Bruininks & G. C. Krantz (Eds.), *Family care of developmentally disabled members: Conference proceedings* (pp. 63–76). Minneapolis: University of Minnesota.

Moroney, R. M. (1981). Mental disability: The role of the family. In J. J. Bevilacqua (Ed.), *Changing government policies for the mentally disabled*. Cambridge, MA: Ballinger Press.

Moroney, R. M. (1983). Families, care of the handicapped, and public policy. In R. Perlman (Ed.), *Family home care: Critical issues for services and policies* (pp. 188–212). New York: Haworth Press.

New York State Office of Mental Retardation and Developmental Disabilities. (1984). *A Survey of Family Support Programs in Seventeen States*. Albany, NY: Author.

Olson, O., & McCubbin, H. I. (1983). *Families: What makes them work*. Beverly Hills: Sage Publishers.

Park, C. C. (1967). *The siege*. Boston: Little, Brown & Co.

Perlman, R., & Giele, J. Z. (1983). An unstable triad: Dependents' demands, family resources, community supports. In R. Perlman (Ed.), *Family home care: Critical issues for services and policies* (pp. 12–44). New York: Haworth Press.

Rosenau, N. (1983). *Final evaluation of family support program*. Macomb-Oakland, MI: Macomb-Oakland Regional Center.

Schilling, R. F., Gilchrist, L. O., & Schinke, S. P. (1984). Coping and social support in families of developmentally disabled children. *Family Relations, 33*, 47–54.

Schilling, R. F., & Schinke, S. P. (1983). Social support networks in developmental disabilities. In J. K. Whittaker & J. Garbarino (Eds.), *Social support networks: Informal helping in the human services* (pp. 383–404). New York: Aldine Publishing Co.

Seltzer, M. M., & Krauss, M. W. (1984a). Family, community residence, and institutional placements of a sample of mentally retarded children. *American Journal of Mental Deficiency, 80*, 257–266.

Seltzer, M. M., & Krauss, M. W. (1984b). Placement alternatives for mentally retarded children and their families. In J. Blacher (Ed.), *Severely handicapped young children and their families: Research in review* (pp. 143–175). Orlando, FL: Academic Press.

Sherman, B. R., & Cocozza, J. J. (1984). Stress in families of the developmentally disabled: A literature review of factors affecting the decision to seek out-of-home placements. *Family Relations, 33*, 95–103.

Skarnulis, E. (1979). Support, not supplant, the natural

home: Serving handicapped children and adults. In S. Maybanks & M. Bryce (Eds.), *Home-based services for children and families* (pp. 64–76). Springfield, IL: Charles C Thomas.

Skrtic, T., Summers, J. A., Brotherson, M. J., & Turnbull, A. P. (1984). Severely handicapped children and their brothers and sisters. In J. Blacher (Ed.), *Severely handicapped young children and their families: Research in review* (pp. 215–246). Orlando, FL: Academic Press.

Steiner, G. Y. (1981). *The futility of family policy.* Washington, DC: The Brookings Institution.

Suelzle, M., & Keenan, V. (1981). Changes in family support networks over the life cycle of mentally retarded persons. *American Journal of Mental Deficiency, 86,* 267–274.

Tapper, H. (1979). Barriers to a family subsidy program. In R. H. Bruininks & G. C. Krantz (Eds.), *Family care of developmentally disabled members: Conference proceedings* (pp. 79–84). Minneapolis: University of Minnesota.

Townsend, P. W., & Flanagan, J. J. (1976). Experimental preadmission program to encourage home care for severely and profoundly retarded children. *American Journal of Mental Deficiency, 80,* 562–569.

Turnbull, A. P., Brotherson, M. J., & Summers, J. A.

(1985). The impact of deinstitutionalization on families: A family systems approach. In R. H. Bruininks & K. C. Lakin (Eds.), *Living and learning in the least restrictive environment* (pp. 115–140). Baltimore: Paul H. Brookes Publishing Co.

Turnbull, A. P., & Turnbull, H. R. (Eds.). (1984). *Parents speak out: Views from the other side of the two-way mirror* (2nd ed). Columbus, OH: Charles Merrill Co.

Upshur, C. C. (1982). An evaluation of home-based respite care. *Mental Retardation, 20,* 58–62.

Wikler, L. (1981). Chronic stresses of families of mentally retarded children. *Family Relations, 30,* 281–288.

Wikler, L., Wasow, M., & Hatfield, E. (1981). Chronic sorrow revisited: Attitudes of parents and professionals about adjustment to mental retardation. *American Journal of Orthopsychiatry, 51,* 63–70.

Zimmerman, S. L. (1979). Families of the developmentally disabled: Implications for research and the planning and provision of services. In R. H. Bruininks & G. C. Krantz (Eds.), *Family care of developmentally disabled members: Conference proceedings* (pp. 87–94). Minneapolis: University of Minnesota.

Zimmerman, S. L. (1984). The mental retardation family subsidy program: Its effects on families with a mentally handicapped child. *Family Relations, 33,* 105–118.

Section
IV

PROGRAMS
AND POLICY ISSUES

Chapter

14

Applications of Family Therapy Theory to Research and Interventions with Families with Mentally Retarded Children

Michael Berger and Martha Foster

RESEARCHERS AND interventionists interested in families with mentally retarded persons need to understand how families function, how they change, and how they are affected by intervention efforts. This chapter is an attempt to bring the conceptualizations of family therapy theory to bear on the question of how best to understand and evaluate the effects of interventions on families with mentally retarded children. In the authors' view, because the family therapy literature offers the most comprehensive thinking at present both about how to change families and how families are affected by intervention (Gurman & Kniskern, 1978, 1981), it is worthwhile to translate this literature for interventionists and researchers concerned with families with mentally retarded persons. Following a discussion of the conceptualizations of family therapy theory with regard to families in general, content areas specific to families with mentally retarded persons are considered; the chapter concludes with

methodological and substantive recommendations for future research.

ASSUMPTIONS OF FAMILY THERAPY

A central assumption of this literature is that families are mutually interactive systems organized in such a way that a change in one part of the system is likely to result in other changes in other parts of the system. Minuchin (1974) puts this elegantly in his description of the web of interconnections between the individual and the family; the same assumption holds for the interconnections between any other subsystem within the family (e.g., spouses, siblings, parents) and the family as a whole, or between any two subsystems in the family.

> The individual influences his context and is influenced by it in constantly recurring sequences of interaction. The individual who lives within a family is a member of a social system to which he must adapt. His actions are governed by the characteristics of the systems and these characteristics

include the effects of his own past actions. The individual responds to stresses in other parts of the system to which he adapts; and he may contribute significantly to stressing other members of the system. The individual can be approached as a subsystem, or part, of the system, but the whole must be taken into account. (p. 9)

This assumption has two important implications for the study of the effects of interventions on families. First, it is arbitrary to assume that an intervention into a subsystem of the family only affects that subsystem. This is, however, a common assumption in intervention research with handicapped children, a literature that most often only assesses the effects of a given treatment on the target child and assumes that the treatment will have no significant effects (positive or negative) on other family members (Bailey & Simeonsson, 1983; Foster & Berger, 1985). Indeed, family therapy theorists would regard such an assumption as not only arbitrary but also as likely to be wrong (Montalvo & Haley, 1973).

Second, in order to change families or members of a family effectively, it is necessary to conceptualize or map family structure so that it is clear which aspects of family structure are maintaining the problem that requires treatment (Bowen, 1978; Haley, 1976; Minuchin, 1974). Hierarchy and boundaries are central concepts used in this literature to conceptualize family structure.

Hierarchy (see Haley, 1976, for a detailed discussion of this concept) refers to the fact that well-functioning families seem to have clear rules about: 1) how decisions are made and, if necessary, altered and 2) which family members or subsystems have the authority to make decisions that are binding on other family members or subsystems. In this culture, family hierarchies tend to be age-graded; that is, adults have the authority to regulate the behavior of young children, whereas young children lack the authority to control their parents' actions. Attention to the hierarchy of the family has, thus far, proved important because the presence and severity of family dysfunction have been linked to the presence of coalitions across hierarchical levels—between, for ex-

ample, a symptomatic child and one parent against another parent, or between a young adult and her grandparents against her parents (Haley, 1976, 1980; Madanes, 1981; Minuchin, 1974; Minuchin, Rosman, & Baker, 1978; Stanton, Todd, and associates, 1982).

Boundaries (see Minuchin, 1974, for a detailed exploration of this concept) concern the rules defining which members of the family can participate in a given subsystem and how they can participate. For example, spouses commonly treat each other in ways that they would not usually treat either their children or their own parents. Similarly, siblings commonly share activities with one another from which they wish to exclude their parents.

Examples of important family subsystems are the spouse subsystem, the parental subsystem (which includes all persons in the family who have responsibility for taking care of children), the sibling subsystem, and the individual subsystem (Minuchin & Fishman, 1981). Because different kinds of competencies are elicited in the different subsystems, it is to the advantage of family members that all these subsystems be able to function. A common dysfunction in this regard occurs in families in which parents are so focused on children that they rarely treat one another as spouses. The frequent habit of one spouse calling the other "Mother, or "Father," rather than by name is an index of how pervasively the spouse subsystem can be dominated by the parental subsystem even though, within a given family, the two subsystems often have the same membership.

In order for all different subsystems to function, subsystem boundaries must be sufficiently clear to permit subsystem members to carry out their functions without undue interference; to allow, for example, spouses to resolve a marital dispute without the input of grandparents or children, or children to settle a quarrel without parental interference. At the same time, subsystem boundaries must be sufficiently open to allow contact between the members of the subsystems and others.

Minuchin (1974) has described two characteristic styles of family behavior with regard to subsystem boundaries in which rigid interactional patterns prevent a flexible integration of the different subsystems. In what he terms the "enmeshed" family, boundaries between different subsystems are nonexistent or are very vague. Transactions between family members are rarely completed because subsystems are subject to frequent interruption from other family members and because there is little agreement about the legitimate authority of any subsystem. Thus, a daughter who has concerns about appropriate dating behavior may not know whether she can talk to her mother, her sister, her grandmother, or anyone about these concerns. Because of the lack of clear subsystem boundaries, it is difficult to tell who is occupying which family role. By contrast, in disengaged families, subsystem boundaries are so rigid that it is nearly impossible to initiate collaborative action across the boundaries. In such families, a child's difficulty may have to escalate to crisis proportions before parents will respond to it. In such families, members inhabit the same physical space, but it is difficult to see how they are connected.

The authors have stressed the issue of rigid family patterns because such patterns have been shown to be associated with the presence and severity of family dysfunction. To give two examples, rigidly enmeshed behavior has been demonstrated to be associated with the presence of a psychosomatically ill child in the family and with the presence of a heroin addict in a family (Minuchin et al., 1978; Stanton et al., 1982).

It is important to keep in mind, however, that neither of the rigid types of family patterns thus described is pathological in and of itself (Minuchin, 1974). Rather, what seems to characterize pathological family behavior is the continued repetition, even in the face of possibilities of change, of the same familial patterns; that is, under stress, enmeshed families become more enmeshed, whereas disengaged families become more disengaged (Bowen, 1978; Minuchin, 1974; Reiss, 1980). Many family therapy theorists, therefore, rather than talking about pathological and nonpathological family styles, distinguish between rigid and flexible family behavior, arguing that, although a number of different family styles are well adapted to particular situations, families are better off if they have a wide range of behavioral patterns and flexibility in using these patterns (Lewis, Beavers, Gossett, & Phillips, 1976; Minuchin, 1974; Reiss, 1980). It is important to recognize also that "normal" families exhibit a very wide and diverse range of behavior (Lewis et al., 1976; McGoldrick, Giordano, & Pearce, 1982; Reiss, 1980; Walsh, 1982).

Finally, two other aspects of family functioning also deserve mention. One is the degree to which families are able to solve problems successfully. Successful problem resolution in families seems to involve the ability of family members to obtain information relevant to the problem, to share that information with other family members, and to tolerate and resolve differences of opinion between family members (Reiss, 1980). With regard to problem solving, one point seems especially relevant to families with a mentally retarded child. This is the frequently reported finding that the presence of a symptomatic child in a family is linked with a family pattern in which parents detour conflicts between them by focusing on the symptomatic child (Foster & Berger, 1979; Haley, 1980; Minuchin et al., 1978; Stanton et al., 1982). Family therapists have also found that altering the context within the family in such a way that parents are able to resolve their differences without focusing on the dysfunctional child results in improvement in the child.

The second aspect is the quality of affect pervasive in the family. A number of studies have shown that the lack of positive affect between family members is associated with family dysfunction (Alexander, 1973; Lewis et al., 1976; Patterson, Reid, Jones, and Conger, 1975). In addition, other studies have shown that, as chronic anxiety increases in a family system, the ability of family members to think clearly and solve problems decreases and the amount of dysfunction in the family system increases (Bowen, 1978; Reiss, 1980).

Thus far, family structure and family functioning have been discussed as if families were static entities.[1] Rather, families are continually pressed to change their patterns of organization. Demands for family change arise both from outside the family (as when professionals indicate that a handicapped adult is now capable of living independently and the parental subsystem must change to accommodate to this increased competence) and from inside the family (when changes in the developmental competence of family members requires the alteration of family rules and subsystem boundaries to allow, for example, more autonomy for adolescents). Recognition that families face constant demands for changes in their organization has focused attention on the notion of the family life cycle, a schema designed to take account of predictable changes in families—changes in membership, family roles, and family tasks (Carter & McGoldrick, 1980; Haley, 1973). Indeed, a number of recent studies have suggested that symptoms in a family member or problems within a family are more likely to arise at difficult transition points in this family life cycle (Bowen, 1978; Carter & McGoldrick, 1980; Hadley, Jacob, Milliones, Caplan, & Spitz, 1974; Haley, 1973, 1980; Hughes, Berger, & Wright, 1978; Walsh, 1978).

To this point, the family has also been characterized as a closed system, isolated from other systems, such as its social network of extended family, neighbors, and friends (Bott, 1971); the network of service systems involved with family members (Hoffman & Long, 1969); or the community. This is, of course, not so. It is more accurate to view the family as part of a complex of interconnected living systems ranging from the biological to the sociocultural (Berger & Jurkovic, 1984; Scheflen, 1980; Spiegel, 1971). Two larger systems are particularly important for families with a mentally retarded child: the family social network and the network of helping agencies. As Berger and Fowlkes (1980) note:

The family social network is the largest group of persons easily accessible to the family of the handicapped child. Further, the network is the group of people with whom family members have the most contact and who have the greatest importance for family members. Most importantly, network members care for family members as people rather than as "the family of a handicapped child." Finally, the network is the group most likely to offer the family the resources it needs, both in terms of direct assistance (e.g., money, babysitting, emotional support) and of indirect assistance (obtaining contacts with persons or institutions known to network members). (p. 23)

Families with a mentally retarded child are likely also to be intensely involved with a number of different service systems because they are unlikely to possess the resources necessary to provide all the training, equipment, and care that such children require in order to develop as normally as possible. Thus, in order to support the development of their child, these families must learn to deal successfully with a number of service agencies. Often, families need to deal with service agencies on an ongoing basis, and often, service agencies function in such a way that it is difficult for families to obtain the services they need (Darling, 1979; Gorham, Des Jardins, Page, Pettis, & Schieber, 1975; Schwartz, 1970). Thus, an important aspect of the functioning of families with a mentally retarded child, an aspect that merits study, is the family's involvement with service agencies (Berger, 1984a; Foster, Berger, & McLean, 1981).

IMPLICATIONS OF FAMILY THERAPY THEORY FOR FAMILIES WITH A MENTALLY RETARDED CHILD

The single most important implication of family therapy theory for intervening with families with a mentally retarded child is the recogni-

---

[1]Over the past decade, family sociologists and demographers have also called attention to the fact that family structures are changing as a result of the increased frequency of divorce and remarriage and changes in the work patterns and child-bearing patterns of women in our culture. Therefore, the notion of "family" in America has become more heterogeneous, complex, and less predictable.

tion that it is impossible to separate interventions aimed at a child from interventions specifically targeted at families: Any intervention with a family member is a family intervention (Montalvo & Haley, 1973). Specifically, this suggests that interventions targeted at individual children need to have a dual focus; namely, what is the effect of the intervention on the child, and what is the effect of the intervention on family structure?

The two-fold focus is particularly necessary if child interventions are not to be iatrogenic; that is, if they are not themselves to be the cause of family difficulty. For example, because early intervention programs for retarded children tend to equate parent involvement with mother involvement (Berger, 1984b; Foster et al., 1981; Turnbull & Turnbull, 1982), it is a not uncommon occurrence for such programs to intensify the closeness in what is already an overly enmeshed mother-child dyad. At times, in such cases, intervention that increases the closeness in the mother-child dyad may also result in greater distance between father and the handicapped child, or between the parents, or between the mother and the other siblings for whom she has less time and energy because of the amount of effort she is spending on the handicapped child (Berger, 1984b; Foster et al., 1979; Harris, 1982).

A dual focus is also necessary for situations in which interventionists intend to work with children in families where family structure is already dysfunctional. For example, in some families, a triangular interactional pattern is created in which parental conflict is detoured and avoided through a focus on the retarded child. This concentrated focus on the child can result in the child remaining more dependent on parents than is warranted by his or her skills. For example, intervention efforts to enable the child to behave more independently at school may fail because a change in the child threatens an established, although maladaptive, family pattern of relating. In short, in families where family structure is dysfunctional, it will be necessary to intervene to change the dysfunctional family patterns in order for the child to benefit.

Content Areas Specific to Families with a Mentally Retarded Child

Because of the paucity of both longitudinal studies of families with mentally retarded children and of comparative studies of families with mentally retarded children and families with "normal" children, it is difficult to know precisely what content areas are especially important to families with a mentally retarded child. However, this section considers some issues that a number of research studies have identified as important.

Social Network Contraction Several studies have found that, following the diagnosis of a handicapping condition, such as mental retardation, parents frequently reduce or cut off contact with members of their social network (Davis, 1967; Farber, 1968; Holt, 1958; Kearns, 1978). This contraction of the family's social network is likely to lead to an increased sense of social isolation for family members that, in turn, increases the family's focus on the handicapped child, making it more likely that the child will become a target for parental anxiety and concern. Reducing contact with the family social network also has the effect of establishing a feedback loop in which initial isolation leads to additional isolation as family members find it more and more difficult to explain the handicapping condition to family members and to explain why the family has withdrawn from the network. In the extreme case, the family ceases to have extended contact with persons who are not connected with the handicapped child, limiting its contact to service providers and parents of similarly handicapped children.

Network contraction is a matter that deserves serious attention from both interventionists and researchers because a number of studies (German & Maisto, 1982; Wortis & Margolies, 1955) have shown that support from the family social network is associated with better adjustment in families with a mentally retarded child.

Need for Assistance in Meeting Pragmatic Demands Wolfensberger (1967), in his magisterial review of the literature on counseling parents of the mentally retarded, noted that, although parents have repeatedly indicated that their major need was for help in dealing with such pragmatic issues as locating, obtaining, and financing services, babysitters, and respite care, professionals in response offered them therapy. More recent studies have supported Wolfensberger's argument. Thus, a critical area for intervention with families with mentally retarded children is the issue of obtaining pragmatic help for tasks of daily living. As noted earlier, one important aspect of this matter concerns dealing with service agencies. Because of the fragmented nature of our service delivery systems, parents (generally mothers) often have to do a huge amount of unpaid work in order to obtain sufficient and coordinated services for their retarded child (Gorham et al., 1975; Schwartz, 1970). Intervention that would increase family members' ability to deal with service agencies (for one such program, see Muir, Milan, McLean, & Berger, 1982) would therefore seem useful. Also useful, in terms of evaluating the effects of interventions on families, would be an assessment of whether the intervention has increased family members' sense of conpetence vis-a-vis service agencies. Wahler (1980) has recently suggested that parental incompetence is linked both to social isolation (thus again suggesting the importance of maintaining social network contact and involvement) and to the perception that contact with service agencies is aversive for the parent.

Time-Limited Concerns A particular time of likely stress for families with mentally retarded children is immediately after the diagnosis of retardation has been given to the family (Wolfensberger, 1967). Other studies have suggested that families with a handicapped child who adjust well to the presence of the child in the family decrease the intensity of their involvement with their child over time (Darling, 1979; Reiss, 1980). Initially following the diagnosis of the handicapping condition, these families are intensely involved with the child. This is a period in which family members are very concerned with understanding the ramifications of the child's handicap,

with constructing an explanation of the origin of the handicapping condition, with interpreting the handicapping condition to other members of the social network, and with obtaining services for the child. However, there then follows a period of consolidation in which the child is obtaining services and family members lessen the intensity of their focus on the child. The authors describe this process because often intervention projects that, of necessity, begin work with families at a particular point in time may misread a time of lessened parental involvement with the child as meaning that the parents do not care for the child. Such misreading may lead to interventionists pushing the parents to become more involved again with the child. If successful, these efforts may have the unfortunate result of reinstating a family pattern that, although previously adaptive, may now be dysfunctional for the family and will hamper the efforts of family members to continue to change (Berger, 1984b; Foster & Berger, 1979; Foster, et al., 1981).

In short, the predictable tasks, problems, and resources available to families in handling these tasks change over time (Berger, 1982; Suelzle & Keenan, 1981; Wikler, 1981). Thus, the interventions that are most helpful to families with a mentally retarded child at one point in time may not be helpful at another time. Similarly, a family structure that is functional at one point in time (for example, a structure in which a mother is intensely involved with a handicapped infant) may be dysfunctional at another point in time (for example, a structure in which a mother remains as intensely involved with a handicapped adolescent). What are needed, therefore, are intervention efforts and research studies that attend both to the changing needs of families over time and to the resources available to families for meeting these changing needs (Kearns & Berger, 1980).

RECOMMENDATIONS

Interventions will be more intelligent if they are based on a comprehensive understanding of clients; therefore, better descriptive, normative research on families with a mentally retarded member is needed. Although the published literature with this population is extensive, there is a lack of controlled, comparative studies; of longitudinal investigations; and of research with families with older and grown children. In addition, the majority of available descriptive studies have been conducted from an essentially individualistic perspective in that the level of analysis has been an individual family member's behavior or perception of the family (most often, that of the mother) (Foster & Berger, 1985; Wolfensberger, 1967).

The perception of an individual is a questionable vantage point from which to study families for several reasons. First, we know that reported and actual behavior are not congruent. Moreover, systems theorists remind us that information about an individual who is part of a system is not valid information about the total system (Scheflen, 1980; Spiegel, 1971). Therefore, one family member's self-report is not an appropriate measure of family affect, function, or structure. The authors are aware of only two observational studies of whole family interaction (Corrales, Kostoryz, Ro-Trock, & Smith, 1983; O'Connor & Stachowiak, 1971), although the research literature on mother-child interaction is somewhat more developed (e.g., Cunningham, Reuler, Blackwell, & Deck, 1981; Kogan, 1980; Terdal, Jackson, & Garner, 1976). The field of mental retardation is not unique in this regard. Except for research with families with an emotionally disturbed member (Jacob, 1975), observational studies of whole family interaction are sparse with other populations as well. Lastly, to the reader of the "family" literature in mental retardation, the number of inconsistencies in findings among different studies is striking. The diversity in findings in the research on siblings' relationships is but one example (Simeonsson & McHale, 1981). To untangle these contradictions, better specification of family characteristics (e.g., demographic factors, family structure, life-cycle stage) and context or setting characteristics (e.g., family's access to and utlization of services) is needed. Multivariate methods that address the interaction among

individual, family, and context variables are the best route for obtaining the kind of specific data about families needed by interventionists.

In terms of intervention research, the authors' major recommendation is that researchers should employ designs that allow for the assessment of the impact of treatments on family members and family subsystems beyond the immediate target of intervention. Medical or educational treatments designed to enhance child functioning may have concomitant positive or negative impact on the marital or sibling subsystems. Although examples from early intervention work were offered above, medical regimes, such as diet programs or physical therapy, also may affect the family system. Conversely, for interventions aimed more directly at parents, such as parenting skills programs or counseling groups, the impact of these on family structure, on the retarded child, and on the siblings should be considered. Although obviously all possible family subsystems cannot be monitored for every intervention, Gurman and Kniskern (1981) offer some guidelines for assigning priority to the assessment of treatment outcomes within different family subsystems. Although their recommendations are directed toward research in marital and family therapy, the authors think they are applicable to any intervention study.

The assessment of the impact of treatment at multiple levels in the family is particularly important because of the need to chart negative as well as positive outcomes. "Deterioration" effects are recognized and studied among psychotherapy researchers (Bergin, 1978), but have received little attention in mental retardation intervention and research.

Second, the diversity among families receiving interventions creates difficulties in matching groups for outcome research. More single-subject designs are needed, as well as greater use of multivariate designs and statistical methods that permit the assessment of the relative contribution of different variables to treatment outcomes.

Third, with any intervention impact study with families, the nature of the treatment needs to be clearly specified. Too many studies have reported vague, global, or unclear descriptions of interventions with families so that it is difficult to determine precisely the nature of the treatment. This concern is nicely discussed by Bailey and Simeonsson (1983) in a recent review of the literature on the impact of early intervention on families. Treatment in the human services fields typically involves the actions of a person interacting with the target of intervention to bring about change. Although specific techniques may be employed (e.g., behavior modification, physical therapy regimes, parent education curricula), these are always mediated by a person or persons. Consequently, the characteristics of the intervenor become a component of the treatment. The question of the impact on treatment outcome of the personal characteristics of the intervenor is a complex and yet unanswered one in intervention research generally. The best source of information about this dimension of treatment is the psychotherapy research literature (Parloff, Waskow, & Wolfe, 1978). Here, at least, such nonspecific factors characterizing the person of the therapist as understanding, respect, interest, encouragement, and acceptance have been found to be as powerful as specific techniques in the determination of treatment outcome.

In general, the psychotherapy research literature offers useful guidelines for intervention research with families with mentally retarded members. Standard operating procedures in this field include:

(1) the study of interactive effects of patient, therapist, treatment, and setting variables; (2) the use

of multidimensional measures of change; (3) the use of multiple vantage points for assessing change (i.e., the assessment of treatment effects, for example, by the consumer, the intervenor, and the researcher); and (4) the use of repeated measures to assess both levels and patterns of change across time. (Gurman, 1983)

This literature can teach us that the meaningful question about intervention outcome is not whether a given treatment works or does not work in a global sense, but rather which specific interventions produce which specific changes in which specific clients under which specific conditions (Paul, 1969).

Lastly, because of the difficulties of large-scale intervention research, the authors think there is considerable merit in collaborative research efforts aimed at pooling data on family interventions across research settings. (The current National Institute of Mental Health collaborative study on depression is an example of this type of enterprise.) The mechanics of such endeavors are organizationally difficult, and they entail precise specification of both family and treatment characteristics and the use of common dependent measures. Moreover, one must be alert to the need to adjust probability estimates if multiple significance tests are performed on the same set of data. However, because the issue of generalization remains a haunting one in mental retardation intervention research, collaborative endeavors that offer the opportunity to study both the generalizability of treatment across settings and the effects of specific treatments on specific family types are particularly attractive.

REFERENCES

Alexander, J. F. (1973). Defensive and supportive communication in normal and deviant families. *Journal of Consulting and Clinical Psychology, 40*, 223–231.

Bailey, D., & Simeonsson, R. (1983, March). *Evaluating the impact of early intervention on families with severely handicapped children: Design issues.* Paper presented at the Conference on Evaluating Early Intervention, Vanderbilt University, Nashville, TN.

Berger, M. (1982). The tasks of the therapists with a family with a handicapped person. In A. Gurman (Ed.), *Questions and answers in the practice of family therapy,* Vol. 2. New York: Brunner/Mazel.

Berger, M. (1984a). Social network interventions with families who have a handicapped child. In E. I. Coopersmith (Ed.), *Family therapy with families with handicapped children* (pp. 127–137). Rockville, MD: Aspen.

Berger, M. (1984b). Systems therapy in special education settings. In M. Berger & G. Jurkovic (Eds.), *Family therapy in context* (pp. 142–179). San Francisco: Jossey-Bass.

Berger, M., & Fowlkes, M. (1980). The Family Intervention Project: A family network approach to early intervention. *Young Children, 35,* 22–32.

Berger, M., & Jurkovic, G. (Eds.). (1984). *Family therapy in context: The practice of systemic therapy in community settings.* San Francisco: Jossey-Bass.

Bergin, A. F. (1978). The evaluation of therapeutic outcomes. In S. Garfield & A. Bergin (Eds.), *Handbook of psychotherapy and behavior change: An empirical analysis* (pp. 217–270). New York: Wiley.

Bott, E. (1971). *Family and social network.* New York: Macmillan.

Bowen, M. (1978). *Family therapy and clinical practice: The collected papers of Murray Bowen, M.D.* New York: Aronson.

Carter, E., & McGoldrick, M. (Eds.) (1980). *The family life cycle.* Long Island, NY: Gardner.

Corrales, R., Kostoryz, J., Ro-Trock, L., & Smith, B. (1983). Family therapy with developmentally delayed children: An ecosystemic approach. In D. Bagarozzi, A. Jurich, & R. Jackson (Eds.), *Marital and family therapy: New perspectives in theory, research, and practice.* New York: Human Sciences Press.

Cunningham, O. E., Reuler, E., Blackwell, J., & Deck, J. (1981). Behavioral and linguistic developments in the interaction of normal and retarded children with their mothers. *Child Development, 52,* 1, 62–70.

Darling, R. (1979). *Families against society.* New York: Sage.

Davis, F. (1967). Family process in mental retardation. *American Journal of Psychiatry, 124,* 3, 96–106.

Farber, B. (1968). *Mental retardation: Its social context and social consequences.* Boston: Houghton Mifflin.

Foster, M., & Berger, M. (1979). Structural family therapy: Applications in programs for preschool handicapped children. *Journal of the Division of Early Childhood, 1,* 52–58.

Foster, M., & Berger, M. (1985). Families with handicapped children. In L. L'Abate (Ed.) *Handbook of family psychology.* Irvington, MA: Dow-Irwin.

Foster, M., Berger, M., & McLean, M. (1981). Rethinking a good idea: A reassessment of parent involvement. *Topics in Early Childhood Special Education, 1,* 55–65.

German, M. L., & Maisto, A. A. (1982). The relationship of a perceived family support system and the institutional placement of mentally retarded children. *Education and Training of the Mentally Retarded,17,* 1, 17–23.

Gorham, K., Des Jardins, C., Page, R., Pettis, E., & Scheiber, B. (1975). Effect on parents. In N. Hobbs (Ed.) *Issues in the classification of children,* Vol. 2 (pp. 154–188). San Francisco: Jossey-Bass.

Gurman, A. (1983). Family therapy research and the "new epistomology." *Journal of Marital and Family Therapy, 9*(3), 227–234.

Gurman, A., & Kniskern, D. (1978). Research on marital and family therapy: Progress, prospective, and prospect. In S. Garfield & A. Bergin (Eds.), *Handbook of psychotherapy and behavior change: An empirical analysis.* New York: Wiley.

Gurman, A., & Kniskern, D. (Eds.) (1981). *Handbook of family therapy.* New York: Brunner/Mazel.

Hadley, T., Jacob, T., Milliones, J., Caplan, J., & Spitz, D. (1974). The relationship between family developmental crisis and the appearance of a symptom in a family member. *Family Process, 13,* 207–214.

Haley, J. (1973). *Uncommon therapy.* New York: Norton.

Haley, J. (1976). *Problem solving therapy.* San Francisco: Jossey-Bass.

Haley, J. (1980). *Leaving home.* New York: McGraw-Hill.

Howard, J. (1978). The influence of children's developmental dysfunctions on marital quality and family interaction. In R. M. Lerner & G. B. Spanier (Eds.), *Child influences on marital and family interaction* (pp. 275–298). New York: Academic Press.

Hughes, S. F., Berger, M., & Wright, L. (1978). The family life cycle and clinical intervention. *Journal of Marriage and Family Counseling, 44,* 33–40.

Jacob, T. (1975). Family interaction in disturbed and normal families: An empirical and substantive review. *Psychological Bulletin, 22,* 33–65.

Kearns, D. (1978). Social networks of parents of the mentally retarded: Characteristics and influences on family functioning. Masters Thesis. Department of Psychology, Wichita State University, Wichita, KS.

Kearns, D., & Berger, M. (1980). Family response to change. *Dimensions, 9*(1), 20–23.

Kogan, K. L. (1980). Interaction systems between preschool handicapped or developmentally delayed children and their parents. In T. M. Field, S. Goldberg, D. Stern, & A. Sostek (Eds.), *High risk infants and children: Adult and peer interactions.* New York: Academic Press.

Lewis, J. M., Beavers, W. R., Gossett, J. T., & Phillips, V. A. (1976). *No single thread: Psychological health in family systems.* New York: Brunner/Mazel.

Madanes, C. (1981). *Strategic family therapy.* San Francisco: Jossey-Bass.

McGoldrick, M., Giordano, J., & Pearce, J. (Eds.). (1982). *Ethnicity and family therapy.* New York: Guilford.

Minuchin, S. (1974). *Families and family therapy.* Cambridge, MA: Harvard University Press.

Minuchin, S., & Fishman, H. (1981). *Family therapy techniques.* Cambridge, MA: Harvard University Press.

Minuchin, S., Rosman, B., & Baker, L. (1978). *Psychosomatic families.* Cambridge, MA: Harvard University Press.

Montalvo, B., & Haley, J. (1973). In defense of child therapy. *Family Process, 12,* 227–244.

Muir, K., Milan, M., McLean, M., & Berger, M. (1982). Advocacy training for parents of handicapped children: A staff responsibility. *Young Children, 36,* 41–46.

O'Connor, W. D., & Stachowiak, J. (1971). Patterns of interaction in families with low-adjusted, high-adjusted, and mentally retarded members. *Family Process, 10,* 229–241.

Parloff, M., Waskow, I., & Wolfe, B. (1978). Research on therapist variables in relationship to process and outcome. In S. Garfield & A. Bergin (Eds.), *Handbook of psychotherapy and behavior change* (2nd ed.). New York: John Wiley & Sons.

Patterson, G. R., Reid, J., Jones, R., & Conger, R. (1975). *A social learning approach to family intervention: Vol. 1. Families with aggressive children.* Eugene, OR: Castalia.

Paul, G. L. (1969). Behavior modification research: Design and tactics. In C. M. Franks (Ed.), *Behavior therapy: Appraisal and status* (pp. 29–62). New York: McGraw-Hill.

Reiss, D. (1980). *The family construction of reality.* Cambridge, MA: Harvard University Press.

Scheflen, A. (1980). *Levels of schizophrenia.* New York: Brunner/Mazel.

Schwartz, C. (1970). Strategies and tactics of mothers of mentally retarded children for dealing with the medical care system. In N. Bernstein (Ed.), *Diminished people*. Boston: Little, Brown.

Simeonssen, R. J., & McHale, S. M. (1981). Research on handicapped children: Sibling relationships. *Child Care: Health, and Development, 7,* 153–171.

Spiegel, J. (1971). *Transactions*. New York: Science House.

Stanton, M. D., Todd, T., & associates. (1982). *The family therapy of drug abuse and addiction*. New York: Guilford.

Suelzle, M., & Keenan, V. (1981). Changes in family support networks over the life cycle of mentally retarded persons. *American Journal of Mental Deficiency, 86,* 267–274.

Terdal, L., Jackson, R., & Garner, A. (1976). Mother-child interactions: A comparison between normal and developmentally delayed groups. In E. J. Mash, L. A. Hamerlynck, & L. C. Handry (Eds.), *Behavior modification and families*. New York: Brunner/Mazel.

Turnbull, H. R., & Turnbull, A. P. (1982). Parent involvement in the education of handicapped children: A critique. *Mental Retardation, 20*(3), 115–122.

Wahler, R. G. (1980). Parent insularity as a determinant of generalization success in family treatment. In S. Salzinger, J. Antrobus, & J. Glick (Eds.), *The ecosystem of the "sick" child*. New York: Academic Press.

Walsh, F. (1978). Concurrent grandparent death and the birth of schizophrenic offspring: An intriguing finding. *Family Process, 17,* 457–463.

Wikler, L. (1981). Chronic stresses of families of mentally retarded children. *Family Relations, 30,* 281–288.

Wolfensberger, W. (1967). Counseling parents of the retarded. In A. Baumeister (Ed.), *Mental retardation: Appraisal, education, rehabilitation*. Chicago: Aldine.

Wortis, H. Z., & Margolies, J. (1955). Parents of children with cerebral palsy. *Medical Social Work, 4,* 110–120.

Chapter

15

Family Roles, Preschool Handicapped Children, and Social Policy

Valora Washington and James J. Gallagher

DURING THE LAST DECADE there has been increasing attention paid to the family that has a member who is handicapped. The presence of a child who is handicapped creates a variety of stressful circumstances that are specifically related to the presence of this atypical member (Gallagher, Beckman, & Cross, 1983).

Yet such families are also affected by larger trends and forces that have an impact on all families in the modern American family. One of the most significant of these changes has been the evolving role of women in the family. It is the purpose of this chapter to focus on the changing status of women in the society, the impact those changes have on the families of young handicapped children, and the range of policy options that might be available to aid such families.

The role of women in our society has changed dramatically in the past 50 years in response to a variety of economic, political, and social influences. Previously, the *nurturant* role of women was firmly based on the fact that women are the childbearers. This orienta-

tion has been altered by three convergent factors: pregnancy control leading to smaller family size, longer life expectancy, and higher female employment rates (Hoffman, 1974). The impact of these basic social changes has been heightened by such short-term factors as economic recessions and the divorce rate—the United States has the highest rate of divorce in the world (Hetherington, 1979). The result is an unprecedented increase in maternal employment rates, a trend that is likely to continue into the 21st century.

There is widespread agreement that the institution of the American family is under a great deal of stress. In order to understand the dynamics of such stress, the authors present a model of family performance, including the allocation of responsibilities in the family. The shift in roles as a result of family crisis is also discussed. Based on this model of family performance, the authors explore the influence of public policy on the family and the surrogate role played by society in aiding the family. Finally, a "decision-matrix" is presented for evaluating some strategies by which government can help families fulfill their child care responsibilities to handicapped children.

For the purpose of this chapter, the family is discussed in generic terms, referring primarily to the traditional nuclear family (two parents and children) and to other family structures as variations of this model.

A MODEL OF FAMILY PERFORMANCE

When any institution as central as the family experiences change and stress, the question is raised about how social policy is influencing, or can influence, the stability and health of that institution. A useful first step in the analysis of changing family roles is to provide a model of family functioning that can provide a basis for explanation and prediction on the nature of family and extra family relationships.

Model Assumptions

1. The family is a dynamic interacting social system designed so that individual members perform distinctive tasks and responsibilities that increase the likelihood of social adaptation to the larger society for each of the family members.
2. The allocation of responsibilities and duties changes as the partners age and as their children mature.

3. If there is chronic manifest dissatisfaction in the division or exercise of these responsibilities, the family system can dissolve.
4. If there is too much external or internal stress on the family, its members can become inefficient and nonfunctional.

Allocation of Responsibilities

For the purposes of this model, the major functions and activities of the family are comprised of nine responsibilities that are allocated in a distinctive fashion by each family unit and its related social linkages. These functions are represented in Table 1, together with the typical allocation of responsibilities by the nuclear family and the societal supports that supplement or supplant these functions. The extended family is a potential source of assistance in each of these nine areas of responsibility.

1. *Health.* The responsibility to sustain the health of family members has rested primarily on the wife, although there are impressive social institutions outside the family that provide health services.
2. *Protection.* Although protecting the physical safety of the family has been mainly assigned to the husband, much of that responsibility is delegated to the larger society through traditional protection agencies, such as fire and police departments.

Table 1. Typical responsibilities of nuclear family

Area of responsibility	Wife	Trend	Husband	Societal assistance
Health	■		☐	Medical and health services
Protection	☐		■	Police and fire
Breadwinner	☐	←	■	Welfare, social security
Household	■	→	☐	Laundry, service providers
Extrafamily social	■	→	☐	Network of friendships, social clubs, recreation, church
Affective support	■	→	☐	Extended family, neighbors, and friends
Child nurturance	■	→	☐	Day care centers, afterschool programs
Morality, standards	☐		☐	Law, religion
Child instruction	■		☐	Schools

☐ Some responsibility.
■ Major responsibility.
→ Trend.

3. *Breadwinner.* An obvious current trend is for this responsibility to shift somewhat to the wife, although husbands still retain the major responsibility for family income.

4. *Household.* There are a wide variety of responsibilities connected with maintaining a physical living space occupied by the family. These include food preparation and selection, laundry, maintenance of home and equipment, and so forth. The wife has traditionally had the major responsibility for household tasks, but in recent years, social pressure has been placed on the husband to assume some of these duties.

5. *Extrafamily social.* There are a variety of responsibilities representing the formal and informal linkages of the family to the larger society. There appears to be a trend to include husbands in this role, although the major responsibliity is still held by the wife.

6. *Affective support.* Responsibilities for both the sexual and emotional satisfaction derived from positive and supportive relationships is assumed to be still with the wife; current trends seem to place more responsibility on the husband than previously.

7. *Child nurturance.* This role provides continued support of the child through a long period of dependency. Although fathers may have recently increased their involvement in child rearing, the mother clearly takes the major responsibility now, as in the past.

8. *Morality and standards.* This role concerns responsibility for the spoken or unspoken rules of conduct followed by family members within and outside the family. There is often a shared responsibility, with the father setting standards in the outside world and the mother setting standards within the family enclave.

9. *Child instruction.* One role of the family has always been the education of children so that they can take their role in the larger society. The schools obviously play a central role in this responsibility. Instruction

within the home, however, largely rests with the mother, although fathers are sharing more of the responsibility.

Another assumption of the model is that, if there are major disagreements among the family members as to how the roles should be allocated or how well they are being conducted, such disagreements will lead to major tensions within the family. Table 2 indicates some expected relationships based on this model.

The Surrogate Role of Society

One of the major functions of the larger society is to play a surrogate role in aiding the family in each of the above roles. As Table 1 indicates, the roles of *health* and *protection* of the family unit are often assumed by organized groups within the community, such as hospitals and police and fire departments. There are a wide variety of services from cleaners to plumbers that aid the family in performing *household* responsibilities. Supporting the *breadwinner* role are supplementary services, particularly for crisis situations, in the form of welfare payments, unemployment funds, and Social Se-

Table 2. Family model relationship assumptions

The perception and expectations of the family members, rather than objective data, will determine the family tone of unhappiness/happiness (i.e., the adequacy of *nurturance* or *breadwinner* roles lies in the eyes of the partner).

The greater the dissatisfaction with the way responsibilities are allocated, the greater the potential for family disharmony.

The greater the stress placed on the family unit (i.e., handicapped child), the more important become the potential resources of the extended family and social support systems.

The importance of each domain to family harmony changes over different stages of family evolution.

The closer the perception of *current* to *ideal* performance of responsibilities by self and partner, the greater the personal satisfaction of the perceiver.

The more support available in a particular domain from outside sources, the less important it is that the partner provides such support.

The more support that is provided by outside sources, the weaker the dependency bonds between immediate family members.

curity. The *extrafamily social* role is supported
by a variety of social and community clubs,
church functions, athletic events, theatre, and
so forth, that provide organized opportunities
for family members to become part of a larger
social unit. Regarding the *affective support*
role, the increased transportation and communication facilities of a modern society extend
the opportunity for a variety of affective contacts, which can bring support and satisfaction
to the individual, although not always strengthening the family bonds. Such *child nurturance*
institutions as day care centers are available,
although this service continues to be unavailable to many parents or expensive when available. The private or public school, by playing a
dominant role in *child instruction,* simultaneously provides "day care" for older children. Reinforcing family *morality and standards* are the major institutions of the law,
religion, and the schools. The extended family
can be either of substantial help or a source of
pressure and stress. Some of these virtues and
benefits are balanced against the additional
stress that comes from a potential lack of concordance in beliefs or practices that either
schools or some extended family members
bring into the family unit.

Paradoxically, the more effective these surrogate services are to the family, the less likely
are individuals to be dependent on large or extended families for survival. Nevertheless, societal and extended family supports make it
more likely that a single parent can provide the
necessary support for other family members.

FAMILY ROLES:
CRISIS AND ADAPTATIONS

The relationship between the family and the
state has centered on how to meet the goal of
caring for dependent members (e.g., children,
handicapped, elderly). The structure of this relationship has been molded by values relating
to what the desired family's role should be in
caring for dependent members and the conditions under which this role should be shared
with, or taken over by, the government.

The Handicapped Child in the Family

The family system that operates on a reciprocal
set of interactions is affected significantly by a
major crisis that strikes any particular member.
Research illustrates that various crises affect
both the family unit and individual family
members, whether the crisis is a chronic illness
(Burr, 1981; Salk, Hilgartner, & Granich,
1972; Simpson & Smith, 1979; Turk, 1964);
unemployment in the family (Cassell, 1976;
Garraty, 1978; Margolis & Farran, 1981;
Thomas, McCabe, & Berry, 1980); or divorce
in the family (Hetherington, 1979; Hetherington, Cox, & Cox, 1978). If we can understand
these crises and their effects, we will have a
better comprehension of how the family system
operates and what public policy can do to support families in crisis.

There appear to be two types of stress that
affect all family members when a handicapped
child is born: the symbolic death of the normal
child that the parent expected (Farber, 1976)
and the chronic sorrow that emerges from day-
to-day problems in caring for the handicapped
child (Olshansky, 1962). The following represents a few key findings on family adaptation to
a handicapped child:

There appears to be an increase in divorce and
   suicide rates in families with handicapped
   children (Price-Bonham & Addison, 1978).
There appears to be a lessening of stress in
   families with available support systems
   (Bristol, 1979; Bristol & Schopler, 1983).
The handicapped child who demands the most
   constant care causes the most stress (Beckman-Bell, 1980; Bristol & Schopler, 1984).
Fathers and mothers both believe that fathers
   should take a more active role in caring for
   the handicapped child (Gallagher, Cross, &
   Scharfman, 1981; Gallagher, Scharfman &
   Bristol, 1984).
The father appears to be more deeply affected
   by the presence of a handicapped child than
   was originally thought (Lamb, 1976).
The mother's attachment to the handicapped
   child depends, in part, on the child's responsiveness to social stimuli (Fraiberg, 1974).

Table 3. Assumptions about the adaptation of families with a handicapped child

The greater the family harmony before the onset of a particular stress (i.e., handicapped child), the more able the family will be to adapt to that stress without major problems.

The greater the parental agreement between family members as to how the allocation of responsibilities should be altered to adapt to the stress, the greater the family harmony.

The greater the agreement on the long-term goals for the handicapped child, the greater the chance for family harmony.

The greater the agreement on short-term treatment goals for the handicapped child, the greater the chance for family harmony.

The greater the number of support sources outside the family perceived to be of help, the greater the chance for family harmony.

The parents' response depends more on the perceptions and values of the parent than the specific problems of the child (Bradshaw & Lawton, 1978; Bristol, 1984).

There are a variety of social support services, such as counseling and respite care, needed to help all members of the family unit to persevere and remain effective. Some of the major assumptions about the adaptations of the family with a handicapped child are provided in Table 3.

PUBLIC POLICY—THE FAMILY AND HANDICAPPED CHILDREN

It is clear that the family crises presented by the presence of a handicapped child can create great stress and pressure on the family unit, causing its dissolution in extreme cases and marked inefficiency and unhappiness in many others. There are serious psychological and fiscal costs to the larger society in such family disruption, and numerous attempts have been made through public policy to ameliorate or eliminate the negative consequences of such crises. Sometimes such policy is specifically targeted to a definable group (i.e., families with a handicapped child, poor children, and so forth). Sometimes the policy is designed to help all citizens and, through such help, affect

positively these crisis-prone families (i.e., graduated income tax).

One key question is the nature of the target group for the policies. Should they be universal, affecting all citizens, or should they be aimed at special subgroups (i.e., the handicapped) for specific purposes? Moroney (1980) advocates a diversity of services along a continuum, ranging from the state assuming a complete responsibility for the handicapped individual (e.g., institutionalization) to total lack of state involvement in family life:

> The needs of families and individuals vary in time, and over time ideally the state would respond to those variations with policies that support families when they need support and substitute for families of their members. (p. 14)

He emphasizes that the conceptualization of services must allow the family to move back and forth along the continuum based on need, rather than on a linear progression from no services to supportive services to substitute services.

One approach to ensuring viable public policy strategies would be to conduct a policy analysis on the specific issue of the needs of families with handicapped children. The purposes of such a policy analysis are: 1) delineate a public issue, 2) develop alternative strategies that are designed to cope with that public issue, 3) design evaluative criteria by which one can weigh the relative merit of the alternatives, and 4) collect data, judgments, expert opinions, and so forth on the relative merit of each of the strategies in each criterion (Gallagher, 1981).

This approach yields a decision matrix of the type shown in Figure 1 that can be presented to decision makers, along with accompanying information and procedures. This decision matrix would make possible a rational decision regarding the relative merit of the strategies in question. In the completed analysis the blank cells would be filled with +'s or −'s, depending on the outcome of the analysis.

Alternative Solutions

The search for the most effective policy decision to meet the needs of handicapped children

Strategies	Cost	Vertical equity	Political feasibility	Preference satisfaction	Evidence of effectiveness
1. State supported day care for handicapped children					
2. Subsidies for main-streaming handi-capped children in day care					
3. Vouchers to parents of handicapped children					
4. Tax credits					
5. Industry supported programs					
6. Status quo					

Figure 1.   Policy analysis matrix for families with handicapped children.

involves a consideration of a variety of possible solutions, each of which would be expected to have its strong and weak points. One of the key decisions in the analysis is to choose a set of strategies that are most likely to receive consideration in the public arena. The following six strategies have received extensive discussion in the professional field.

1. *State supported child care of developmental programming for handicapped children.* This strategy would provide special programs with trained personnel to the families of handicapped children from birth to age 5. There is already in existence a national network of demonstration centers supported by the U.S. Department of Education through the Handicapped Children's Early Education Act. The comprehensive law, 94-142, the Education for All Handicapped Children Act, also provides for the use of federal funds for special education for handicapped children earlier than traditional school age. This strategy would provide support for all such children, rather than the small number now being served through the demonstration programs.

2. *State subsidies for mainstreaming handicapped children in day care.* Instead of providing services that tend to separate handicapped children from normal children, state subsidies could be provided to day care centers that are willing to accept handicapped children as part of their enrollment. Such subsidies could provide the additional resources and help that would be needed by a day care center to provide for the special needs of handicapped children. This strategy would be

expected to prepare the handicapped child for a greater acceptance in the mainstreamed public school.

3. *Vouchers to parents of handicapped children.* The voucher concept has received considerable attention in a number of different versions and settings, including the purchase of services from such institutions as public schools and rehabilitation agencies (Coons & Sugarman, 1978). The parents would receive a voucher or check that could be used to purchase services for their handicapped children at any eligible setting of their choice. Such a system would place more power and decision making in the hands of the parents, allowing them to choose the type of environment they find most effective for their own child.

4. *Tax credit for parents of handicapped children.* The philosophy underlying tax credits for child care expenses has already been recognized at the federal level. Nearly 4 million Americans use this tax credit for child care at a cost of a billion dollars (Moore, 1982). This strategy proposes a much more substantial tax credit, perhaps up to one-half the cost of handicapped child care during the preschool years.

5. *Industry support for handicapped child care.* This strategy is based on the concept that a manufacturing concern or business has a major stake in the welfare and well-being of its employees. When employees have a handicapped child, they are subject to special pressures and tensions that can reduce their job satisfaction and increase tension in the workplace. Industries might provide special provisions for the handicapped child within an existing child care arrangement already supported by the industry, through the purchase of child care slots in existing centers and family day care homes for their employees, or through a cash subsidy for child care arrangements made by the employees themselves. In turn, the industry would receive

tax benefits for participating in the program.

6. *Status quo.* Any consideration of strategies or solutions must include, as a type of baseline, the status quo; one may decide to leave the situation alone on the grounds that it is being adequately taken care of at the present time. The status quo essentially represents the current availability of resources for preschool handicapped children in some communities in some areas of the country. There rarely is comprehensive coverage of services in any major metropolitan area or state. In most instances, parents are left on their own to find and negotiate services for their children, a particularly difficult problem when it is necessary that both parents work.

This set of strategies described above does not, of course, include the full range of possibilities, but it represents most of the solutions under current consideration.

Criteria for Strategy Choice

The decision matrix presented in Figure 1 lists the alternative solutions and the proposed criteria by which each of these solutions can be compared. The particular choice of these criteria is left to the analyst and provides a basis for an evaluation of the adequacy of the analysis itself. Those criteria listed here have received substantial credibility through past use.

1. *Cost.* One of the universal factors in reviewing any potential or existing public policy is the issue of cost. How much funds are needed to carry out each of the proposed strategies? As in other decision making, it is not always the cheapest strategy that turns out to be the best. Some balance between costs and the other factors is usually considered.

    One of the basic dilemmas of families of preschool handicapped children is that those families most in need of support can least afford to obtain it. If one would estimate an annual expense of $4000 for developmental programming for handicapped children, such an expense would constitute about 47% of the total income of the average single-parent mother, while only representing 13% of the incomes of high-income families! For families at the poverty level, such provisions could amount to 60% of the total family income. Clearly, the provision of special preschool services for their handicapped children is prohibitive for low-income families.

2. *Vertical equity.* Many social policies are intended to provide special help to persons who are at the bottom of the economic ladder often through little or no fault of their own (poverty, handicapping conditions, and so forth). The principle of vertical equity, *the unequal treatment of unequals in order to make them more equal,* is designed to provide assistance to low-income families to help them more adequately meet the needs of their families.

3. *Political feasibility.* This criteria must always be considered in terms of informed or experienced judgment. It is unlikely that total agreement would be obtained on the political feasibility of any of the strategies, but some consensus can be obtained. Regardless of the amount of specific data on the costs or benefits of a strategy, there is a point at which some judgment must be applied as to whether the policy is so politically unacceptable that it endangers the political careers of those public figures who espouse it.

4. *Preference satisfaction.* Does the policy itself provide the individual receiving services the maximum amount of choice? For example, if there is only one type of service available, such as an institution for handicapped children, then the parents have little or no opportunity to choose what they think would be the best solution for their child. A policy that affords the parents a choice between alternative services would presumably yield much greater parent preference satisfaction.

5. *Past evidence of success.* Some of these suggested strategies have been tried in other places, at other times, and thus have

a track record in terms of adequacy of performance or implementation. Some may reveal special problems in the process of implementation that would cause decision makers to pause before choosing it, whereas others may have a history of successful implementation to recommend them. In the consideration of alternative strategies, some history of past performance of these strategies seems essential.

Analysis of Strategies

In this section, an example of a policy analysis is provided, as each of the strategies in Figure 1 is matched against the criteria shown in there.

Strategy 1: State Supported Developmental Programming for Preschool Handicapped Children In considering this strategy, an important issue is its high level of projected cost. Table 4 shows the potential public cost for North Carolina, which has an estimated 400,000 children of preschool age (0–5). Assuming that 10% of a given age group meet the criteria of being handicapped (Martin, 1974), then there would be 40,000 handicapped children. If all of the handicapped children expected in this age group were served at an estimated cost of $4,000 per child and the total cost was paid by public funds, then this programming would cost $160 million dollars per year, a substantial sum of money representing about 4%–5% of the existing state budget.

As Table 4 indicates, if one scales down the number of children expected to be served to 50%, then the cost would be $80 million dollars; if 30% were served, then the cost would be $48 million dollars. Similarly, if only a portion of the cost were expected to be paid by public funds, with the rest assumed either by private sources or by the citizens directly involved, then the amount necessary from public resources would be dramatically reduced. Thus, if 50% of the children of this age group were served and 50% of the costs were provided by public funds, then the total amount required from the state treasury would be $40 million dollars or roughly 1% of the state budget, a more likely or plausible figure to many people. This strategy would not be responsive to *ver-*

Table 4.   Potential costs[a] of child care for preschool handicapped children[b] in North Carolina

Percentage of handicapped children served (%)	Total public expenditures (Thousands of dollars)		
	100% of costs paid by public funds	50% of costs paid by public funds	30% of costs paid by public funds
100	160,000	80,000	48,000
50	80,000	40,000	24,000
30	48,000	24,000	14,400

[a]Median cost of programming for preschool handicapped children is $4,000.
[b]Number of all children age 0–5 in North Carolina is estimated to be 400,000; 10% of these children, or 40,000, are estimated to be handicapped.

tical equity because it would propose that the money would go equally to families in all income levels.

Although it is difficult to measure *political feasibility,* there has been wide public acceptance of providing services to handicapped children as their right for the past 20 years, and it seems likely that such a proposal would not be politically damaging to the proposer. Whether there was *preference satisfaction* or parental choice in services to be provided would be determined by how the program was implemented. Conceivably, a variety of settings could be supported, with the parents being allowed to choose which of these services would be most appropriate for their child.

Program effectiveness for such services has been discussed by a number of evaluation studies (Reaves & Burns, 1982). These evaluation reports suggest strong parental satisfaction with the preschool services provided in the demonstration programs for handicapped children described earlier; there is also some evidence that less segregation is necessary for the handicapped child who has received these services when he or she enters public school. The long-term effectiveness and efficiency of such preschool programs remain to be determined.

Strategy 2: State Subsidies for Mainstreaming Handicapped Children in Day Care   By providing some additional monies to existing day care providers who take handicapped children, the *cost* of this strategy should be sub-

stantially less than that of Strategy 1, which envisions establishing full services for handicapped children in a separate setting. The criterion of *vertical equity* would not be met unless the subsidies were scaled to parental income. The *political feasibility* would seem to be moderately good in the sense that, for a modest sum of money, we as a society would be providing what seems to be needed services for citizens who have a serious family problem that is not of their own making.

In terms of *preference satisfaction* the parents would be limited in their choice to those day care centers that would agree to participate in the state program and would be eligible for the provision of services. With regard to *program effectiveness,* there have been studies available to suggest that mainstreaming handicapped children in regular day care programs can be done without a major disruption of the program and with apparently reasonable success (Suarez, 1982).

Strategy 3: Vouchers to Parents of Handicapped Children   The provision of vouchers to parents of handicapped children would *cost* a substantial amount if the full cost were borne by the public. Typically, vouchers have covered less than the full cost—perhaps half the cost—of the particular service. In this case, the cost would be in the range of $80 million dollars as seen in Table 4, or $40 million dollars if one expected the vouchers to be used by only half of the eligible parents. Vouchers would seem to be responsive to *vertical equity* because they would provide more proportionate aid to families in need. Further, they have to enable needy families to increase their effective income by allowing the mother to be employed, rather than having to care for a dependent handicapped child at home. The *political feasibility* of the voucher concept has been reviewed by Levin (1980). It has had a mixed history in providing options for parents and in producing better child care programs through the mechanism of competition between service providers. One assumption of the voucher system is that it would produce a healthy competition analogous to the free enterprise system.

In terms of *preference satisfaction,* vouchers would, in theory, provide maximum flexibility for the parents who would not be forced to purchase any particular service but would be able to spend their money on the service most desirable from their standpoint. In terms of *program effectiveness,* there have been few true tests of such strategies because the vouchers rarely reach the level of financing necessary to provide reasonable support. Such vouchers would almost inevitably have to be supplemented by other monies in order to meet the full cost of the programs. The *political feasibility* of the voucher system is doubtful. It represents a major shift in service delivery and would be opposed by a number of influential groups.

Strategy 4: Tax Credit Services for Preschool Handicapped Children   Since 1976, the federal income tax code has provided a tax credit of 20% of work-related day care expenses, up to a maximum of $900 annually. By 1982, this tax credit is estimated to have saved $1 billion dollars for working parents. The *cost* of such a program would involve minimal administrative expenses and would depend substantially on the percentage of money used as a tax credit.

In terms of *political feasibility,* providing such tax credits is a hidden expense, rather than a visible one, and thus would seem to have substantial popularity with legislative bodies. Tax credits do not fulfill the criteria of *vertical equity,* because only wage earners are entitled to them. However, it is possible to equalize the tax credit for wage earners by allowing a higher percentage of expenses to be used as a tax credit by low-income families than by high-income families. The other disadvantage is that this policy is one of reimbursement, rather than payment at the time services are provided. In other words, the money has to be spent by the family before they receive credit for it in their next year's tax return.

In terms of *preference satisfaction* the tax credit seems to get high marks. It would give a wide degree of flexibility to the taxpayer (Haskins, 1979). Although the tax credit plan has in the past received good public support, its *program effectiveness* in this particular domain remains untested.

Strategy 5: Industry-Supported Services for Handicapped Children   The *cost* of this program would be difficult to estimate because it depends on how many industries would join in cooperating and providing these services for their employees. If the program were merely to include handicapped children in existing child care programs in industry, the costs would be rather limited. If the industry provided monies for their employees to seek child program support as one of their fringe benefits, then the *preference satisfaction* would be likely to be very high, because the parents would then have the flexibility of choosing their own solution. The principle of *vertical equity* would not be well served by this strategy, however, because only industry employees would be eligible for the service. Those who are unemployed or who are not in certain industrial settings would gain little or no benefits from such services. The *program effectiveness* of such industry-supported efforts has been of a mixed character in the past and would likely receive heavy political scrutiny. There would be doubts raised regarding the *political feasibility* of such a program as it would seem to favor certain industries and enterprises over others and would provide a very uncertain umbrella for parents of handicapped children.

Strategy 6: Status Quo   The most specific advantage of proceeding with the status quo is that of *cost.* One would obviously not have to incur those additional expenses that would be part of each of the competing strategies. The substantial problem of the status quo is its current uneven distribution of services and the total unavailability of services under certain conditions and circumstances. The principle of *vertical equity* is being ill served by the status quo because many low-income families have a difficult time providing for their handicapped children, and *preference satisfaction* is not served when there are no effective services available at all. The *program effectiveness* of existing efforts is as uneven as the distribution of services themselves, with some programs receiving high marks and others low ones. It has essentially been the failure of the status quo to provide comprehensive services that has given rise to the need to consider alternative strategies that might be reasonably applied.

FINAL WORD

The changing style of the American family creates a number of special problems, particularly when there is an additional presence of the handicapped child. The available strategies proposed here would each, in their own way, provide policies that would have some degree of acceptance and support. The need or preference of both parents to work would be met by most of these strategies. As is seen in this review, the proper public policy strategies to cope with such problems are not easy to determine, but it is the purpose of such an analysis to display the major options available and present the positive and negative elements of each strategy as completely as possible.

Such analyses will not eliminate controversy; nor should they. They should, however, point out the consequences and implications of various policies as clearly and as quantitatively as possible so that both citizens and policy-makers can make the most reasonable decision on preferred policies on the basis of as much information as is available at the time.

REFERENCES

Beckman-Bell, P. (1980). *Characteristics of handicapped infants: A study of the relationship between child characteristics and stress as reported by mothers.* Unpublished doctoral dissertation, University of North Carolina, Chapel Hill, NC.

Bradshaw, J., & Lawton, D. (1978). Tracing the causes of stress in families with handicapped children. *British Journal of Social Work, 8,* 181–192.

Brenner, M. H. (1976, October). *Estimating the social costs of national economic policy: Implications for mental and physical health and criminal aggression.* Testimony before Joint Economic Committee 94th Congress, US Government Printing Office.

Bristol, M. M. (1979). *Maternal coping with autistic children: The effects of child characteristics and interpersonal support.* Unpublished doctoral dissertation, University of North Carolina at Chapel Hill, NC.

Bristol, M. M. (1984). Family resources and successful adaptation of autistic children. In E. Schopler & G. Mesibov (Eds.), *Families of autistic children* (pp. 289–310). New York: Plenum Press.

Bristol, M. M., & Schopler, E. (1983). Coping with stress in families of autistic adolescents. In E. Schopler & G. Mesibov (Eds.), *Autistic adolescents* (pp. 251–278). New York: Plenum Press.

Bristol, M. M., & Schopler, E. (1984). A developmental perspective on stress and coping in families of autistic children. In J. Blacher (Ed.), *Review of research on families of severely handicapped children: Research in review* (pp. 91–141). New York: Academic Press.

Burr, C. (1981). *Public policies affecting chronically ill children and their families.* Nashville: Center for the Study of Families and Children, Vanderbilt University.

Cassell, J. (1976). A sociological model of adaptive functioning: A contextual development perspective. In N. Carlson (Ed.), *The contexts of life: A socioecological model of adaptive behavior and functioning.* East Lansing, MI: Institute for Family and Child Study.

Cherlin, A. (1979). Work life and marital dissolution. In G. Levinges & O. C. Moles (Eds.), *Divorce and separation.* New York: Basic Books.

Coons, J. E., & Sugarman, S. D. (1978). *Education by choice: The case for family control.* Berkeley, CA: University of California Press.

Farber, B. (1976). Family adaptations to severely mentally retarded children. In M. Begab & S. Richardson (Eds.), *Mentally retarded in society* (pp. 247–266). Baltimore: University Park Press.

Fraiberg, S. (1974). Blind infants and their mothers: An examination of the sign system. In M. Lewis & L. A. Rosenblum (Eds.), *The effect of the infant on its caregiver* (pp. 215–232). New York: John Wiley & Sons.

Gallagher, J. J. (1981). Models for policy analysis: Child and family policy. In R. Haskins & J. Gallagher (Eds.), *Models for analysis of social policy: An introduction* (pp. 37–77). Norwood, NJ: Ablex.

Gallagher, J. J., Beckman, P., & Cross, A. H. (1983). Families of handicapped children: Sources of stress and its amelioration. *Exceptional Children, 50*(1), 10–19.

Gallagher, J. J., Cross, A., & Scharfman, W. (1981). Parental adaptation to a young handicapped child: The father's role. *Journal of the Division for Early Childhood, 3,* 3–14.

Gallagher, J. J., Scharfman, W., & Bristol, M. M. (1984). The division of responsibilities in families with preschool handicapped and nonhandicapped children.

Journal for the Division of Early Childhood, 8(1), 3–11.

Garraty, J. A. (1978). *Unemployment in history.* New York: Harper & Row.

Gil, D. (1973). *Violence against children: Physical child abuse in the United States.* Cambridge, MA: Harvard University Press.

Haskins, R. (1979). Day care and public policy. *Urban and Social Change Review, 12,* 3–10.

Hetherington, E. M. (1979). Divorce: A child's perspective. *American Psychologist, 34,* 851–858.

Hetherington, E. M., Cox, M., & Cox, R. (1978). The aftermath of divorce. In J. Stevens, Jr., & M. Matthews (Eds.), *Mother-child, father-child behaviors* (pp. 149–176). Washington, DC: National Association for the Education of Young Children.

Hill, M., & Corcoran, M. (1979, November). Unemployment among family men: A ten-year longitudinal study. *Monthly Labor Review, 102,* 19–23.

Hoffman, L. W. (1974). The employment of women, education and fertility. *Merrill-Palmer Quarterly, 20,* 99–119.

Lamb, M. (1976). The role of the father: An overview. In M. Lamb (Ed.), *The role of the father in child development* (pp. 1–70). New York: John Wiley & Sons.

Levin, H. (1980). Educational vouchers and social policy. In R. Haskins & J. Gallagher (Eds.), *Care and education of young children in America* (pp. 103–132). Norwood, NJ: Ablex.

Margolis, L. H., & Farran, D. C. (1981). Unemployment: The health consequences for children. *North Carolina Medical Journal, 42*(2), 849–850.

Martin, E. (1974). Thoughts on mainstreaming. *Exceptional Children, 41,* 150–153.

Moore, E. (1982). Day care: A black perspective. In E. Zigler & E. Gordon (Eds.), *Day care: Scientific and social policy issues* (pp. 413–444). Boston: Auburn House.

Moroney, R. M. (1980). *Families, social services, and social policy: The issue of shared responsibility* (NIMH Monograph Series. DHHS Publications No. (ADM) 80-846). Washington, DC: US Government Printing Office.

Olshansky, S. (1962). Chronic sorrow: A response to having a mentally defective child. *Social Casework, 43,* 190–192.

Price-Bonham, S., & Addison, S. (1978). Families and mentally retarded children: Emphasis on the father. *The Family Coordinator, 3,* 221–230.

Reaves, J., & Burns, J. (1982). *An analysis of the impact of the HCEEP: Final report for SEP.* Washington, DC: Roy Littlejohn Associates.

Salk, L., Hilgartner, M., & Granich, B. (1972). The psychological impact of hemophilia on the patient and his family. *Social Science and Medicine, 6,* 491–505.

Simpson, O. W., & Smith, M. A. (1979). Lightening the load for parents of children with diabetes. MCN: *The American Journal of Maternal Child Nursing, 4,* 293–296.

Suarez, T. (1982). Planning evaluation of programs for high risk and handicapped infants. In C. Ramey & P. Trohanis (Eds.), *Finding and educating high risk and handicapped infants* (pp. 193–215). Baltimore: University Park Press.

Thomas, L. E., McCabe, E., & Berry, J. E. (1980). Unemployment and family stress: A reassessment. *Family Relations, 29,* 517–524.

Toffler, A. (1971). *Future shock.* New York: Random House.

Turk, J. (1964). Impact of cystic fibrosis on family functioning. *Pediatrics, 34,* 67–71.

Chapter

16

Case Management for Families of Developmentally Disabled Clients

An Empirical Policy Analysis of a Statewide System

Ann E. MacEachron, Denise Pensky, and Barbara Hawes

FAMILIES WHO HAVE a developmentally disabled member living at home have historically received few support services to assist them in providing care or to enable them to prevent or delay out-of-home placement. As discussed by Krauss (Chapter 13 in this volume), it is only recently that comprehensive programs of family support services have been conceptualized, initial statewide attempts of implementation have begun, and research to examine the needs of families and the effectiveness of support services in meeting these needs has been forthcoming. The newness of these services, coupled with the trend to establish comprehensive community-based systems of care in the last two decades, has often led to the conclusion that the path between need, conceptualization, fiscal support, and implementation is relatively direct. However, in this dec-

ade fiscal austerity at the national, state, and local levels for the human services has led to cutback management, retrenchment of current services, and few or no resources to develop and maintain new services. One major question, therefore, is how to meet the obvious need for family support services within severe budget constraints.

The purpose of this chapter is to report the efforts of one state to redirect its limited resources to serve families with a developmentally disabled member living at home. Although this continuing effort encompasses a range of support services, the focus of this chapter is on case management services for two reasons. First, case management is an example of a service that is recommended for clients living in a number of different residential settings from families to institutions. The decision

This research was supported by the New York State Office of Developmental Disabilities. The opinions of the authors are their own and do not necessarily reflect those of any organizations.

as to who should receive this service, given budget limitations, reflects the priority of family support services within the context of competing demands. Second, the primary basis for decision making for this service was to be grounded on an empirical policy analysis of who was already receiving and who should receive case management services. This study, therefore, illustrates how research may be applied directly to the shaping and provision of family support services.

CASE MANAGEMENT

Case management emerged nationally as an important client service in the 1970s as community services expanded and as large-scale deinstitutionalization began. The President's Panel on Mental Retardation emphasized, as early as 1962, the requirement of a "continuum of care" to ensure that the often long-term service needs of mentally retarded persons would be met. The concept of services integration (Argranoff & Pattakos, 1979; Gans & Horton, 1975; Hogan & MacEachron, 1980; Intagliata, 1982; Redburn, 1977) was a complementary response to these problems. For coordinating direct services to individuals, the concept of case management was of particular importance (Aiken, Dewar, DiTomaso, Hage, Zeitz, 1975; Baerwald, 1983; Beatrice, 1981; Dombrowick, 1979; Hogan & MacEachron, 1980; Intagliata, 1982; Magrab & Elder, 1979; Neufeldt, 1977; Ross, 1980). Moreover, specific service integration mechanisms for services to developmentally disabled persons were mandated by Congress in the 1975 Developmental Disabilities and Bill of Rights Act (PL 94-103) and in the Developmental Disabilities Amendments of 1978 (PL 95-602). The 1975 Act mandated a strong requirement for comprehensiveness and continuity through an habilitation plan, follow-along services, and coordination services. The 1978 Amendments further specified case management as a priority service for developmentally disabled persons.

Within New York State, where the present study was conducted, the legislation that created the Office of Mental Retardation & Developmental Disabilities (OMRDD) in 1977 also mandated it to develop a comprehensive integrated system of services that would serve the full range of needs of the mentally retarded and developmentally disabled person. A regional model, consisting of 20 regions across 62 counties, was identified as the framework to meet the legislative mandate. One of the three staffing areas allocated for the regions was Individual Case Management and Advocacy. This case management emphasis was congruent with national legislation and practice at that time. A survey of all 50 states (Fritz, Wright, & Snipes, 1978) indicated that at least 34 states had a case management system, and at least 11 states provided the core functions of information and referral, assessment, service plan development, services coordination, monitoring and tracking, direct service provision, and follow-up. Not only was the presence of case management widespread by 1978, but comprehensive systems were also common in such states as California, Florida, Illinois, Maryland, Missouri and Pennsylvania, as well as New York State.

The development of the case management service systems has been complicated by conflicting mandates. In New York State, for example, the established legal responsibility for OMRDD to serve all developmentally disabled individuals within a comprehensive community service network continues to be constrained by budget allocations that provide case management staff resources to serve only specific groups, particularly deinstitutionalized clients placed in the community. Former residents of the Willowbrook Developmental Center, identified under the judicial mandate of the Willowbrook Consent Decree and called "class clients," are mandated to receive a 1:20 case manager to client ratio. For all other clients, or nonclass clients, only two residential settings have allocated staffing ratios: Clients living in foster family/personal care homes are allocated a ratio of 1:30, and clients living in community residences receive a ratio of 1:35. The majority of these nonclass clients left institutional care since 1975. Given the tradition of allocating resources to serve primarily deinstitutionalized clients, developmentally disabled persons living with their families among other groups have not been included specifically in these staff allocations. Exclusion from these budgeted allocations has severely limited the availability of case management for families. Moreover, because the main purpose of case management had been to maintain the community placement of deinstitutionalized clients and to prevent readmission to developmental centers, the past success of deinstitutionalization and the current decreased rate of deinstitutionalization placements raised the question of whether or not case management services should be reduced substantially or redirected to other client groups. The increasing federal and state budget constraints were sufficiently severe to suggest an alternative possibility that the resources for case management should be reduced and then reallocated to direct rather than support services. The question, therefore, was whether a state case management system should continue to exist, and if so, to whom should limited and reduced resources be allocated?

From a public advocacy and policy perspective in the early 1980s, case management was beginning to be identified nationally and statewide as a core service within the concept of family support services (Human Services Research Institute, 1984; National Association of State Mental Retardation Program Directors, 1979). This service was seen as especially helpful for families with disabled children under the age of 5 who may need assistance in gaining access to clinical and habilitative services, for families with young disabled adults who may need transitional assistance from the educational system to the adult system, and for families with older disabled adults who may need help to establish permanent out-of-home care in the least restrictive and cost-effective environment. This family support service perspective on case management offered a strong alternative rationale for this service, but only if the system could be shifted from serving primarily deinstitutionalized clients to more persons living with their families. To accomplish this shift, however, required more than a log-

ical and normative rationale. Layoffs of state employees had already begun, including a substantial number of case managers, to meet budget constraints. More layoffs were planned within the next year. In addition, consistent with the national trend of demanding "hard facts" to document current and proposed service patterns within specified budget limits, any proposed continuation of resources or redirection of resources required an empirical and analytical rationale. Because time and the need to collect data were of the essence, 6 months in 1983 were allotted to implement and complete this empirical policy analysis.

THIS STUDY

This chapter is based on a series of studies (New York State OMRDD 1983; 1984a; 1984b) initiated to obtain immediate information on actual case management service practice and the effects of proposed changes in current practice. Previous reviews of OMRDD case management services (New York State Board of Social Welfare, 1980; New York State OMRDD Case Management Steering Committee, 1982) had identified thirteen functions that case managers may perform: outreach, resource identification, intake, discharge/termination, assessment, individual program development, linking, monitoring, advocacy, coordination, recordkeeping, support or crisis intervention, and follow-up. Both reviews acknowledged that many factors, including client need, may influence which clients receive these core functions and with what intensity. However, then and now, there were no studies in the field of developmental disabilities that provided quantitative evaluations of case management service delivery at the client, case manager, and systems levels of analysis. The major research questions of this study were, therefore:

1. Who receives case management services, in what amount, and of what kind?
2. What predicts the amount of service received: client characteristics, case manager characteristics, regional office charac-

teristics, or service characteristics, such as residential placement, class status as defined by the Willowbrook Consent Decree, or case manager to client ratios?

The first question focused on prevailing professional practice in the delivery of state case management services. Prevailing practice information would not only suggest standards of equity for service delivery but also which groups of clients were overserved or underserved. Differences in service received would thus provide for an empirical evaluation of equity of delivery of service: 1) to clients in residential care settings, rather than to family clients; 2) to all class clients and only some nonclass clients; and 3) to clients in some residential settings who are co-served by both state and voluntary agency case managers and thus are likely to receive substantially more service. The extent of such descriptive differences were expected to highlight how case management resources could be redistributed to provide more services to clients living with their families. The second question was asked to discover which factors were associated with the delivery of case management services and thus which might be altered to change the system and to rationalize the administration of this statewide support service.

In general, answers to these research questions were directed toward clarifying the role of state case management services by providing a rich description of what services exist now and by assessing which factors account for how much service clients receive. No attempt was made to determine the effectiveness of case management services both because the complexity of the longitudinal research design that would be required was inconsistent with the time-frame limits on gathering information and because no specific measures of case management effectiveness exist. Morever, because no empirical studies had yet examined the parameters of a statewide case management system, the choice of other than a descriptive study would have been premature. From a policy perspective, a descriptive study of the entire case management system was judged to be an important first step in rationalizing decisions regarding the continuation of the system, the determination of client priority for service, especially for clients living with their families, and the determination of case manager ratios to match these priorities.

Methodology

Sample In March of 1983, a one-third random sample from 477 state case managers was selected from each case management unit of the 20 regional Borough/District Developmental Service Offices (B/DDSOs) of the New York State Office of Mental Retardation and Developmental Disabilities (OMRDD). The 157 state case managers who responded, a 97% response rate, provided information for all clients in their caseloads. This procedure resulted in information on 4,738 clients, or 32% of the 14,871 clients receiving state case management services at that time.

The state case managers also provided information on clients who were co-served by voluntary agency case managers in community residences and Intermediate Care Facilities for the Developmentally Disabled (ICFs/DD). The voluntary agency case managers provided information on the same instruments for 286 clients in 35 agencies, or 27% of clients served in community residences or ICFs/DD and who were potentially co-served by the state and voluntary agency case managers in the original sample. These clients were served by 85 case managers.

Information on the organizational structure and administration of all state case management units, as well as their 63 case management subunits was collected from the unit and subunit administrators. Detailed information on the samples, populations and measures is available elsewhere (New York State OMRDD 1983; 1984a; 1984b).

Client Measures Information was requested for the client's age, gender, level of intellectual functioning, and level of care. Level of intellectual functioning was measured on a 5-point scale: 1=normal (IQ above 69), 2=mild (IQ 55–69), 3=moderate (IQ 40–54),

4=severe (IQ 25–39), and 5=profound (IQ under 25). Level of care or functional disability was measured in six global areas: self-care skills, communication skills, mobility skills, independence capacity skills, self-direction skills or behavior problems, and medical care problems. Each of these areas was measured on a 4-point scale: 1=independent—does the task or seeks the service without prompting, 2=supervision—does the task with verbal or written prompts, 3=assistance—often needs physical hands-on aid or prompts to do the task, and 4=total support—staff must do the task or be involved throughout the task. These six level of care measures formed an additive scale (Cronbach's alpha = .86), ranging from independence (scores 6–7), supervision (scores 8–12), assistance (13–18), to total support (scores 19–24).

Case management service characteristics included the caseload size of the client's case manager (staffing ratio), the client's residential placement, the client's class/nonclass status in regards to the Willowbrook Consent Decree, the number of years clients received case management services, and the number of years clients were served by their current case managers. In addition, the extent to which other agencies perform case management activities for the client was evaluated on a 4-point scale, ranging from not at all (score of 1) to a substantial amount (score of 4). Lastly, the amount of travel time from the case management office to the client's residence, day program, and other agencies was measured on a 4-point scale: 1=less than 15 minutes, 2=15–30 minutes, 3=31–60 minutes, and 4=over 60 minutes.

The dependent variable was the case manager time spent per client during a year's time, the usual time cycle in which all case management functions occur. Each case manager was given detailed instructions on how to summarize time spent for the past year (April 1982 to March 1983). These instructions included the definition of case management functions (see Table 1), as well as a list of 42 behavioral activities associated with these functions. Under the function of linking, for example, the following activities were listed: refer problem for resolu-

tion to appropriate staff or alternate service providers, arrange for service required as a result of the program planning team meeting, and accompany client to programs/ services. The case managers estimated the time they had spent on each function in hours and minutes. These estimates were then added together to provide an overall amount of time spent during the past year. The amount of time spent on all case management functions was adjusted as follows: 1) taking the percentage of time spent on each client relative to all other clients in that case manager's caseload and 2) multiplying the percentage of time by an adjusted number of hours a case manager could work in a year. The OMRDD Office of Employee Relations (New York State Department of Civil Service, 1981) reported that employees take an average of 42.9 days or 343.2 hours of annual leave. On average, therefore, case managers work 1,736.8 hours per year.

Case Manager Measures Self-reported background data included the case managers' education, years in current job title, job title and salary grade, years of experience in developmental disabilities, current caseload size, number of hours they worked in a week, number of hours typically spent on direct case management to clients, and number of hours spent traveling to perform case management. Case managers were also asked whether or not they typically performed each case management function, as well as such other activities as supervision of other case managers, survey/certification work, administrative inservice training, administrative paperwork, public education, outreach, and resource identification.

Case Management Unit Measures These measures included the number of clients in each type of residential placement who receive state case management services, the supervisor to case manager ratio, the typical case manager to client ratio, and whether or not the supervisor also had a caseload. The administrators also assessed the actual and ideal importance of eleven criteria for assigning clients to caseloads on a five-point scale ranging from not at all important (score of 1) to very impor-

Table 1.   Definitions of case management functions

Function	Definition
Intake/discharge	Determining a client's eligibility for services or termination of those services no longer needed or desired
Assessment	Ascertaining a client's developmental level and specific needs for service
Individual program plan development	Planning for a written plan of needs and goals for the individual client
Recordkeeping/recording	Maintaining comprehensive written records regarding intake information, strengths and needs assessments, goal and routine service planning, staff action, client progress, and case reviews
Linking	Referral for new services as outlined in the Individual Program Plan, including arranging for services at generic agencies, accompanying client to agencies, assisting in completing of forms or other activities that ensure that the client is linked to new services.
Support/crisis intervention	Helping the individual and/or his or her family with unanticipated problems
Coordination	Serving as a focal point for service coordination among diverse providers of service required by an individual, including health, education, vocational training, job placement, follow-up residential services, recreational services, transportation services, financial and legal guidance, and protection from exploitation
Monitoring and follow-up	Ensuring that the client is receiving appropriate services as outlined in their Individual Program Plan and the periodic reassessment of the individual client's progress
Advocacy	Protecting and upholding the rights of clients

tant (score of 5), and the actual and ideal degree of case management coordination with seven other agencies on a five-point scale ranging from not at all integrated (score of 1) to very integrated (score of 5).

Analysis   The first part of the analysis was to describe the characteristics of clients, case managers, and case management units. All group differences were analyzed by chi-square, Student's t-test, or one-way analysis of variance using the Scheffe test for multiple comparisons and eta-squared for estimating the strength of association. All comparative results presented in this report were significant at the .001 level of probability. The second part of the analysis used hierarchical multiple regression procedures with effects coding of the independent variables and with case manager time spent for the 4,738 clients as the dependent variable. Each of the measures described above was a potential predictor of case manager time spent per client during a year. Inclusion

in the equation began with client characteristics that explained 4% or more of the variance in time spent ($r = .20$); case manager characteristics that met the same criterion were then included; lastly, all case management unit and subunit measures were included and retained if they accounted for more variance.

There were two major limitations of the study. First, the data on case manager time spent and functions performed were collected retrospectively. However, the consensus of case managers and of a state technical advisory committee was that the retrospective estimates were quite accurate because: 1) case managers had worked with their clients an average of 2 years and 2) the work cycle for case management responsibilities is a year's time. Thus, because of the case managers' longevity of serving each client and their ability to summarize a complete cycle of work, this retrospective study was viewed as a more accurate means of obtaining data than of attempting a year-long prospective study. Second, the non-random selection of clients co-served by state and voluntary agency case managers brings the necessity of caution to any generalization. The client characteristics of co-served clients in this sample, however, did not differ significantly from other clients living in community residences and ICFs/DD.

Results

Clients The average age of clients was 36 years. The majority of the clients were males (54%), most had a diagnosis of mental retardation (95%), and between 2% and 15% of the clients had other diagnosed developmental disabilities. The average level intellectual functioning was moderate, or an IQ between 40 and 54: seven percent of the clients were assessed at a normal level, 48% were assessed at a mild/moderate level, and 45% were assessed at a severe/profound level. The average level of care required was supervision: Eleven percent were independent, 44% needed supervision, 32% needed assistance, and 13% needed total support.

Almost a fifth (17%) of the clients had a Willowbrook class status, and the remaining 83% were nonclass clients. About three-quarters (71%) of clients lived in residences within OMRDD's residential continuum of care (that is, the extent to which more core services are provided in each successive level of the continuum); of these, 8% were in independent living or supportive apartments, 15% were in community group homes, 19% were in family foster care, 11% were in foster personal care homes providing health services, 15% were in small community-based Intermediate Care Facilities for the Developmentally Disabled (ICFs/DD), and 3% were in ICFs/DD over 30 beds in size. In addition, 26% of the clients lived with their families and 3% lived in other settings, such as residential schools or nursing homes. Lastly, level of care need was related to the sequence of the continuum of care ($R^2 = .20$, $Eta^2 = .22$) and with the client's age ($R^2 = .10$, $Eta^2 = .12$). As level of care needs increased, clients were more likely to live in residential settings with more core ser-

vices, and younger clients were more likely to have higher levels of care needs. Within this context, clients living with their families needed an assistance level of care on average and, when placed within the continuum of residential care, had the same average level of care needs as clients living in ICFs/DD. Case management services to clients living with their families, therefore, focused on clients whose needs were substantial.

On average, clients had received state case management services from the regional office unit for 6 years and from their current case managers for 2 years. Clients received an average of 50 hours of state case management or the equivalent of a 1:35 case manager to client ratio. This 50 hours of service was distributed among the case management functions as follows: Twenty-two percent of the time was spent on support, 21% on monitoring, 15% on recordkeeping, 15% on development of the Individual Program Plan (IPP), 7% on intake/discharge, 6% on linking, 6% on coordination, 4% on advocacy, and 4% on assessment on average. All clients had case managers who traveled to their residence, and 83% of the clients had case managers who traveled to their day program. Travel to other agencies was less likely; relatedly, interagency coordination of case management activities was rated as minimal on average.

Nonclass Clients Living with their Families Nonclass clients living with their families were on average younger than all other nonclass clients in this study (22 versus 41 years of age) and less likely to have a diagnosis of mental retardation (88% versus 97%), although their average level of intellectual functioning was the same on average (moderate) and their average level of care needs was equivalent to clients in ICFs/DD. In addition, 60% of the clients living with their families were over the age of 17, and among these clients, 42% were aging-out of children's services (ages 18 to 24)—two of the three main age groups particularly apt to need case management services.

On average, the family client had received state case management services for 4 years and from his or her current case manager for 1 year. Family clients received an average of 38 hours annually of case management services or the equivalent of a 1:46 case manager to client ratio. In comparison with other nonclass clients, family clients received fewer hours of service on average than clients living in independent settings (49 hours), foster family care (57 hours), foster personal care (55 hours) and other settings (46 hours). Clients living with their families, however, received an equivalent amount of service on average as clients living in community residences (38 hours) and in ICFs/DD (39 hours).

The average percentage of time spent on each case management function did not differ significantly for family clients as compared to other clients, except that family clients received a greater emphasis on intake/discharge functions (14%) and less emphasis on monitoring (15%) than did other clients. Although interagency coordination of case management was at the same minimal level as for other clients, case managers spent more time traveling to family homes and to agencies than for other clients.

In sum, although clients living with their families had substantial need of case management service in terms of level of care and age factors, the amount of service they received was much less than for clients in most other residential settings.

Clients with Class Status   A comparison of class and nonclass client characteristics in this sample indicated significant mean differences in terms of gender (63% male versus 53% male) and average level of intellectual functioning (severe versus moderate). These were no significant mean differences for age, type of diagnosis, or level of care needs.

The majority of class clients lived in ICFs/DD (51%) or generally under the auspice of the OMRDD residential continuum of care (92%). Only 6% of class clients lived with their families.

There were no significant mean differences for the number of years clients received case management services, for the number of years clients were served by their current case man-

agers, or for their case manager's travel time or interagency coordination. However, class clients received more hours annually of state case management services than did nonclass clients (79 versus 45 hours, or the equivalent of 1:21 versus 1:39 case manager to client ratio). Even so, with the exception of the support or crisis intervention function (13% versus 24%), the relative percentage of time spent on each function was equivalent for class and nonclass clients.

In sum, class clients appeared to receive a substantial amount of service primarily because this amount was mandated under the judicial mandate of the Willowbrook Consent Decree.

Co-Served Clients   On average, clients in community residences co-served by both state and voluntary agency case managers were mildly to moderately retarded, required a supervision level of care, and were 37 years of age. Co-served clients in ICFs/DD were moderately to severely retarded on average, required an assistance level of care, and were 36 years of age. This sample of co-served clients was similar to other clients in these settings.

In community residences, class clients received more hours of case management services on average than did nonclass clients from state case managers (70 versus 33 hours, or the equivalent of a 1:25 versus 1:52 case manager to client ratio) but not from the voluntary agency case manager (65 versus 106 hours, or the equivalent of a 1:27 versus 1:16 case manager to client ratio). On average, class clients received the equivalent of a 1:13 ratio from both the state and voluntary agency case managers, whereas nonclass clients received the equivalent of a 1:12 ratio from both case managers.

In ICFs/DD, class clients received more hours of case management services than did nonclass clients from both the state case manager (77 versus 28 hours, or the equivalent of a 1:22 versus 1:62 case manager to client ratio) and the voluntary agency case manager (191 versus 84 hours or the equivalent of a 1:9 versus 1:21 case manager to client ratio). On average, class clients received the equivalent of a 1:6 ratio from both the state and voluntary agency case managers, whereas nonclass clients received the equivalent of a 1:16 ratio from both case managers.

In sum, joint case management efforts for class and nonclass clients in each residential setting resulted in a substantial amount of case management services being provided. Moreover, state and voluntary agency case managers of these co-served clients performed all case management functions. There was no specialized set of functions that a state or voluntary agency case manager performed exclusively. These clients therefore appeared to receive more services because they were served by two case managers.

Case Managers State case managers generally earned more than did voluntary case managers ($20,000 versus $15,000), were somewhat more likely to have a bachelor's degree (96% versus 89%), had spent more years in their current job title (4 versus 2 years), and had spent more time in the field of developmental disabilities (8 versus 5 years).

State case managers had a larger caseload on average than did voluntary agency case managers (30 versus 17 clients). State managers were also more likely to spend their total work time on direct case management services (47% versus 26%). Lastly, state case managers were much more likely to work full-time than were voluntary agency case managers (98% versus 80%).

For state case managers only, higher civil service level and salary were associated with level and type of education: sixty percent of those with bachelor's degrees were at the lowest civil service levels for case management, 69% of those with a master's degree were at the intermediate civil service levels (14% had a Master of Social Work degree, whereas 55% had another type of master's degree), and 87% at the supervisory civil service levels had a master's degree (78% had a Master of Social Work degree, and 19% had another type of master's degree).

Regional Case Management Units and Subunits Fifteen of the twenty regional case management units consisted of multiple subunits: Ten units were subdivided on the basis of

geographic or county areas alone, four units were subdivided on the basis of both geography and case management core functions, and one unit was subdivided only on the basis of function. Interestingly, each case management unit had equivalent case manager travel time no matter how it was structured and regardless of the geographic size or population density of its area. In addition, even with most regional case management units divided into multiple subunits, each unit and almost all subunits provided a complete range of case management functions for clients in all residential settings.

Within units, the average supervisor to case manager ratio was 1:6.3, but ranged from 1:2.8 to 1:12. The previous budget allocation for supervisor to case manager ratios was established at a 1:10 ratio. The range of supervisory ratios was related, however, to how supervisors were deployed: Twelve of the subunits (19%) had supervisors who carried other than case management responsibilities in the regional office, 40 subunits (63%) had a full-time supervisor, and 11 subunits (18) had more than one full-time supervisor. Of those subunits with one full-time supervisor, 55% of the supervisors had a caseload. Of those subunits with more than one supervisor, 82% of the supervisors had a caseload. Among supervisors with active caseloads, there appeared to be a tradeoff between size of their caseload and the number of case managers supervised. Supervisors who did not carry a caseload supervised an average of nine case managers. Supervisors with a caseload under the size of 21 clients supervised an average of six case managers. Supervisors with a caseload of 21 or more clients supervised an average of four case managers.

All unit and subunit supervisors rated the importance of eleven criteria for assigning caseloads. On average, the most important criteria were the current caseload size of the case manager and the experience or expertise of the case manager. The three least important criteria were the client's level of disability, the case manager's fluency in languages other than English, and the safety of the client's neighborhood. Criteria of intermediate importance were the availability of the case manager at the time of assignment, the need for interagency coordination, the type of residence where a client lives, the Willowbrook class status of the client, and the degree of family involvement. When asked to assess the ideal importance of these criteria, the importance of several criteria increased, but generally the relative rank order among criteria did not change.

All unit and subunit supervisors also rated the extent of interagency coordination for case management. Coordination with voluntary agencies was reported to be quite high, but moderate with the Office of Vocational Rehabilitation and the State Education Department, low with the Department of Social Services, the Office of Mental Health, and the criminal justice system, and none with the Department for Youth. The ideal ratings maintained the same rank order, but suggested that more integration with all agencies was desired.

Prediction Model As reported earlier, each client received an average of 50 hours of state case management services in a year. Given the above descriptive information, the second major concern of this study was this question: What predicted the amount of case management services delivered to clients? Among all the client, case manager, regional office, and service characteristics described as potential predictors, only four variables contributed to increasing the amount of variation explained in the number of case management hours received. As shown in Table 2, the following four predictors explained 35% of the variation: caseload size of the case manager, percent of work time the case manager spent on case management services over all clients, the client's residential placement, and the client's Willowbrook class status. These predictor variables accord well with the rank order of caseload assignment criteria as assessed by supervisors. The current caseload size of the case manager was ranked as the supervisor's most important criterion; the other three predictors were ranked as moderately important. Client disability received a low supervisory ranking, and in this prediction model, no client characteristics were predictive of the amount of service received.

Table 2. Multiple regression model of number of annual hours of case management received with effects coding of the independent variables ($N = 4,718$ clients)

Predictors	Unstandardized Beta
Constant	50.1
Caseload size of case manager	
11–20	32.9
21–30	5.1
31–40	– 5.6
41–50	–14.5
51+	–18.0
Residential continuum of care	
Independent/supportive apartments	5.6
Community residence	– .5
Foster family care	7.7
Foster personal care	7.6
ICF/DD under 30 beds	– 5.9
ICF/DD over 30 beds	– 7.1
Development center	– .8
Family	– 4.1
Other	– 2.5
Percent case manager time on all case management activities	
95% or more	5.2
Less than 95%	– 5.2
Willowbrook class status	
Class	.9
Nonclass	– .9
	$R = .59$
	$R^2 = .35$

A review of the magnitude of effect for each predictor in Table 2 indicates that the caseload size of the case manager has the greatest influence on the amount of case management services received by clients. As with the predictor regarding the percentage of case manager work time allocated to case management, common sense would suggest that case managers have more time to deliver services when they serve fewer clients and when they have more work time available to provide these services. Because these variables are also subject to clear management, budget, and judicial mandates, the amount of service received by clients may be guided closely by such mandates. The relatively weak effect of Willowbrook class status demonstrates the saliency of these two predictors. Once the judicial mandates of a 1:20 case manager to class client ratio and of a case manager working full-time on direct case management services for class clients were accounted for by these two predictors, class status only meant an hour more for client service during a year. Added to the fact that client characteristics did not predict the amount of client service received, the direct influence of these two case manager predictors gains importance in developing intervention strategies. Lastly, a client's residential placement was also associated with the amount of service received. With the exception of clients living with their families, clients living in residences at the more independent end of the continuum of residential care in which fewer core services are provided generally received more state case manager services than did clients at the lower end of the continuum. Clients living in more independent settings were also likely to live in residences for which there were established case manager ratios, such as foster family/personal care and community residences. In contrast, clients living with their families, who are more likely to need coordinative service assistance because they lack other service resources and who had substantial level of care needs, were likely to receive relatively fewer hours of case management services than clients at the more independent end of the residential continuum.

Discussion

One of the most important findings of this study was that the delivery of case management services is predictable by a small rather than large number of factors. Case management, as with many family support services, is often thought to be an incredibly complex set of services to describe and manage. Indeed, the potential list of influential factors ranges from all possible client characteristics to all possible case manager, delivery system, and service provision characteristics. The results of this study show, however, that over one-third of the variability in amount of case management services received by clients could be accounted for by only four factors: the caseload size of the case manager, the percentage of case manager work time spent on case management, the cli-

ent's residential setting, and the client's Willowbrook class status. This finding suggested clear directions to reshape the current system without an increase of resources allocated to it by establishing eligibility for service, case manager ratios, and case manager deployment to include service provision to families.

The historical emphasis on residential setting and class status for establishing service eligibility and case manager to client ratios was consistent, but not perfectly so, with the empirical description of how these services were actually provided. The empirical description offered both a more precise description, as well as a basis to project the potential future effects of respecifying these historically based criteria. To generate the resources required to serve family clients within current budget limits required readjustments in both the service eligibility criteria and case manager to client ratios. These readjustments, however, needed to be congruent with service levels already provided to clients within the system. Thus, the average amount of current service received by clients was used as a standard of equity and as a guideline to minimize the actual amount of service delivery change for current clients.

Under the standard of equity, the range of eligible residential settings in which nonclass clients might live was extended beyond family foster care and community residences to include both families and ICFs/DD. This broader range of eligible residential settings could be justified by increasing the state case manager ratio for class clients in ICFs/DD and for nonclass clients in community residences, as well as by targeting the provision of case management services to critical time periods. First, for clients in foster family/personal care, the current practice of serving all clients at a 1:30 ratio was retained to stay in compliance with the regulations for these programs. Second, for class clients, the findings that the characteristics of class and nonclass clients did not differ significantly and that over half of the class clients live in ICFs/DD (and consequently receive substantial joint case management services from the state and residential case managers) led to a shift of resources agreed on by the Willowbrook Court. All class clients were to continue to receive a 1:20 state case manager-to-client ratio; however, for class clients living in ICFs/DD, the state case manager ratio was to be changed from a 1:20 to a 1:40 ratio. Third, because case management services were traditionally viewed in this state as assisting the client in making a successful community transition, the duration of service was precisely defined to meet just this purpose. During the first year only of their community placement, 100% of the deinstitutionalized clients living in community residences and 70% of the clients in ICFs/DD may receive case management services; thereafter, 30% of the community residence clients and 20% of the ICFs/DD clients may be expected to receive state case management services. By calculating the number of clients to be deinstitutionalized during the next 5 years who would require service, and by estimating and balancing the number of clients living with their families who may need this service, these percentages were arrived at by professional consensus of high-level clinicians and administrators as defining the most critical time periods for substantial case management services. Because the ICFs/DD program provides a comprehensive system of habilitative services, the percentage of eligible clients after a year's placement was smaller than for clients living in community residences. Complementary changes were also made in the case manager to client ratios. The ratio for clients in community residences was increased from 1:35 to 1:40; although this change was less than historically allocated, it was more generous than what was typically provided in actual practice (average of 1:46, median of 1:48). The ratio for clients in ICFs/DD was to be newly established at 1:50, the approximate amount of service actually provided (average of 1:45, median of 1:64). Given these changes in eligibility and staffing ratios, the proposed staffing ratio of 1:40 for families was based on what families currently received (average of 1:42, median of 1:53) but also was adjusted to be richer than current practice to allow for case manager assignments to other than direct case management services to clients (e.g., resource identification and community education).

Rather than treating these staffing ratios as absolutes, flexibility could also be added by considering all case manager ratios for nonclass clients as the average amount of service to be provided over a year's time by all case managers in each region, rather than the amount required to be given to each client. Using an average ratio allows for variations in service intensity, depending on the skills of the case manager and the needs of the client, that can be balanced against the availability of other services. A focus on average caseload size for each residential setting would also suggest that the regression model of hours spent per client could be used as a management and advocacy tool at the local level. For example, one use would be to compare the regression model's estimated hours spent with the actual number of hours spent by case managers on clients in this residential setting. The predicted number of hours for a nonclass client living with his or her family and receiving a 1:40 ratio is about 45 hours. If clients were to receive substantially fewer or greater hours than this amount, a professional rationale could be requested to justify the discrepancy.

Another use of the regression model is to budget, sequence, and assess the feasibility of different case mixes for case managers' caseloads. Each case manager works an average of 1736.8 hours a year. A case manager who served 35 nonclass clients living with their families (35 clients X 45 hours per client on average at a 1:40 ratio = 1,575 hours a year) and 5 clients in personal foster family care (5 clients X 67 hours per client on average at the ratio of 1:30 = 335 hours a year) would be overextended by 173 hours or 4 weeks of work over a year's time. When the estimated total is greater than the hours available for the case manager in a year, the supervisor may decide to plan an alternative case mix or retain this case mix given the needs of the clients served relative to other clients on average.

Because unit and subunit characteristics of the regional case management offices were not predictive of the amount of case management services received by clients, this suggested that the structure of these units and subunits could be organized by general guidelines consistent with the empirical results. Regional offices should utilize no more than three subunits or no more subunits than the number of counties they serve to promote accessibility for clients and to save case manager travel time, to decrease the amount of supervisory personnel required for multiple subunits, and to emphasize full-time administrative and clinical supervision without caseload responsibilities. When there is a small number of case managers in a subunit, the recommended caseload for supervisors is as follows: Supervisors of one to four case managers will carry a caseload of over 20 clients, and supervisors of five to seven case managers will carry a caseload of less than 20 clients. These guidelines were based on current practice and on the actual budgeted allocation of a 1:10 supervisor to case manager ratio. By specifying the circumstances when an absolute 1:10 ratio would not be required, additional flexibility is given to management.

As with regional office characteristics, the characteristics of case managers did not predict the amount of service received by clients. The study findings also indicate that all case managers, regardless of educational background or certification, perform the full complement of case management functions, rather than specializing in one or several functional areas. The implication of these findings was that it would be possible to rationalize case manager qualifications within civil service title series by utilizing a general case management title series, rather than by specifying only social work or another profession as the single profession allowed to perform case management. That is, utilization of a general case manager title series would allow for a flexible system, with a mix of professionals, for the delivery of regional and local case management services.

CONCLUSION

From a policy perspective, this study occurred at a time when the client service of case management either required a new rationale for existence based on a redirection of populations to be served or face the reduction and transfer of resources to other higher priority services. A rich description of this system of services was fundamental to understanding what actually existed and then to suggesting where intervention and redirection of resources might be most efficacious. Factors clearly linked to the amount of client services received were viewed as the principal statewide intervention points, whereas other factors were assigned to local management and professional control. The precise nature of each change, however, was a collaborative decision-making process among high-level administrators and professionals within the agency and among control agencies responsible for the budgeting and monitoring of services. Together, it was possible to reform and stabilize a system of services—to deemphasize state case management services to clients in successful community placements with a corresponding redirection of resources to clients living with families—congruent with current needs and to focus on a broader population of clients without additional resource expenditure.

The reform process of this statewide case management system, within a zero-based budgeting resource context at best and a severe cutback management context at worst, suggests that the implementation of a broad array of statewide family support services may be difficult to achieve unless there is consensus among normative, empirical, and management rationales. Although the normative value of providing support services to families could not be doubted, the means to do so had to be demonstrated empirically with specific management guidelines for the entire system. It was not enough to demonstrate that the needs of currently served family clients were similar to the needs of clients in ICFs/DD, although this did substantiate the need for service. Further requirements for implementation included empirical evidence of how this reform would result only in a shift of resources and with no harm to all categories of previously served clients, of how to determine case mix and caseload size, of how to administer regional case management offices, and of how to administer civil service title series for case managers.

From a research perspective, this initial descriptive study provides the groundwork for additional studies by indicating the principal client, case manager, management, and service characteristics implicated in the system management of case management. Although either more characteristics or more sophisticated measures may be necessary, three broad directions for future research would be useful. First, and most important, the linkages with and contingencies of case management provision with other family support services need to be explored. Does case management enhance or impede the delivery of other family support services, does the provision of one family support increase or decrease the demand for other support services, and does case management or any other family support service prevent or delay out-of-home placement? Second, research is required to examine the similarities and critical differences in the management and financial structures of each family support service to determine if efficiencies in either scale or pooling joint resources could be gained. A related concern, of course, is the analysis of which services other than family support services could be cut back to provide other more needed services. This concern requires the empirical integration of needs assessment data with service demand and cost analyses. Third, the use of longitudinal and experimental research designs is necessary to determine what the long-range effectiveness of case management is, and under which client, family, and service situations case management is a necessary service. The achievement of this objective, however, is dependent on the normative or policy definition of case management effectiveness, a definition that does not yet exist. Pragmatically, therefore, emphasis on the first two objectives seems more feasible and more likely to influence decisions regarding which family support services to provide, to whom, and in what quantities. Indeed, the word "pragmatic" is critical to understanding the bridge between research and family support services. Research that is to assist in the development, implementation, and evaluation of family support services not only needs to be focused directly on these services and on the families who receive them but also on the broad range of potential factors that could be manipulated to design a cost-effective and manageable service to families.

REFERENCES

Agranoff, R. (1977). Coping with the demands for change within human service administration. In W. F. Anderson, B. J. Friedan, & M. J. Murphy (Eds.), *Managing human services*. Washington, DC: International City Management Association.

Agranoff, R., & Pattakos, A. (1979). Dimensions of services integration, policy management, organizational structure. *Human Services Monograph Series, 13*.

Aiken, M., Dewar, R., DiTomaso, N., Hage, J., & Zeitz, G. (1975). *Coordinating human services*. San Francisco: Jossey-Bass.

Baerwald, A. (1983). Case Management: Defining a concept. In L. Wikler & M. P. Keenan (Eds.), *Developmental disabilities: No longer a private tragedy* (pp. 219–223). Washington, DC: American Association on Mental Deficiency.

Beatrice, D. F. (1981). Case management: A policy for long-term care. In J. J. Callahan & S. S. Wallack (Eds.), *Reforming the long-term care system* (pp. 121–162). Lexington, MA: Lexington Books.

Dombrowick, A. (1979). *Case management/service integration: A conceptual design*. Madison, WI: Wisconsin Division of Community Services, Office of Regional Support.

Fritz, J., Wright, R., & Snipes, E. (1978). *Case management for the developmentally disabled: a feasibility study report*. Raleigh, NC: North Carolina State University, Center for Urban Affairs and Community Services.

Gans, S., & Horton, G. (1975). *Integration of human services: The state and municipal levels*. New York: Praeger Publishers.

Hogan, M. F., & MacEachron, A. E. (1980). *Plan Evaluation Guide*. Downsview, Ontario: National Institute on Mental Retardation.

Human Services Research Institute. (1984). *Supporting families with developmentally disabled members: A review of the literature and results of a national survey*. Boston, MA: Author.

Intagliata, J. (1982). Improving the quality of community care for the chronically mentally disabled: The role of case management. *Schizophrenia Bulletin, 8*(4), 655–674.

John, D. (1977). Managing the human service system: What have we learned from services integration? *Project Share Monograph Series*.

Magrab, P. R. and Elder, J. O. (Eds). (1979). *Planning services to handicapped persons*. Baltimore: Paul H. Brookes Publishing Co.

National Association of State Mental Retardation Program

Directors. (1979). *The minimal array of services essential for mentally retarded persons: An analysis of consumer and provider opinions.* Arlington, VA: Author.

Neufeldt, A. (1977). Coordination simply stated. *Deficience Mentale/Mental Retardation.* 27(2), 3–6.

New York State Board of Social Welfare. (1980). *Case management: Issues and models.* Albany, NY: Author.

New York State Office of Mental Retardation and Developmental Disabilities, Case Management Steering Committee. (1982). *Case management in the New York Office of Mental Retardation and Developmental Disabilities: A report to the commissioner.* Albany, NY: Author.

New York State Office of Mental Retardation and Developmental Disabilities. (1983). *Case management time and effort study: Second interim report.* Albany, NY: Statewide Services, OMRDD.

New York State Office of Mental Retardation and Developmental Disabilities. (1984a). *Case management time and effort study: Third interim report.* Albany, NY: Statewide Services, OMRDD.

New York State Office of Mental Retardation and Developmental Disabilities. (1984b). *Case management time and effort study: Final report.* Albany, NY: Statewide Services, OMRDD.

New York State Department of Civil Service. (1981). *1980 Leave Survey Report.* Albany, NY: Author.

President's Panel on Mental Retardation. (1962). *National Action to Combat Mental Retardation.* Washington, DC: Government Printing Office.

Redburn, S. (1977). On human services integration. *Public Administration Review, 37,* 349–356.

Ross, H. (1980). *Proceeding of the conference on the evaluation of case management programs (March 5–6, 1979).* Los Angeles: Volunteers for Services to Older Persons.

Section

V

SUMMARY
AND CONCLUSIONS

Chapter

17

Research with Families of Handicapped Persons

Lessons from the Past, Plans for the Future

Peter M. Vietze and Deborah L. Coates

PROFESSIONALS INTERESTED IN children's development have traditionally focused on how socialization practices and parental attitudes influence the behavior and development of children. Until recently, a unidirectional model of influence was assumed in understanding parent-child relationships. It was thought that variation in child behavior was influenced by parental behavior. For example, numerous studies have explored the effects of parental discipline techniques on children's aggressiveness, dependency, and morality (Baumrind, 1967; Chamberlin, 1974; Hoffman, 1963; Nevius, 1972; Sears, Maccoby, & Levin, 1957; Winder & Rau, 1962). Other studies have investigated the relationship between parental control and cognitive development, achievement, creativity, and social competence (Armentrout, 1971; Baumrind & Black, 1967; Gecas, 1971; Healey, 1974; Hess & Shipman, 1965; Sprehn, 1973). Mixed results have been reported for studies evaluating the mechanisms of parent-child relationships and the influence

of parents on their children. Nevertheless, it has been assumed that some aspects of parental behavior account for variance in the child's behavior.

In much of this research, the focus on parent attitudes and behavior is often based on retrospective accounts (e.g., Sears, Maccoby, & Levin, 1957) or on prospective studies of mother-child interaction (e.g., Hess & Shipman, 1965; Lewis & Goldberg, 1969; Moss, 1967). It is only recently that child development researchers have taken a serious interest in the role of fathers in the development of their children (Parke, 1981). This newer interest in fathers has taken advantage of the lessons learned from earlier interest in mother-child relations. Currently, there is an increasing focus on how the family as a whole affects the child living in the family (Lamb, 1981; Parke & Sawin, 1980; Seligman, 1984).

During the last 15 years, there has been a shift in focus from how parents cause their children to act to how children's behavior and characteristics affect the parent's behavior (Bell, 1971; Lewis & Rosenblum, 1974). Research on the effects of the child on the caregiver has begun to emerge. Often, this research focuses on children who were known to be at risk for developing handicaps, or on children known to be handicapped. There is now general agreement that parents and children exert mutual influence on one another's behavior and that this mutual influence is often expressed in the child's development and behavior. This view has led to the development of some new but limited methods and techniques for studying children's development in the context of bidirectional and multidirectional transactions between the child and the environment. Nevertheless, this research relied on available methods rather than on devising methods to fit the research questions posed. Although the study of how children's handicaps affect families and how families affect children with handicaps has been important for understanding the context of handicapped children's behavior and development, as the foregoing chapters demonstrate, these processes are still a long way from being understood. One of the reasons for this is that family functioning is extremely complex and therefore difficult to study.

To illustrate the complexity of studying children in the context of the family, it is important to distinguish when in the life cycle of a family a child with disabilities becomes a member. Does a first-born child who is retarded or otherwise handicapped affect the family differently than if the child with disabilities is last of five children? What is the effect on the family of a child's being identified at birth as being handicapped or at risk for mental retardation as compared with the designation occurring when the child is 5 years old? Are there different ways to go about studying families of these two varieties? These are among the many questions that led to the conference on which this book is based. The conference was planned to stimulate discussion of issues, research concepts, methods findings, and designs relevant to research on families with a retarded or handicapped member. The ultimate goal is to provide information necessary to increase the quality of life for persons with mental retardation and their families.

THE CHANGING FAMILY

The first task of improving quality of life is to understand how the family itself is changing. Despite the fact that many people have a fixed concept of what constitutes a family, the concept of family has changed and continues to change. Farber (Chapter 1, this volume) reviewed some of the past changes and suggested that cultural and social demands on the family may have differential impact on persons with mental retardation. He also indicated that researchers should try to anticipate the future status of the family and should try to produce research findings for the future family. One of the biggest problems for families with a retarded child is that they do not know how to handle the uncertainty of the future. Interventionists need to learn how to prepare families for uncertainty. Farber also pointed out that as the traditional external pressures that kept families together disappear (e.g., economic necessity or religious sanctions), new structures for family support must take their place—notably affective bonds. How does having a child with handicaps affect the formation of these bonds?

Societal expectations create unusually strong pressures for families with retarded members. The family is expected to look normal, and any deviation from what is considered normal may be judged as a failure for the family. Generally, more is expected of families with retarded children with regard to child-rearing skills. The major question that Farber poses is whether a family with a retarded member differs from other families with atypical members or families with no atypical members. This may be the most basic question that can be asked about families with retarded members. It has been asked in many different ways throughout this volume and it will take years of further research until the answer is known.

How is the family changing as a social institution? Are there changes in the demographic characteristics of families? According to Norton (1983), there are a number of noteworthy trends in family structure in the United States. First, the family is diminishing in size. This is the result of a number of trends including decreasing fertility, increasing divorce rate, decreasing marriage rate for women, and delayed childbearing. In addition, there seems to be a new human life course emerging with more transitions than previously existed. This is primarily due to the prevalence of divorce and remarriage that often brings with it second families with children.

Another important trend in the demography of the family is that larger numbers of children live in one-parent homes (usually with their mothers) and below the poverty line. Half of the black children in the United States live in one-parent homes that are usually maintained by the mother. Unfortunately, how these demographic trends affect children with mental retardation is not known since researchers do not have any recent complete demographic or epidemiological studies of children with mental retardation who are living in families in the United States (Rowitz, 1985).

Having reviewed how the concept of the family might be changing and how the demographics of families seems to be changing in the United States, it is now important to ask the question of how and if having a child with handicaps or mental retardation changes the family. In fact, researchers may not really have an accurate concept of what a "normal" family is. They also may not know what the appropriate responses are to having a child with handicaps in the family. It is most likely that there are different appropriate responses at different stages of development. How different is the family with a retarded child from other families in crisis or from "normal families"? Some of the chapters in this volume have answered this question to the extent possible with the knowledge extant.

FAMILIES OF HANDICAPPED CHILDREN

What are families with mentally retarded children like? In Chapter 2, Iris Tan Mink presented some data that described empirical taxonomies of families with retarded children. Two

sets of families were studied: 115 families with severely retarded children, and 218 families with educable mentally retarded children. Two slightly different typologies were revealed by the multivariate analyses for the two groups. It is important to note that these classification schemes need replication. A number of alternative analytic strategies are possible with the sample of EMR families without collecting new data. Dividing the group in half randomly and developing typologies on each subsample and then trying to fit each sample into the other typology is one alternative. Another is to develop a typology on half the sample and then perform discriminant analysis, trying to replicate results on the other half. Certainly one problem of empirical analyses such as this one is that if different parameters are established for the analysis, it is possible that different results may emerge. Thus, if fewer clusters are desired in a cluster analysis, then the results may be different from an analysis in which more clusters are desirable.

Mink raises the issue of how these typologies will hold up over the life cycle. This is an extremely important problem since a functional family at one stage may be dysfunctional at a later stage. Service providers might also find it useful to examine how these typologies fit families without retarded or handicapped children. Furnishing information for service providers and the families themselves regarding coping strategies may lead to less stressful transitions across the life stages.

In an area of research in which activity has been somewhat limited, the knowledge base usually begins building with empirical investigation in scattered topics. Thus, research on families with children with handicaps has enjoyed some interest in recent years but, as yet, an organized body of knowledge cannot be identified. It is often the case that a theory can bring some order to such a set of findings and that such theory is typically borrowed from other disciplines. Family life cycle theory has emerged from the field of sociology, and in Chapter 3, Turnbull, Summers, and Brotherson have applied aspects of this theory to families with mentally retarded members. Perhaps the most important aspects of this application are that of recognizing transitions in the family life cycle and understanding how families with retarded members adapt to these transitions. The impact of having a family member with a disability is often viewed as being stressful, and the success with which the family copes with the stress may determine the quality of life for the member with a disability and the family itself. Increased knowledge of how families adapt to the stress of life transitions and how such transitions are bridged given the presence of a member with a handicap or disability will greatly facilitate intervention efforts designed to ease these transitions.

In the field of family research, there has been a great deal of emphasis on family process and functioning, and much attention on parents. The role of the children in the family has often been seen only as the target of parental behaviors and concerns. How the children in a family interact specifically is often overlooked. In families in which there are no chronically disabled children, only the exigencies of daily living and life stress act to differentially affect the nonaffected children. However, in families in which at least one of the children has a chronic disability or handicap, the other children take on important roles. The other children in the family may be affected differently depending on the specific disability of the affected sibling. One review of the research on siblings of children with handicaps (Simeonsson & Bailey, Chapter 4, this volume; Simeonsson & Simeonsson, 1981) suggested that there are no differences among various disabilities in their reactions to a sibling's handicap. It also appears that the siblings who are closer in age to the affected child may have difficulty in adjusting to their sibling's disability. Finally, there does not seem to be a relationship between the type of disability and whether the sibling will react positively or negatively. An important suggestion by Simeonsson and colleagues is that the type of reaction will be mediated by the unaffected sibling's perception of his or her own competence.

Some of the most important information about family functioning can be gained only from direct observation of families in interaction. Brody and Stoneman (Chapter 11, this volume) apply their observational methods to studies of sibling interaction in various social and environmental contexts. Their results suggest that the types of activities, presence of other children, which parent might be present, age spread, social roles, and the gender composition of the children in the family are among the important contextual variables that must be considered in studying sibling interaction. They conclude that the fact that a child with handicaps is among the children in a family should not overshadow the fact that they are siblings.

It is illuminating that the major focus of studies of siblings with handicaps is on the nonaffected sibling's reaction rather than some more positive aspect of the relationship. Anecdotal reports from persons who have siblings with handicaps suggest that the siblings taught one another. The sibling with handicaps learned skills from the unaffected sibling, while the latter learned a variety of less tangible social and emotional lessons from the sibling with handicaps. This may be a feature of family functioning that is less likely to be studied by traditional family researchers but should be on the agenda of scientists studying families with handicapped members.

PARENTING OF HANDICAPPED CHILDREN

As mentioned earlier, much of the focus of family research has been on attitudes and behavior of parents in relation to the children. In the past, mothers have occupied the central place in this research. However, during the past decade, a curiosity has developed concerning the role and influence of fathers in the development of children. Pedersen (Pedersen & Robson, 1969) and Parke (Parke & Sawin, 1976) have been among the most articulate researchers. They stressed the importance of considering the father's role in understanding child development. It has only been very recently that fathers have been examined in relation to their children with handicaps. Research on fathers' roles in infant development has sometimes concluded that the father has influence indirectly through the mother. The father is there to support the mother and serve as a back-up parent (Pedersen, Anderson, & Cain, 1980). There has, until recently, been a question about whether fathers were adequate caregivers for their infants. Findings suggest that the fathers tend to play with their children while mothers are the real caregivers. More recently, this view has been challenged by findings and theory (Lamb, 1981; Parke, 1981). When the father's role in the family with a handicapped or retarded child has been considered, fathers have been characterized as being withdrawn from the family in many cases and of being uninvolved in caregiving of the affected child. Bristol and Gallagher's review of the sparse literature on fathers and their handicapped or chronically ill children suggests that most examinations of such studies focused on negative outcomes, and their methods rarely allowed for the possibility of positive outcomes (Bristol & Gallagher, Chapter 5, this volume). They advise the reader to proceed with care in designing interventions for fathers of children with handicaps.

Little attention has been paid to fathers in general, and even less has focused on fathers of youngsters with handicaps so that attempts at intervention with fathers may disrupt family systems irreparably. In Chapter 6 of this volume, Parke reviews much of the extant literature on father influence in child development and relates this to both retarded and at-risk infants. He also questions research efforts that rely on single methodologies to study family systems. Despite the recent popularity of the views that children also affect parents and that the relations between parent and child are reciprocal, there appears to be little research on fathers that has taken this approach. The view that fathers withdraw from their children with disabilities, or are more severely affected than mothers by having a child with disabilities suggests that the impact on the father of having such a child is an important area to be studied.

One of the most understudied topics in the area of families and mental retardation concerns parents who themselves have mental retardation. In a recently published book (Thurman, 1985), the issue of children of parents with handicaps is addressed, focusing on a variety of parental disabilities including mental retardation. In Thurman's book, Zetlin, Weisner, and Gallimore (1985) indicate that few studies of parents with mental retardation have been conducted. This topic is made more sensitive because it is related to the reproductive behavior of persons with mental retardation, which in itself is a difficult issue. The fact that some persons with mental retardation may be as sexually active as nonretarded persons may have contributed to the pressure to house the former in institutions (Greenspan & Budd, Chapter 7, this volume). Proof of this explanation is beyond the scope of this discussion which focuses on persons with mental retardation as parents.

The major problem with mentally retarded persons functioning as parents relates to the fact that they are generally seen as lacking competence in many domains of life, and that being an adequate parent may also stretch the limits of their competence. At another level, interventionists must be concerned that, because of the demands of parenthood, children of parents with mental retardation may also be at risk for mental retardation due to socioenvironmental deprivation. As Greenspan and Budd (Chapter 7, this volume) point out, one of the classic reports on the malleability of intelligence (Skeels & Dye, 1939) studied how institutionalized retarded women cared for young children and led to the latter not becoming retarded themselves. It may be, these authors go on to speculate, that one difficulty in sanctioning persons with mental retardation as parents has to do with the inability to clearly specify the criteria for adequate parenting. Perhaps, if there could be a consensus on such criteria, it would be easier to provide parents with mental retardation with services so that their children would develop optimally. Unfortunately, there is not enough information available to do this. Greenspan and Budd (Chapter 7, this volume) note that there is little if any research that utilizes naturalistic observational methods to study the parenting behavior of persons with mental retardation. The Zetlin et al. (1985) study reported an ethnographic account of 13 families in which one or both parents were retarded. These authors indicate that one of the most important features of these families was the degree to which the extended family of these parents with mental retardation provided support and assistance to them in raising and caring for their children. It is clear from their study that research on parents with mental retardation must also take the total ecology of these families into account.

A number of other important issues in this area must be addressed by researchers in the future including the styles of parenting of persons with mental retardation, how these parents view their normally developing children, and what sorts of comparison groups should be included in research on parents with mental retardation. If researchers are to obtain an accurate picture of how parents with mental retardation function in parental roles. They must observe them and their children directly. This is probably the most crucial need in understanding more about this neglected subject.

Because the move to mainstream persons with mental retardation and handicaps has become one of national and international significance, a new issue has gained prominence. What happens to children with mental retardation and handicaps whose parents cannot adequately care for them? This question might also apply to the children of persons with mental retardation. Fortunately, there are many families who are eager to adopt children with mental retardation. This raises theoretical as well as practical issues that have yet to receive sufficient scientific attention.

Glidden (Chapter 8, this volume) has conducted some preliminary investigations to study the process of how families who adopt children with mental retardation adapt to this set of circumstances. This topic intersects with issues of how any adopted children fit into families and how families adapt to having children with mental retardation. In another chapter from Thurman's (1985) book on children of parents with handicaps, Coates, Vietze, and

Gray (1985) present two alternative paradigms for families with handicapped parents. One paradigm considers families in which the parent was handicapped when the child was born (congenital disability), and the other paradigm (adventitious disability) refers to families in which the parental disability occurs after the children are present in the family. In the congenital disability paradigm, the family system develops de novo with the advent of the first child. The adventitious disability paradigm applies when the disability occurs in a family that already has an established system of functioning. In studying families who adopt a child with mental retardation or handicaps, these two paradigms could also be used conceptually since the child who is adopted comes into a family system that is already established. Glidden (Chapter 8, this volume) points out that the existential aspects of adopting a child with handicaps are much different from those in biological families with children with handicaps. For example, in adoptive families, the parent has chosen the child and presumably is prepared for the experience of raising a child with handicaps. This is not the case in biological families with handicapped children. Studies of families who have adopted children with handicaps can do much to illuminate some of the processes of parenting a child with handicaps and the family process in general. Here too, the direct observation of parents and their children is essential if interventionists are to understand how families function and adapt in the presence of a child with handicaps.

FAMILY SYSTEMS AND THE ECOLOGICAL PRESS

One of the recurring themes in this volume is that having a child with handicaps in the family is a stressor. Farran, Metzger, and Sparling (Chapter 9, this volume) present one model that suggests how various stressful events have an impact on families with handicapped children. An important ingredient in their analysis is the stress that comes from the family's perception of the situation. This is a new approach in the study of stress in families, as most other stress models focus on objectively defined stressors. Wikler (Chapter 10, this volume) describes how Reuben Hill's ABCX model as elaborated by McCubbin & Patterson (1983) can be adapted to families with mentally retarded children. Both of these accounts rely heavily on the view that the family is a complex social system in which perturbation has varied and far-reaching consequences for each family member and for the family as a whole. This is a very different view of the family and stress than earlier perspectives that saw life stresses as simple additive stimuli often with only momentary impact. Combining these two perspectives (Farran et al., Chapter 9, and Wikler, Chapter 10, this volume) with the transactional perspective suggested by Sameroff and Chandler (1975) leads to a very complex and sophisticated multivariate view of how the presence of a child with handicaps in the family is affected by and affects not only the family itself but also the social environment in which the family exists. Kaiser and Fox (Chapter 12, this volume) also adopt an ecological view of the family as seen through a behavior analytic framework. Their contribution allows the evaluation not only of how the family and its ecology influence one another, but also how experimental treatments might be applied to the family with a handicapped child.

It is evident from these authors that in order to fully understand how the family with a handicapped child functions, it is necessary to consider the interactional components of the family as well as the transactions between the family and the ecological niche in which it exists. This highlights the problem of measurement since measurement of interaction in the family is difficult enough (Vietze & Anderson, 1981; Yarrow & Anderson, 1979), and measurement of the process of transaction between the family and its social niche has yet to be adequately developed. The challenge of an ecological/transactional approach to studying families is a sizeable one. Researchers do not have handy methods to empirically represent the process of transactions among family members across time, nor do they have easy ways to represent the impact of environmental events

or stressors as they affect the family. Nevertheless, the future research in the arena of families and their transactions with internal and external stressors will make the ensuing years of study exciting and illuminating ones. It can be expected that the scientists approaching these topics will develop new methods and techniques that will permit greater understanding of how a child with handicaps affects and is affected by variation and variability in his or her family and social environment.

PROGRAMS AND POLICY ISSUES

One of the goals of engaging in scientific endeavor is to effect change in treatment or intervention and to influence social policy, which in turn affects treatment. In the field of mental retardation, there have been conflicting forces on various levels of society regarding the treatment of individuals with handicaps. Moreover, programs and policies that affect families of children with handicaps often conflict with one another as a result of the way in which resources have been allocated. For example, it is sometimes the case in some states that responsibility for children with handicaps belongs to the education bureaucracy, while that for families is under the social service system. The fact that these two bureaucratic structures may have different requirements and criteria for services may mean that services offered by one system preclude the services offered by the other. This means that treatment of the family and treatment of the child are in direct conflict.

Berger and Foster (Chapter 14, this volume) review the tenets of family therapy theory and suggest how such theory can be applied to families with retarded children. They point out that the most important aspect of family therapy theory is that interventions focused on the child cannot be separated from interventions aimed at the family. Unfortunately, there are many outmoded service delivery systems that are incapable of dealing with either the family or the child. One possible conclusion from this is that a family focus may be necessary in all service delivery designed to meet the needs of children. Another recommendation by Berger and

Foster is that in conducting intervention research, the nature of the intervention must be clearly specified. This is not always done in intervention research. In addition, it might be added that the impact of different components of the intervention should be evaluated so that more specific subsequent interventions might be proposed.

The above principles must also be applied to statewide service delivery systems such as family support programs. In order to know what services are needed by families with handicapped children, scientific inquiry must be framed to indicate those needs. According to Krauss (Chapter 13, this volume), such data must be collected longitudinally in order to discover how family support programs affect families over time. It is clear that as children develop, the needs of the family change, and services must be provided to meet those changing needs. This notion is connected to the view of the family as a dynamic social system that changes throughout the life cycle. Krauss also suggests that specific family characteristics may be related to the family's need for support services. Research into the demography of families with retarded members will reveal how demographic patterns predict use of service programs and will subsequently facilitate planning of such programs.

The development of methods for policy analysis is an important step in linking research on families with retarded members to provision of treatment programs and service delivery systems. Until recently, there has been little effort to develop policy in the area of human services for families of children with mental retardation using data specifically relevant to the particular policy. Thus, many policies relevant to children with handicaps and their families have been developed using incomplete or inadequate data.

One approach to the use of data to develop a policy that affects families of children with handicaps is presented by MacEachron, Pensky, and Hawes (Chapter 16, this volume). In their study, they used a multivariate empirical approach to develop a policy for the delivery of case management services using data already available in a statewide data base. The focus of the study was on the amount of case management services rather than on the quality of the service received by the clients. The quality of services could also have been analyzed, but a slightly different approach would have been necessary. This empirical approach indicated that a small number of variables were effective predictors of outcome—amount of case management services. The four effective predictors were size of caseload, client's residence, client's "Willowbrook class status," and the percent of time spent on case management by the case manager. This study led to a change in policy that did not require an increase in resources. The approach taken here depended on the existence of a useable data base for the state in question (New York), and points to the usefulness of such a data base. Other service delivery systems could carry out similar types of analyses to develop or reshape policies relevant to families with handicapped members.

In their chapter, Washington and Gallagher (Chapter 15, this volume) present a model of family performance and describe how this model can be used to evaluate policy decisions that affect families of children with handicaps. It is important to note that in any policy analysis, certain assumptions are made on which the analysis is based. If any of those assumptions are faulty, the analysis may not be valid. Nevertheless, the importance of this approach is that systematic use can be made of data derived from individual studies for the development of government policies affecting families. Through such an approach, alternatives can be explored, and better informed decisions may be made. It is evident that research of this kind is extremely important if interventionists are to apply data on families of children with handicaps to decision-making about services. It is also worthy to note that policy analyses of this kind may also point to the need for more basic information on families and family functioning.

SUMMARY AND CONCLUSIONS

The foregoing discussion has reviewed the chapters in this volume, emphasizing some of the important issues discussed. It has attempted to include some of the ideas that came out in discussions following each presentation at the Conference on Families with Mentally Retarded Children on which this volume is based, as well as some ideas that are presented in the preceding chapters. A number of succinct themes emerged from the various chapters and are briefly described here. The author sees these themes as contrasts since he believes that they represent different forces in the scientific literature underlying the study of families with handicapped or retarded members.

The first set of contrasts seems to reflect evaluative assumptions held by researchers studying families with handicapped members. The issue of whether families with a handicapped member are deficient or whether they are merely different when compared with families without such a member emerged often at the conference. It may be that these families are not different from other families but have responded to the member with handicaps in an appropriate way—the way that any family responds to any perturbation. Whether research should focus on the strengths of the family or on the weaknesses of the family in its adaptation to the member with handicaps was also discussed a number of times. The assumptions made by the researcher in this regard may well shape the kinds of results reported. And finally, the issue of whether whatever stress is brought about by the presence of a member with handicaps is negative or whether it is an opportunity has also emerged at various points in the foregoing chapters.

The second set of contrasts could easily be applied to many other research areas and might concern the methodology and design of the research itself. First, the issue of experimental versus correlational analysis has been raised, and, along with this, whether random assignment to treatments can be carried out. These two issues depend on the nature of the study being conducted. However, as with any scientific study, experiments with random assignment will lead to more definitive conclusions and more precise inferences about the processes being investigated. Whether to compare the target group (families with handicapped members) to other families has also been asked a number of times. Although it may be illuminating to have some sort of comparison group, it is difficult to say what sort of comparison group is appropriate. Again, the nature of the investigation may dictate whether to have a comparison group, and, if so, what kind. Several chapters pointed out the need to study the family over time. This necessitates longitudinal investigation. At this stage of the development of this area of study, such large investments of time and resources may not be as fruitful as carefully conducted cross-sectional studies. If there are longitudinal questions being asked, then longitudinal designs are in order. Finally, the question of whether microanalysis or macroanalysis is the best approach to understanding families has been voiced by some. As reflected in the variety of approaches presented, both are probably important and necessary.

Finally, some contrasts having to do with the focus of research as contributing to policy were expressed. The issue of whether individual needs should be addressed as opposed to the general needs of families with handicapped members was raised a number of times. It is not easy to focus on one side of this issue without also taking the other into account. Whether to approach the issues studied from the perspective of one culture or to take a broader cross-national view is another issue that is also difficult to decide. Scientifically, researchers are interested in all families with handicapped members. However, different national cultures may have different approaches to serving people with handicaps. A cross-national perspective would be a strength in providing insights for policy development but might make for confusion scientifically if it is not carried out with care. Are short-term outcomes or long-term outcomes necessary? The answer to this issue may have major impact on policy development. The results of analysis of early intervention programs lead to different policy decisions depending on which view is taken. Finally, whether to focus on the person with handicaps or the family as the outcome may also lead to different and conflicting policy decisions.

It is evident that the contrasts just described that have emerged from this collection have no easy answers. The answers may come from the future studies that these and other scientists will conduct. The National Institute of Child Health and Human Development is committed to continued support for research on families of children with handicaps and mental retardation. This research will contribute to the future health and well-being of all families.

REFERENCES

Armentrout, J. A. (1971). Parental child-rearing attitudes and preadolescents' problem behaviors. *Journal of Consulting and Clinical Psychology, 37,* 278–285.

Baumrind, D. (1967). Child care practices anteceding three patterns of preschool behavior. *Genetic Psychology Monographs, 75,* 43–88.

Baumrind, D., & Black, A. E. (1967). Socialization practices associated with dimensions of competence in preschool boys and girls. *Child Development, 38,* 291–328.

Bell, R. Q. (1971). Stimulus control of parent or caretaker behavior by offspring. *Developmental Psychology, 4,* 63–72.

Coates, D. L., Vietze, P. M., & Gray, D. B. (1985). Methodological issues in studying children of disabled parents. In K. S. Thurman (Ed.), *Children of handicapped parents* (pp. 155–180). New York: Academic Press.

Chamberlin, R. W. (1974). Authoritarian and accommodative child-rearing styles: Their relationships with the behavior patterns of two-year-old children and with other variables. *Journal of Pediatrics, 84,* 287–293.

Gecas, V. (1971). Parental behavior and dimensions of adolescent self-evaluation. *Sociometry, 34,* 466–482.

Healey, R. E. (1974). *Parental behavior as related to children's academic achievement.* Unpublished doctoral dissertation, Catholic University of America, Washington, D.C.

Hess, R. D., & Shipman, V. C. (1965). Early experience and the socialization of cognitive modes in children. *Child Development, 36,* 869–886.

Hoffman, M. L. (1963). Parent discipline and the child's consideration for others. *Child Development, 34,* 573–588.

Lamb, M. E. (1981). *The role of the father in child development* (2nd ed.). New York: John Wiley & Sons.

Lewis, M., & Goldberg, S. (1969). Perceptual-cognitive development in infancy: A generalized expectancy model as a function of mother-infant interaction. *Merrill-Palmer Quarterly, 15,* 81–100.

Lewis, M., & Rosenblum, L. (Eds.). (1974). *The effect of the infant on its caregiver.* New York: John Wiley & Sons.

McCubbin, H., & Patterson, J. (1983). Family stress adaptation to crises: A double ABCX model of family behavior. In H. McCubbin, M. Sussman, & J. Patterson, (Eds.), *Social stresses and the family: Advances and developments in family stress theory and research.* New York: The Haworth Press.

Moss, H. A. (1967). Sex, age and state as determinants of mother-infant interaction. *Merrill-Palmer Quarterly, 13,* 19–36.

Nevius, J. R. (1972). *The relationship of child-rearing practices to the acquisition of moral judgments in 10-year old boys.* Unpublished doctoral dissertation, University of Southern California, Los Angeles.

Norton, A. (1983, November). *Demography of the family.* Paper presented at the NICHD conference on Research on Families with Retarded Persons, University of North Carolina Conference Center, Rougemont, N.C.

Parke, R. D. (1981). *Fathers.* Cambridge, MA: Harvard University Press.

Parke, R. D., & Sawin, D. B. (1976). The father's role in infancy: A re-evaluation. *The Family Coordinator, 25,* 365–371.

Parke, R. D., & Sawin, D. B. (1980). The family in early infancy: Social, interactional and attitudinal analyses. In F. A. Pedersen (Ed.), *The father-infant relationship* (pp. 44–70). New York: Praeger Publishers.

Pedersen, F. A., Anderson, B., & Cain, R. (1980). Conceptualization of father influences in the infancy period. In M. Lewis & L. Rosenblum (Eds.), *The social network of the developing infant* (pp. 45–66). New York: Plenum Press.

Pedersen, F. A., & Robson, K. S. (1969). Father participation in infancy. *American Journal of Orthopsychiatry, 39,* 466–472.

Rowitz, L. (1985). Proposal for information networks in mental retardation. *Mental Retardation, 23,* 1–2.

Sameroff, A. J., & Chandler, M. J. (1975). Reproductive risk and the continuum of caretaking casualty. In F. D. Horowitz, E. M. Hetherington, S. Scarr-Salapatek, & G. Siegel (Eds.), *Review of child development research* (Vol. 4, pp. 187–244). Chicago: University of Chicago Press.

Sears, R. R., Maccoby, E. E., & Levin, H. (1957). *Patterns of child rearing.* Evanston, Il: Harper, Row, Peterson.

Seligman, M. E. P. (1984). *A comprehensive guide to understanding and treating the family with a handicapped child.* New York: Grune & Stratton.

Simeonsson, R. J., & Simeonsson, N. E. (1981). Review of research on handicapped children: Sibling relationships. *Child Care, Health and Development, 7,* 153–171.

Skeels, H. M., & Dye, H. B. (1939). A study of the effects of differential stimulation on mentally retarded children. *The Journal of Psycho-Asthenics, 44,* 114–136.

Sprehn, G. C. (1973). *Correlates of parent behavior and locus of control in nine to twelve-year-old males.* Unpublished doctoral dissertation, Emory University, Atlanta.

Thurman, K. (1985). *Children of handicapped parents.* New York: Academic Press.

Vietze, P. M., & Anderson, B. J. (1981). Styles of parent-child interaction. In M. Begab, H. C. Haywood, & H.

Garber (Eds.), *Psycho-social influences in retarded performance* (pp. 255–286). Baltimore: University Park Press.

Winder, C. L., & Rau, L. (1962). Parental attitudes associated with social deviance in preadolescent boys. *Journal of Abnormal and Social Psychology, 64,* 418–424.

Yarrow, L. J., & Anderson, B. J. (1979). Procedures for studying parent-infant interaction: A critique. In E. B. Thoman (Ed.), *Origins of the infant's responsiveness* (pp. 209–244). Hillsdale, NJ: Lawrence Erlbaum Associates.

Zetlin, A. G., Weisner, T. S., & Gallimore, R. (1985). Diversity, shared functioning and the role of benefactors: A study of parenting by retarded persons. In K. S. Thurman (Ed.), *Children of handicapped parents* (pp. 69–96). New York: Academic Press.

Index